Pharmaceutical Marketing
Principles, Environment, and Practice

Mickey C. Smith, PhD
E. M. "Mick" Kolassa, PhD
Greg Perkins, PhD
Bruce Siecker, PhD

informa
healthcare

New York   London

Informa Healthcare USA, Inc.
52 Vanderbilt Avenue
New York, NY 10017

© 2010 by Informa Healthcare USA, Inc. (original copyright 2002 by The Haworth Press, Inc.)
Informa Healthcare is an Informa business (cover design by Anastasia Litwak)

No claim to original U.S. Government works
Printed in the United States of America on acid-free paper
10 9 8 7 6 5 4 3

International Standard Book Number-10: 0-7890-1583-8 (Softcover)
International Standard Book Number-13: 978-0-7890-1583-9 (Softcover)

Library of Congress Cataloging-in-Publication Data

Pharmaceutical marketing : principles, environment, and practice / Mickey C. Smith, et al.
    p. cm.
  Includes bibliographical references and index.
  ISBN-13: 978-0-7890-1583-9 (Soft : alk. paper)
  ISBN-10: 0-7890-1583-8 (Soft : alk. paper)
  1. Drugs--Marketing.
  2. Pharmaceutical industry.
  I. Smith, Mickey C.

HD9665.5 .P525 2002
615'.19'0688--dc21   2002022045

Visit the Informa Web site at
www.informa.com

and the Informa Healthcare Web site at
www.informahealthcare.com

To Molli, my favorite wife
E. M. Kolassa

Dedicated to my wife, Glenda, and son, Sean
Greg Perkins

My efforts herein are dedicated to the U.S. pharmaceutical industry and pharmacy profession, and to Beverly A. Siecker, my favorite pharmacist, business associate, wife, and best friend.
Bruce Siecker, RPh, PhD

This, the last of my books in the series on pharmaceutical marketing, is dedicated to Mary K. Hopkins Smith, RN, PhD. The first in the series would not have come about without her forbearance. This final book is due to her persistence and the same forbearance.
Mickey Smith, RPh, PhD

We would like to acknowledge Linda Rike, Marilyn Biondi, Peg Marr, and Amy Rentner, who made production easy.

CONTENTS

SECTION II: PRODUCT

SECTION VI: CONCLUSION

ABOUT THE AUTHORS

Dr. Mickey Smith is Director of the Center for Pharmaceutical Marketing and Management at the University of Mississippi School of Pharmacy. He is the author of more than twenty books and editor of the *Journal of Pharmaceutical Marketing & Management* (Haworth) and the *Journal of Research in Pharmaceutical Economics* (Haworth).

Dr. E. M. "Mick" Kolassa is the coordinator of the program in pharmaceutical marketing and management research in the Research Institute of Pharmaceutical Sciences at the University of Mississippi. He is a former Vice President of the Strategic Pricing Group in Boston and former Director of Pricing and Economic Policy at Sandoz Pharmaceuticals. Dr. Kolassa is the author of *Elements of Pharmaceutical Pricing* (Haworth).

Dr. Greg Perkins is Senior Vice President of Global Regulatory Systems at Solvay Pharmaceuticals. He has worked for four pharmaceutical companies over 27 years. His experience encompasses regulatory affairs, clinical research, quality assurance/control, and compliance. His achievements embrace a diversity of accomplishments ranging from the OTC conversion of Actifed to participating in the development of the first two drugs for AIDS, Retrovir and Hivid.

Dr. Bruce Siecker is President of Business Research, Inc. An advisor to drug manufacturers, wholesalers, reverse distributors, pharmacies, and associations, he conducts client-sponsored research on business and professional issues; offers regulatory and programmatic compliance audits, investigations, and training programs; and provides Channel Clicks, a client trend-spotting service.

Preface

As this book was being prepared, several factors were much in my mind. Certainly it would be the last in a series of five pharmaceutical marketing books I have published over a period of more than thirty years. I have been in the "drug business" for more than forty years (if you begin counting with my first job as a soda jerk in, literally, a corner drugstore). And, of course, there is the new millennium.

Looking back on thirty years of publishing and forty years of experience, I have begun saying recently that most of the things I knew about pharmaceutical marketing over the years that made me so smart are not true anymore. That sort of self-deprecation often makes for good conversation, but the fact is that the principles of marketing are as true today as they were when they appeared in that first book published in 1968. What changed, and had to change, was the application of the principles.

In this book, my co-authors and I go back to the principles. Then we attempt to describe the environmental factors that affect their application. Finally, we offer examples of the application of pharmaceutical marketing principles in response to those environmental factors.

The primary intended audience for this book consists of two groups: those with an academic background in business but with little knowledge of or experience in the pharmaceutical field and those with an academic background in pharmacy or other medical science but with little or no formal training in marketing. The ideal reader would be one who has just taken or hopes to take his or her first position in the pharmaceutical industry. That first job need not be in one of the many facets of the company's marketing activities. Indeed, it is my personal belief that everyone who is employed in the pharmaceutical industry, from retail pharmacy clerk to laboratory scientist, should have a basic understanding of how marketing affects the company for which he or she works as well as society as a whole.

I believe that a secondary audience should include anyone who would regulate, criticize, invest in, or otherwise be indirectly involved in the workings of the industry. Journalists, politicians, regulators, consumer advocates, educators, stockbrokers, and leading health professionals all have a stake in the efficient and effective workings of the pharmaceutical market, and a systematic attempt at understanding it might be time well spent.

Missing from this book are many of the technical aspects of pharmaceutical marketing—no formulas for perceptual mapping, no guidelines for the use of secondary market research audits, no pricing models, no formulas for outcomes assessment. There is, however, a literature appendix that can serve as a good beginning in locating such details.

The book does include a bit of history, but I have intentionally placed it at the end. I believe it is important to understand how the industry reached its present configuration for all the obvious reasons. ("He who does not remember history is doomed to repeat it.") I feel as well that newcomers to the industry should have some idea of the efforts of the people who make their marketing jobs possible today.

This book is based on the premise that marketing follows certain principles, that pharmaceutical marketing is affected by a variety of environmental influences which lead to a rich array of marketing practices. These practices are presented to demonstrate how the successful application of marketing principles—with appropriate adaptation to environmental forces—can lead to success in the marketplace. Failures will also be presented.

Given the nature of this wonderful and complex industry and its enormous potential for both good and ill, I suggest that preparation for a career therein must include more than mastery of the subject of marketing (or, for that matter, chemistry or pharmacology or pharmaceutics). A context is necessary and can best be obtained from sources such as Dubos's *The Mirage of Health*, proceedings of Congressional hearings—even harshly critical and often one-sided treatments such as Mintz's *The Therapeutic Nightmare*. A partial list of available literature appears in the appendix.

There is also value in giving some attention to the literature of "social marketing," with contraception being a notable example. With or without the label, marketing principles are applied in many fields of endeavor (cf. Ries and Trout's description of the marketing of religion in their book *Positioning, the Battle for Your Mind*).

Finally, it is the abiding belief of the author that good marketing leads to good medicine. Exceptions exist, but when the system works, bad marketing never succeeds for long—and neither does bad medicine.

Mickey C. Smith

SECTION I:
INTRODUCTION

Chapter 1

General Principles

Mickey Smith

"Marketing is the process of planning and executing the conception, pricing, promotion, and distribution of ideas, goods and services to create exchanges that satisfy individual and organizational objectives."[1] The foregoing definition was approved by the American Marketing Association in 1985. Other definitions exist, of course, and some are especially helpful. One professor defined marketing as "the creation and delivery of a standard of living."[2] This macro view is echoed in another definition: "a fundamental social process which . . . evolves within a society to facilitate the effective and efficient resolution of the society's needs for exchange of consumption values."[3] Such macro views are particularly relevant for an industry in which the products are so closely tied to the well-being of individual members of society as well as to society as a whole. Nevertheless, it is at the micro level that we find the more traditional views of marketing. McCarthy and Perreault, two of the best-known marketing scholars, define micro marketing as "the performance of activities which seek to accomplish an organization's objective by anticipating customer or client needs and directing a flow of need-satisfying goods and services from producer to customer or client."[4]

Levitt summarized some of the "genuine wisdom" coming from the ranks of marketing professors. Competitive success, he reports, has but a few, deceptively simple requisites:

1. The purpose of any business is to get (or create) and then keep customers.
2. To achieve that purpose, one must produce and deliver desired goods and services at a cost consistent with the customer's evaluation and do so in a successfully competitive way.
3. To survive, one must produce a profit regularly.
4. Doing these things requires clarity of purpose, clever planning, and clear communications.
5. A system of rewards for success and sanctions, along with methods of correction for failure, is essential.[5]

The reader is urged to remember the phrase "deceptively simple."

Marketing activities have a pervasive influence on almost all aspects of our everyday life. Marketing analysis is the reason for the availability of automobiles in more than one color. The distributive portion of marketing accounts for the availability of fresh oranges in Michigan and Maine literally within hours of their harvesting in Florida or California. The influence of marketing on package development has been the cause of fantastically convenient prepackaged, precooked foods.

Further reason for study of marketing lies in its contribution to the cost of the goods we buy. It has been estimated that marketing costs account for as much as one-half of the selling price of all the goods we purchase. As consumers, then, we should have some understanding of the nature of these costs so that we might better determine whether we are receiving good value for our marketing investment.

Marketing principles are a worthwhile field of study because they are principles, and an inherent quality of any principle is its applicability in more than one situation. Thus, the principles of pharmaceutical marketing, while presented here mainly from the producer's point of view, will bear application throughout the industry.

THE EVOLUTION OF MARKETING

Marketing has always existed. The first marketing transaction might be said to have set a poor precedent—when Adam and Eve traded the Garden of Eden for a bite of an apple. Some would have us believe that marketing practices have not improved much in ethical standards since the serpent promoted that first deal.

Trading or bartering seems to have existed throughout history, though usually engaged in on a limited scale. Marketing as a major force in society is, however, rather recent. It could not become truly important until humans had passed the point at which their productivity exceeded their immediate needs for survival. This evolutionary development occurred at different times in different parts of the world. For this reason, the level of marketing competence is not uniform worldwide, although the rapid spread of international trade seems to be correcting this.

Marketing might be said to follow increased production, which follows specialization. In the United States, for example, early history found settlers eking out an existence on the few acres of land they were able to clear. As these people became more proficient at farming, it became apparent that some were more accomplished tobacco growers than others. Their neighbors, however, might excel at growing corn or wheat. Soon a system of barter sprang up. Tobacco was traded for corn, corn for wheat, and wheat for rice. Soon it became more efficient for individuals to specialize in that which they did best. Since this was already their best line of work, their efficiency increased even more, and, as the practice of specialization spread, total output of all types of goods increased.

One of these specialists must certainly have been a wagon maker, for, to find adequate trading facilities, producers had to transport their goods beyond the immediate trading area. The problem of transportation was mitigated somewhat by the adoption of a medium of exchange—money. It was no longer necessary to transport the entire productive output to each potential customer. In some cases, specialists arose who would buy all of the output of one farmer for a number of buyers, hence the development of wholesalers.

The last major part of the marketing process has been a result of the rapidly developing technology of mass production and the evolution of efficient means of mass communication and rapid transit. In the United States, it now seems possible to produce enough of almost any product. It has been the task of the promotion portion of marketing to

1. make the public aware of the availability of the product and
2. inform the people of the desirable characteristics of the product, with an aim of increasing sales.

THE DEVELOPMENT OF PHARMACEUTICAL MARKETING

Among the specialists who emerged during the development of this country were the forerunners of our modern pharmaceutical manufacturers. The peddlers of the Revolutionary War were the forerunners of our present-day detail men, purveying their herbs and remedies to physicians and patients alike. The developing nation spawned the Lillys, the Squibbs, the Parkes, and the Dohmes who founded the firms that lead the industry today.

Retail or community pharmacy as a specialty did not come into its own until after the Civil War, whereas drug wholesaling actually preceded it in terms of its importance as a separate marketing institution.

Sonnedecker points out that pharmaceutical manufacturing in the United States has been repeatedly stimulated by wars.[6] Particularly since the Civil War, the special demands of wartime conditions have spawned rapid development of the pharmaceutical industry. The most important period has been that of World War II. Indeed, in many respects, the early and middle 1940s mark the beginning of pharmaceutical marketing as we now know it.

It is difficult to separate cause and effect, but there seems little doubt that the widespread use of the sulfas, the development of penicillin, and, ultimately, the arrival of the "wonder drugs" brought about the near explosions of therapeutic advances that occurred in the second half of the twentieth century. So rapid was the technological progress that marketing has been hard-pressed to keep up.

There was, in fact, little real incentive for rapid progress in the development of the technology of marketing. Even during the Depression years pharmaceutical sales were good. In the years following World War II, a booming economy was coupled with unusually productive pharmaceutical research, producing a period of unparalleled prosperity for the industry. Because of the nature of the products, those which were successful usually found use by literally millions of people. The product failures, however, were impressive in the magnitude of their failure.

Because of the general success of the industry, more and more firms attempted to gain a foothold in pharmaceuticals. Competition increased proportionately. It was no longer possible to depend upon product development for sales. The wholesalers and retailers who had grown with the manufacturers became more demanding as well as more sophisticated. Price became a means of competition. These and other developments forced the pharmaceutical industry to provide a marketing technology to match its research and development (R&D) capabilities.

Those charged with the organization and functioning of effective pharmaceutical marketing departments found themselves in an industry with some unique characteristics and problems. The most dramatic difference between this industry and others producing goods for general use was the unusual method by which the decision to purchase was made. The consumer had no choice regarding the individual product he or she purchased. This decision was made by a third party—the physician. As a consequence, the industry found itself concentrating its promotional activities on 400,000 men and women who decided the purchases of 250 million people.

The products themselves are unusual. At the same time they are helping save lives and reduce human misery, they can also do harm if misused. Many are dangerous. As a consequence, pharmaceutical marketing finds itself the most heavily regulated of any industry. Both the retailers and the decision makers must be licensed. Manufacturers and wholesalers must be registered. Distribution, which most industries strive to make as wide as possible, is limited by law to certain outlets. Because of their involvement with health, drugs take on a special character. Discussion of health matters tends to be both personal and emotional. As a consequence, pharmaceutical marketing is open to strong and immediate criticism for any mistake.

Despite its peculiarities, however, the industry still functions under the same set of basic market restraints as any other. The same functional principles must be applied, albeit in unusual circumstances. The same functions must be performed whether the product is an injectable anticancer agent or a "revolutionary breakthrough in household detergents."

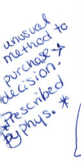

THE SOCIAL FUNCTIONS OF MARKETING

Returning to the concept of macro marketing, we wish to focus on the ways marketing makes possible great effectiveness and efficiency in advanced economies. Figure 1.1 shows that both supply and consumption are

Production sector

Specialization and division of labor result in heterogeneous supply capabilities.

Marketing needed to overcome:

SPATIAL SEPARATION	Producers and consumers are separated geographically. Producers tend to cluster together by industry in a few concentrated locations, while consumers are located in many scattered locations.
SEPARATION IN TIME	Consumers may not want to consume goods at the time they are produced, and time may be required to transport goods from producer to consumer.
SEPARATION OF INFORMATION	Producers do not know who needs what, where, when, and at what price. Consumers do not know what is available from whom, where, when, and at what price.
SEPARATION IN VALUES	Producers value goods and services in terms of costs and competitive prices. Consumers value goods and services in terms of economic utility and ability to pay.
SEPARATION OF OWNERSHIP	Producers hold title to goods and services that they themselves do not want to consume. Consumers want goods and services that they do not own.
DISCREPANCIES OF QUANTITY	Producers prefer to produce and sell in large quantities. Consumers prefer to buy and consume in small quantities.
DISCREPANCIES OF ASSORTMENT	Producers specialize in producing a narrow assortment of goods and services. Consumers need a broad assortment.

Consumption sector

Heterogeneous demand for form, time, place, and possession utility to satisfy needs and wants.

FIGURE 1.1. Marketing Facilitates Production and Consumption (*Source:* Adapted from William McInnes, A Conceptual Approach to Marketing, in *Theory in Marketing,* Second Series, eds. Reavis Cox, Wroe Alderson, and Stanley J. Shapiro [Homewood, IL: Richard D. Irwin, 1964], pp. 51-67.)

heterogeneous and affected by troublesome heterogeneities and separations. The role of marketing is to overcome both. It is generally agreed that this is accomplished by performance of the universal functions of marketing: buying, selling, transporting, storing, standardization and grading, financing, risk taking, and market information. Success in such performance provides economic utility and, we believe, better health and a better quality of life.

A brief look at these functions can demonstrate the importance of each:

- Buying involves finding and evaluating goods and services. For retailers and wholesalers, this is done on behalf of their customers.
- Selling is the most "visible" function and includes all forms of promotion, although management consultant Peter Drucker has written:

> There will always, one can assume, be a need for some selling. But the aim of marketing is to make selling superfluous. The aim of marketing is to know and understand the customer so well that the product or service sells itself. Ideally, marketing should result in a customer who is ready to buy.[7]

- Transportation involves physical movement of goods and provides place utility.
- Storing means holding goods until customers need them—a major activity in the channels of distribution.
- Standardization and grading sort goods in a variety of ways so that the customer need not do so. Regulatory agencies require much of this activity.
- Financing brings the money necessary to discover, develop, produce, and deliver the goods.
- Risk taking covers the uncertainties that are especially inherent in pharmaceuticals.
- Market information involves collecting, analyzing, and distributing information needed to plan, carry out, and control marketing activities.

Not all marketing functions must be performed by every firm, but every function must be performed. The ways in which this works are portrayed in Figure 1.2. Individually, each company will attempt to modify its "marketing mix" (the combination of goods, services, promotion, and distribution that it offers) to make it distinctive. Because of this relationship, the usually happy result is a combination of products and services that approximates the needs of the marketplace as closely as possible.

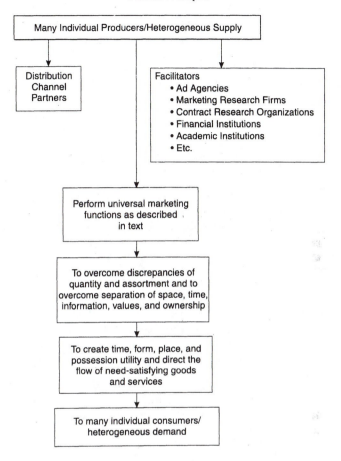

FIGURE 1.2. Marketing System Model (*Source:* Adapted from E. Jerome McCarthy, *Basic Marketing* [Burr Ridge, IL: Richard D. Irwin, 1981], p. 26.)

The efforts of marketing practitioners to match as closely as possible the marketing mix of their companies with the needs of consumers has led to the development of a way of thinking known as the "marketing concept." The marketing concept states what seems obvious now but was not always practiced: it is easier to change the products and activities of the individual manufacturer to fit the market than it is to convince the entire market to use the products and services as the individual marketer prefers them. The marketing concept further requires that all of the resources of the firm be organized into a total system aimed at meeting the needs of the customer. Those firms

(handwritten margin note: firms strive to be @ the right place @ the right time)

which once prided themselves on their production expertise now find that marketing know-how is perhaps more important. Any firm wishing to serve its market adequately will strive to direct marketing activities so that the right product is sold in the right quantity at the right place at the right price at the right time. Since the products with which we are dealing in this industry affect peoples' health, some of these factors assume even greater importance than that attached to the stimulation of sales.

THE RIGHT PRODUCT

Few industries feel so keenly the need to have their products meet such rigid specifications as the drug industry. A few micrograms difference in the composition of the active ingredients of a tablet may not only injure the sales curve but the patient as well.

One of the most desirable developments in recent years in the pharmaceutical industry has been the increased role played by the marketing department in the development of the right product. The specific subdivision of marketing that bears the major responsibility for aiding in this development is marketing research. This functional area is charged with determination of not only the therapeutic activity needed for diseases (diseases whose incidence also must be determined) but also the dosage form, package, and price most likely to be acceptable to both prescriber and patient.

(handwritten margin note: mkt research)

Current practice in modern pharmaceutical companies finds medical research working hand in hand with marketing research in selecting product characteristics that best suit patient characteristics. It is a tribute to the production technology of the industry that neither of these research efforts often finds itself faced with the roadblock of inability to produce that which is needed.

THE RIGHT QUANTITY

The quantity characteristics of pharmaceutical products are closely related to the packaging. In certain situations, the packaging of the drug can determine its effectiveness. At other times, the packaging can be so unusual as to serve as a form of promotion. The quantity and type of packaging for an analgesic, for example, may range from the bottle of 100 tablets sent to the community pharmacy to the drum of 5,000 individually wrapped tablets designed for unit-dose dispensing in the hospital. Again, the right quantity is an important marketing characteristic of a product, but it has parallel value in relation to public health.

THE RIGHT PLACE

For prescription drugs, the problem of place would seem to be an easy one. Prescription drugs must be dispensed by a physician or pharmacist; therefore, the place is prechosen. It is not that simple, however. Efforts toward fulfilling the requirements to distribute prescription drugs as efficiently as possible have been the reason for the development of the complex distribution channels that include wholesalers, retailers, hospitals, clinics, and government installations. These establishments are influenced by both the needs and the desires of patients. Further, the location of the patients and the establishments in the channels of distribution will affect plant location, warehousing, development of sales territories, and transportation of the product.

A further responsibility of marketing in the consideration of the problems of "place" is the maintenance of good business relations with the other elements of the distribution channels. Thus, retailers, wholesalers, and hospitals all must be familiar with the distribution policies of the manufacturer. Extremely important in maintaining good trade relations will be the nature of the returned-goods policy of the manufacturer, efficiency of invoicing and issuance of credit, and good communications regarding the availability and nature of all of the company's products. Most (but not all) drug manufacturers have a director of trade relations or a director of distribution in their marketing departments whose job it is to see that the establishments on whom the manufacturers must depend for distribution understand and, in general, agree with their distribution policies.

THE RIGHT PRICE

Price is an integral part of the marketing mix. Although needed drugs will probably be purchased regardless of price, within limits, insofar as other products are substitutable, those bearing an excessive price tag may find themselves without a market.

As we shall see throughout this text, one of the many unique characteristics of the drug industry is the undesirability of its products; that is, with few exceptions, patients would prefer not to purchase a prescription. They would prefer to purchase a new dress, a ticket to a movie, or a dinner in a fine restaurant. Further, they are usually ill when the prescription is necessary. These factors combine to make prescription drugs unpopular and prescription drug prices even more unpopular. As a consequence, drug prices are regularly publicly criticized. Sometimes community pharmacists receive the complaints. At other times the industry as a whole is criticized. In this context, there is no right price—only a "too high" price (or a "soaring" price).

Obviously, if drugs continue to be produced by private-sector industry, they will have to have a cost. As Theodore Levitt has observed, "Eating is a requisite, not a purpose of life. Without eating life stops. Profits are a requisite of business. Without profits, business stops."[8] Regardless of whether drugs are paid for by the patient, an HMO, a managed care agency, or some government agency, it is a part of the task of the marketing department to determine what that price should be. In practice, not one price, but several prices, will be set for a given product. The price per capsule for a given antibiotic might differ

1. as sold in varying quantities,
2. as sold to retailers,
3. as sold to the wholesaler,
4. as sold to hospitals,
5. as sold to physicians, or
6. when sold in foreign countries. ← *emmerging markets push for ↓ prices.*

Many business reasons, some more valid than others, go into the determination of price. The marketing department would want to know, among other things,

1. expected sales of the product,
2. price of competing products,
3. cost of R&D, and
4. nature of the market.

As we shall see in later chapters, some drugs are actually priced at a level that incurs a loss to avoid placing a financial burden on the limited number of persons requiring them.

THE RIGHT TIME

Availability of the drug product when it is needed is a further responsibility of marketing management and is closely related to the place function. The injection of adrenalin must be available in the hospital emergency room when the patient is there, not several hours later.

Another dimension to the timing problem is also the responsibility of marketing. This is the determination of the optimal timing for the introduction of a new pharmaceutical product. Obviously, the time for the introduction of a safe, effective cure for any life-threatening condition is immediately. For other types of drugs, the decision may not be so clear-cut. The introduction of the oral contraceptive, for example, required a special social atmosphere that did not exist even ten years earlier. A new product for the treatment of frostbite would not logically be presented during the summer months.

SPREADING THE WORD

Even though marketing succeeds in its basic task, which we defined to include right product, quantity, place, price, and time, it is still theoretically possible for the product to fail as a marketable item. The potential area of failure could be described broadly as communications. The part of the marketing communications process most familiar to us is advertising. This is the most visible and, perhaps, exciting form of communication. However, if marketing is performing efficiently, communication will be a two-way process.

The minimum amount of information that must be communicated by the manufacturer is the availability of a product. Obviously one does not purchase a product one does not know exists. Physicians are engaged in what Alderson calls a "vicarious search": with a knowledge of the needs of their patients, they search the characteristics of available products for the patients (who are not equipped to judge) for that which most closely approximates the answer to their patients' problems.[9] Although physicians are engaged in this relatively active and educated search process, there is a strong possibility that they will not become aware of a given product unless someone (usually, but not always, the manufacturer) has made a formal effort to communicate to them its availability.

We would not expect the producer of an expensive new product to limit this communication to a terse "Utopiotic is now being marketed by Rhemstrand Pharmaceuticals." The marketer will wish to tell doctors what makes the product worth their prescriptions, to explain its proper use, and, for the patients' good, to point out the inherent dangers in the use of the product. Drugs have been described as a "two-edged sword," with the benefits of therapy always offset to some degree by risk. The sale of a product should not be so important that a manufacturer tries to conceal the potential side effects of a drug. However, to safeguard the public against such shortsighted thinking, the Food and Drug Administration (FDA) has promulgated regulations aimed at ensuring that complete information on the use of each drug reaches physicians.

MARKETING MANAGEMENT

We have outlined in the preceding pages a number of major responsibilities of marketing. Almost none of these responsibilities can be fulfilled by marketing alone. Preparing the right product, for example, requires the co-operation of the production and R&D departments. Setting a price requires the knowledge of the finance division. Yet marketing is the key to the delivery of all of the "right" things. How does this all come about?

Successful coordination of all of the activities of the firm requires a certain type of thinking on the part of the top management. There are two prerequisites: the ability and willingness to identify clear-cut company goals and the understanding and acceptance of the need for a coordinated focus of all corporate activities on the pharmaceutical market. A statement of corporate goals can range from vague general statements to a detailed description of the specific aims of the company in terms of sales, profits, and return on investment. Some such definite target is a necessity to give direction to the activities of all of the firm's departments, and all of these activities, in the most modern philosophy of management, should be guided by the evaluation by the marketing department of the needs of patients and physicians. Levitt puts it this way: "There can be no effective corporate strategy that is not market oriented (i.e., seeing its purpose as creating and keeping customers). All other truths on this subject are merely derivative."[10]

THE SOCIAL POSITION OF PHARMACEUTICAL MARKETING

Drugs affect and alter health. By their very nature they play a prominent role in society. The drug industry consequently also plays a prominent role. The president of one of the largest pharmaceutical manufacturers has defined this role to include the following:

1. Discovery and development of new drugs
2. Rapid and safe development of these drugs into useful therapeutic tools
3. Production and distribution of safe and efficient existing drugs

This role is admirably fulfilled by most members of the pharmaceutical industry (at all levels). Nevertheless, the health field is ripe for exploitation. Those who are ill make easy prey for all manner of quacks, counterfeiters, and outright crooks. The vulnerability of the sick has led to the development of an extensive network of regulatory devices, self-imposed by the industry and enacted by government agencies, for the protection of the public.

Although the term has been used almost generically, an "ethical" pharmaceutical industry jealously guards the reputation of its members—both individually and collectively—by adherence to industry-wide codes of ethics. The unethical and the unscrupulous are controlled by the most extensive set of laws and regulations imposed on any industry, ranging from restrictions on the content of manufacturers' advertising to requirements that the distribution of prescription drugs at the community level be limited to licensed health professionals.

Principles of marketing can be applied to any industry, but the pharmaceutical industry provides enough paradoxes and unique facets to test the mettle of any marketing student. The industry is as modern as the many new drugs it produces, and its role in society is as important as that of any other industry. These facts combine to make the study of the industry's marketing a fascinating and worthwhile topic.

For any consumer, an understanding of basic marketing principles is desirable. Marketing contributes both cost and value to all products. The marketing costs of pharmaceuticals have been criticized by some. The value added by pharmaceutical marketing practices has, perhaps, not been explained adequately. One of the purposes of this text will be to discuss these aspects of marketing.

Chapter 2

General Environment

Mickey Smith

INTRODUCTION

The difference between data and information is that while data are a crudely aggregated collection of raw facts, information represents the selective organization and imaginative interpretation of these facts.[1]

One of several recognized approaches to the study of marketing as well as to marketing decision making is the environmental approach. This paints the marketing executive as the focal point of numerous environments within which the firm operates and which effect the outcome of marketing programs. Such an approach is used in this book and is portrayed in Figure 2.1.

As we hope to demonstrate at various times in the book, interesting parallels exist between medicinal systems and marketing systems. In this instance, we begin with the observation that the human organism is affected internally as far down as the single cellular level as well as being affected externally by factors as immense as global warming (see Figure 2.2). For the practitioner of pharmaceutical marketing, it is important to know that the pharmaceutical industry affects, but is subject to, a variety of internal and external pressures that alter in an important way the marketing activities of its members, both individually and collectively. In many respects the pharmaceutical manufacturer is "in the middle," for even though the patient is the focus of attention, the manufacturer is subject to the changes in characteristics of the society, the industry, and the patient.

Business derives its exercise from the environment. Thus, it should monitor its environment constructively. To do so the business should scan the environment and incorporate the impact of environmental trends on the organization by reviewing the corporate strategy on a continual basis.

In this chapter we examine the environmental components shown in Figure 2.1, starting with the patient.

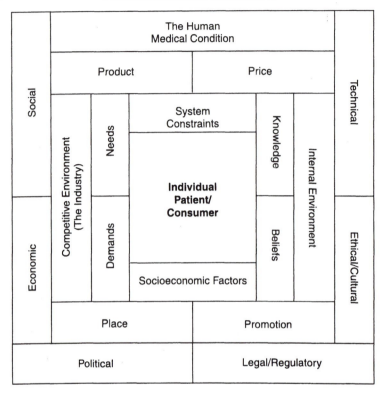

FIGURE 2.1. Pharmaceutical Marketing Environments

PATIENTS AND CUSTOMERS: THE INNER CIRCLES

Except in an emergency situation, nothing happens in the pharmaceutical industry until an individual initiates some kind of action. Symptoms are an important, but not essential, cue to action. The reverse is true as well. Symptoms are often ignored or consciously left untreated. The reasons are as complex as any other aspect of human behavior. Who the patients are and why they behave as they do are the focus of this section.

Who Are These People?

William Osler wrote, "It is much more important to know what sort of patient has a disease than what sort of disease a person has." This is especially true for pharmaceutical marketing.

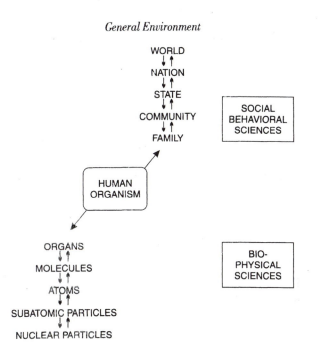

FIGURE 2.2. Dual Position of Humans in Nature (*Source:* Adapted from Nathan B. Talbot, Concerning the Need for Behavioral and Social Science in Medicine, in *Views of Medical Education and Medical Care,* ed. J. H. Knowles [Cambridge: Harvard University Press, 1968], p. 20.)

The most basic kind of market research consists of identifying potential consumers of one's product. For the pharmaceutical industry that is virtually everyone. For an individual product things become more specific. At the most basic level, a pharmaceutical marketer must identify a group within the population in the most general terms. Fortunately, though often overlooked, statistics, which are virtually cost free, are available to aid in this process.

Some very pedestrian population characteristics can and do have an important impact on the research, development, and marketing success of pharmaceutical products. A few examples follow:

- *Age:* Certainly ample evidence suggests that older people use more medicines, as do the very young. The proportion of elderly in the total population is growing.
- *Gender:* Women use more medication, proportionately, than do men. They also live longer, on average, than do men. They also bear chil-

dren with certain attendant medication use. (They also tend to serve as the purchasing agent for the family, if any.) Thus, they may buy things for others to use.

- *Race:* Some illnesses are race specific, with some significant variations in incidence and severity of illness by race. African-American males, for example, have a much higher than average incidence and prevalence of hypertension and prostate cancer.
- *Marital status:* This characteristic affects purchasing patterns. It has also been demonstrated that married people are more likely to take their medicines appropriately.
- *Education:* This is associated with reading and understanding labels and verbal instructions regarding general health, symptoms, and medication use.
- *Economic status:* This is still an important variable in decisions such as if or when to seek medical care and whether to use a prescription or over-the-counter (OTC) medication.
- *Ethnic/religious characteristics:* In a culture as diverse as that of the United States, these can be important in the understanding and use of medications. The obvious example of use (or nonuse) of oral contraceptives by Roman Catholics has been diluted by reported actual practice, but different primary language is an issue, as are differing cultural views of the meaning of illness and the response to illness.

The foregoing and other such variables are relatively easy to assess on a national basis. They can and should be thoroughly understood before beginning any market strategy. Again, they are necessary but not sufficient.

The Mattson Jack Group (St. Louis, MO) suggests that there is an advantage in using patient-based models to do market forecasting. Patient-based models, they argue, allow for

- population changes (i.e., the sorts of things just mentioned);
- changes in incidence, prevalence, and excess mortality;
- changes in diagnosis and treatment rates;
- identification of current needs;
- disease subtypes; and
- other, nondrug therapies.

They point out that patient-based models allow for a better picture of the entire market for a disease. It should be obvious, however, that the Mattson Jack proposal goes beyond simple demographics. Further, it does not mention specifically the items contained in the second internal section in Figure 2.1, yet all of these are important in any total market assessment and strategy formulation.

The crux of any strategy formulation effort is market definition. The problem of identifying competitive product and market boundaries pervades all levels of marketing decisions. Such strategic issues as the basic definition of a business, the assessment of opportunities presented by gaps in the market, the reaction to threats posed by competitive actions, and the decisions on major resource allocations are strongly influenced by the breadth or narrowness of the definition of a market. A large market has a variety of submarkets or segments that vary substantially. One of the crucial elements of marketing strategy is to choose the segment or segments that are to be served. This, however, is not always easy. There can be different methods of dissecting the market. Deciding which method to use may pose a problem. Segmentation is aimed at increasing the scope of business by closely aligning a product or brand with an identifiable customer group.

Segmentation criteria will vary depending on the nature of the market. In marketing, one may use simple demographic and socioeconomic variables, personality and lifestyle variables, or situation-specific events (such as use intensity, brand loyalty, attitudes, etc.) as the bases of segmentation. For prescription drugs, such factors as nature of the illness and types of third-party payment become important (see Table 2.1).

Study of the size and character of the market obviously involves more than mere nose counting. The demographic data that may be necessary for any evaluation of the consumer market for prescription drugs must include, among other factors, the gender, age, and income of the population. For other types of products a great many other considerations, such as occupation, religion, education status, and mobility must also be considered.

From the manufacturer's viewpoint, gender is an important demographic characteristic. It has been shown that women comprise somewhat more than their expected half of the population, and this trend is expected to continue.

TABLE 2.1. Bases for Pharmaceutical Customer Segmentation

Consumer Markets

1. Demographic Factors (age, income, sex, etc.)

2. Socioeconomic Factors (social class, stage in the family life cycle)

3. Geographic Factors

4. Psychological Factors (lifestyle, personality traits)

5. Consumption Patterns (heavy, moderate, and light users)

6. Perceptual Factors (benefit segmentation, perceptual mapping)

7. Brand Loyalty Patterns

8. Medical Condition

Perhaps even more important, as far as the manufacturer is concerned, is the finding that women account for significantly more than their share of the health care market, prescription drugs included. The obvious special interest in the sexual makeup of the population by the manufacturers of such drug products as estrogen, vaginal creams, and oral contraceptives would seem to require little elaboration.

Data on age are of interest in a general way to all of industry. The relative proportion in each age category is important, not only for purposes of forecasting demand for an individual class of prescriptions (e.g., antispasmodic for infant colic), but also to help direct research efforts. Particularly important trends for the pharmaceutical industry are found in the infant to nineteen-year-old and sixty-five-plus age categories. Not only do these groups offer specialized product development opportunities, but they are the two categories most frequently considered in the development of government health care programs. Both of these considerations must enter into the long-range planning of pharmaceutical manufacturers. A further consideration is that these two segments of the population demand proportionately more health care than do other segments of the population.

income steers treatment/drug choice by consumer.

Because level of income determines the total available monies for expenditure on drug products, this statistic becomes extremely important. A further consideration is the importance of income levels in determining the type and level of health care purchases. For example, the greater the affluence of a given family unit, the more likely it is for members to seek medical attention (with the potential of resultant prescriptions) for increasingly minor ailments. Those in the lower income brackets may lean more heavily toward self-medication for such things as colds and aches and pains. (It should be noted that programs such as Medicaid may confound intuition in this regard, so market research is essential.)

What Do These People Want?

Over four decades ago, psychologist Abraham Maslow noted that people typically try to fulfill some kinds of needs only after other, more primary needs have been satisfied.[2] He identified five different need categories that can be arranged into a vertical hierarchy, with the most primary at the bottom step and those of the highest order at the top. According to this psychologist, an individual normally tries to satisfy the most basic needs first and, satisfying these, is then free to devote attention to the next on the list. This list follows:

Maslow's heirarchy of needs....

- *Self-actualization need:* This is the desire to achieve to the maximum of one's capabilities, and although it may be present in everyone, its fulfillment depends upon prior fulfillment of the more basic needs.

- *Esteem needs:* People need both self-esteem, a high evaluation of self, and the esteem of others in our society. Fulfillment of these needs provides a feeling of self-confidence and usefulness to the world; failure to fulfill these needs produces feelings of inferiority and helplessness.
- *Belongingness and love needs:* Affectionate relations with individuals and a place in society are so important that their lack is a common cause of maladjustment.
- *Safety needs:* In modern society these are more often reflected in terms of economic and social security rather than physical safety.
- *Physiologic needs:* This group includes hunger, thirst, sleep, and so forth. These are the most basic needs, and until they are satisfied other needs are of no importance.

At first glance it would seem that pharmaceuticals solve only the physiologic needs. New developments in prescription drugs, however, give promise of meeting more and more of the other needs. Certainly many other products currently offered in pharmacies are designed to meet these needs. Interestingly, recent developments help us understand that pharmaceuticals, rather than exerting their power at the *bottom* of the list, may actually be most important at the *top*.

A cover story in *Business Week* referred to a "New Era of Lifestyle Drugs."[3] Triggered by the unprecedented public interest in, and media coverage of, Viagra, this article (and scores of others in supermarket tabloids) called attention to the potential of future drugs to enhance the quality of life for "healthy" people faced with anxiety, obesity, memory loss, and, of course, hair loss. Quality-of-life issues are not new (the oral contraceptive fit this category), but treatment with this specific aim is comparatively new.

What is the ultimate motivation in life? Our minds are filled with Darwinian notions of survival, but survival needs are primary needs: they are basic needs, but they are not the ultimate needs in life. The ultimate need, the most far-reaching, comprehensive motive in life, is self-fulfillment or self-actualization. As with most profound ideas, however, self-fulfillment is much easier to recognize after it is described than it is to define in precise terms.

Philosophers and theologians have argued about the meaning of life for centuries, and we surely do not want to join that argument. Yet an important, unanswered question remains: What do people do when they have satisfied their physical safety, belonging, and status needs? What do they pursue *then?* The answer is often, but disappointingly not always, self-actualization, the complete fulfillment of all their human capacities. This means enlarging and enhancing themselves. It means extending their personal identities, their individuality, their uniqueness.

It is easy to see that most of us are busy trying to fulfill more basic needs than self-fulfillment most of the time. We all spend most of our lives trying to stay alive and healthy, to be secure, to maintain relationships with our family and friends, and to get some respect and recognition for who we are as people. Most consumers' minds are occupied with their efforts to stay well, get along with people, and look good while doing so. It takes a lot of time, experience, and maybe even some wisdom just to meet those basic needs. So most people do not really get to the point where they can pursue self-actualization until they have a few decades behind them. Pursuing this kind of need satisfaction is much more typical of the mature consumer than of younger people who are still striving for the more basic things in life.

A reference to elderly people may conjure up images in people's minds of poverty and destitution, loneliness and ill health. In fact, nothing could be further from the truth. Only a very small fraction of elderly consumers in society fit that stereotype. Yet most people think that way because elderly people in such unfortunate circumstances get most of the media attention. They certainly deserve our concern, but marketers should not generalize the image to the entire group.

We can point out one rather surprising statistic that may help dispel some of the misconceptions about mature consumers: by the year 2000 more than half of all disposable personal income in this country was in the hands of people over fifty years of age! These are precisely the people most likely to have reached a place in life where they can, and do, pursue fulfillment of their self-actualization needs.

It is also well to note that self-actualization can refer to getting the most out of the life one has, even if it is impaired. With that view, the pharmaceutical industry in the latter part of the 1980s began earnest study of the role of their products in the "quality of life" of the chronically ill. Indeed, this attribute has become a part of both clinical trials and promotional themes.

Although it is very useful, if not absolutely necessary, to examine the hierarchy of needs, we are not confined to only a vertical view. We can look at consumer needs from a cross-sectional point of view as well. From this horizontal perspective, no single category of demands consistently takes precedence over the others. What is more, this approach permits us to identify more categories and to specify them more precisely. These needs are not classified according to the sequence in which consumers approach them. Instead, that classification is based on the kinds of concerns and activities that consumers associate with them. So these categories of needs are more often closely associated with particular types of consumer products, services, brands, and outlets.

In Table 2.2, fifteen fairly distinct categories of consumer needs are listed, followed by a brief description of each. For each needs category, several kinds of related pharmaceutical goods and services are identified.

TABLE 2.2. Consumer Needs and Pharmaceutical Markets

Need	Description	Product/Service
Achievement	Accomplish difficult feats; perform arduous tasks; exercise one's skills, abilities, or talents	Steroids, Ritalin, vitamins, appetite suppressants, tranquilizers
Independence	Be autonomous; be free from the direction or influence of others; have options and alternatives; make one's own choices and decisions; be different	Compliance aids, seizure medicines, patient-controlled analgesics, home diagnostics, all OTCs
Exhibition	Display one's self; be visible to others; reveal personal identity; show off or win the attention and interest of others; gain notice	Rogaine, OCs, appetite suppressants, oral contraceptives
Recognition	Seek positive notice of others; show one's superiority or excellence; be acclaimed or held up as exemplary; receive social rewards or notoriety	Steroids
Dominance	Have power or exert one's will on others; hold a position of authority or influence; direct or supervise the efforts of others; show strength or prowess by winning over adversaries	P&T committees, physician prescribing
Affiliation	Associate with others; belong or win acceptance; enjoy satisfying and mutually helpful relationships	RPh/professional organizations, senior citizens' clubs
Nurturance	Give care, comfort, and support to others; see living things grow and thrive; help the progress and development of others; protect one's charges from harm or injury	Mothers as advocates/surrogates for children, geriatrics
Succorance	Receive help, support, comfort, encouragement, or reassurance from others; be the recipient of nurturant efforts	RPh counselor, MD satisfaction
Sexuality	Establish one's sexual identity and attractiveness; enjoy sexual contact; receive and provide sexual satisfaction; maintain sexual alternatives without exercising them; avoid condemnation for sexual appetites	Sexual dysfunction, beta-blockers, oral contraceptives
Stimulation	Experience events and activities that stimulate the senses or exercise perception; move and act freely and vigorously; engage in rapid or forceful activity; saturate the palate with flavor; engage the environment in new or unusual modes of interaction	Nonsedating antihistamines, caffeine, CNS stimulants, flavors—Cholybar, Ceclor

TABLE 2.2 *(continued)*

Need	Description	Product/Service
Diversion	Play; have fun; be entertained; break from the routine; relax and abandon one's cares; be amused	Alcohol, antidepressants, minor tranquilizers
Novelty	Seek change and diversity; experience the unusual; do new tasks or activities; learn new skills; be in a new setting or environment; find unique objects of interest; be amazed or mystified	New dosage forms, self-monitoring, "little, different, yellow, better"
Understanding	Learn and comprehend; recognize connections; assign causality; make ideas fit the circumstances; teach, instruct, or impress others with one's expertise; follow intellectual pursuits	PDRs for consumers, counseling, PPIs/antipsychotics, Ritalin
Consistency	Desire order, cleanliness, or logical connections; control the environment; avoid ambiguity and uncertainty; predict accurately; have things happen as one expects	Laxatives
Security	Be free from threat of harm; be safe; protect self, family, and property; have a supply of what one needs; save and acquire assets; be invulnerable from attack; avoid accidents or mishaps	Patient medication profiles

Source: Adapted from Robert B. Settle and Pamela L. Alreck, *Why They Buy* (New York: Wiley, 1986), pp. 339-366.

Note: CNS = central nervous system; OC = oral contraceptive; OTC = over the counter; P&T = pharmacy and therapeutics; PDR = *Physicians' Desk Reference;* PPI = patient package insert.

The list of goods and services in Table 2.2 certainly is not all-inclusive or exhaustive, but the products and services identified are typical of goods that serve each kind of demand. No one-to-one association exists between different wants and various consumer goods; obviously they overlap to some degree. Yet this list of collateral demands is more fine-tuned than the five-category need hierarchy. Thus, we can legitimately make some generalizations about what goes with what—about the most common products and services associated with each type of demand. It is easy to recognize the utility in doing so: by examining the different needs and the kinds of consumer goods most often used to meet them, one can identify the most appropriate needs on which to base a promotional appeal strategy for a particular product or service.

Demands lead to behavior, and various models of consumer behavior are available. We have chosen to use as a framework the model developed by Andrew Twaddle.[4] It is simple but comprehensive and is based on the concept that sickness is a decision-making career. Twaddle's premise is that illness is an altered state of well-being about which an individual makes a series of decisions (see Figure 2.3).

Has a Change from Normal Occurred?

Trying to define "normal" for society is not really necessary for the present discussion. Normal, for our purposes, and for those of the patient, is whatever the patient perceives it to be. For that reason, of course, the characteristics of normality vary from individual to individual.

In any case, changes from normal can take several forms. The most typical one is what we usually call symptoms. For most people pain is not normal, nor is constipation. Thus, these symptoms represent a change from normal. Another kind of change is altered capacity—for instance, the inability to cut the grass without becoming winded. This kind of change may, of course, be attributed to something other than illness, such as aging. (In-

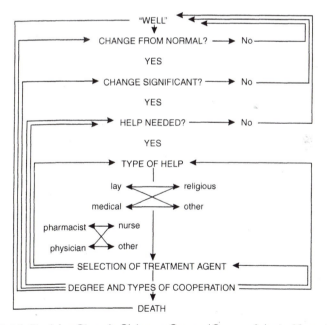

FIGURE 2.3. Decision Steps in Sickness Career (*Source:* Adapted from Andrew C. Twaddle and Richard M. Hester, *A Sociology of Health* [St. Louis, MO: C. V. Mosby, 1977], p. 124.)

deed some such changes should be so attributed, but stereotyping can result in misdiagnosis.)

It should be obvious that some people enter the health care system without experiencing any change from normal. Many hypertensive patients, for example, are diagnosed as ill even though they are asymptomatic. Such patients begin their sickness careers as a result of routine checkups or screening programs.

Drug manufacturers and public health proponents also are concerned with helping people decide that a change has occurred. Cancer's "seven danger signals" have been described in terms of deviations from normality, while some commercials for nonprescription drugs describe, or at least imply, physical changes that should (or should not) occur in a normal individual.

The role of tolerance threshold should be obvious. Some people stoically bear levels of pain that would send others immediately for help. Some variations in response to pain have also been demonstrated.

Symptoms are likely to be defined as serious in direct relationship to their unfamiliarity to the patient or to the degree to which they seem threatening. Mechanic has also found that symptoms which persist or recur tend to be viewed as serious.[5]

Assumptions about cause include a component of ambiguity. The seriousness attached to back pain, for example, may differ depending on whether the patient believes it is due to muscle pain or to a kidney disorder (Doan's Pills would make a good case study). The same is true for assumptions about a prognosis. Symptom seriousness appears to be related directly to the length of time the symptom is expected to last, to the degree of incapacity expected to be associated with it, and to the degree to which death is thought to be a likely outcome.

Interpersonal influence often takes the form of what has been referred to as the "lay referral system"—that is, the network of friends and relatives who are consulted when a symptom is experienced. It should be apparent that the influence of these significant others is, in turn, a function of the degree to which they are influenced by their personal perceptions of the factors under discussion.

It is well-known that many symptoms are experienced routinely by the population, yet many never do anything to relieve these symptoms. Some studies have shown that social stress from other life crises may be a trigger to action. A person who has lived with intermittent bouts of stomach pain, stimulated by a divorce action, suddenly decides to seek medical care.

Tractability apparently affects perception of seriousness, in that conditions perceived as untreatable are likely to take on the identity of disabilities rather than of sickness. Physical manifestations (visible to the patient and to others) are likely to result in attaching great seriousness to symptoms. The same is true for the way a patient handles symptoms. Grimaces and groans by the patient, whether voluntary or involuntary, are likely to lead to a greater level of severity being attached to the condition by those around him or her.

It should be clear from the foregoing that health decisions are complex, subjective, often emotional, and subject to influence by others.

Significance of the Change

Among the factors that appear to enter into the patient's decisions concerning symptoms are the following:

1. Extent of interference with normal activities or characteristics
2. The clarity of the symptoms
3. The tolerance threshold of the symptomatic person
4. The familiarity and seriousness of the symptoms
5. Assumption about cause
6. Assumptions about prognosis
7. Interpersonal influence
8. Other life crises of the symptomatic person
9. Assumptions about treatability
10. Physical manifestations
11. Impression management

This list is not necessarily exhaustive, and the evidence supporting the impact of each factor is sometimes equivocal. Nevertheless, evidence in each case suggests that these factors play some (usually unquantitative) role in the complex decision-making process of the patient as he or she pursues a sickness career.

It has also been found that the more a condition inconveniences an individual (or sometimes those with whom he or she relates), the more likely it is to be viewed as significant. The same is apparently true for symptom clarity—the more obvious the meaning of the symptom, to the patient or to those around the patient, the more significance attached to it.

Need for Help

We have shown that a number of often related factors are involved in the decision that a symptom is significant. Even having made that decision, however, it is by no means universally true that the patient will decide to seek aid as opposed to self-treatment or even capitulation to the illness.

Type of Help Needed

Once the decision to seek help has been made, the patient is still faced with a decision as to type of help needed. Although the physician is our society's model for primary care, the physician is by no means the only alternative. Other examples are dentists, podiatrists, optometrists, chiropractors, clinical psychologists, and many other nonphysician health care providers. Choice of type of help will be a function of social, cultural, economic, educational, emotional, geographic, and legal factors.

Selection of Treatment Agents

For prescription drugs it is still accurate to state that most selection decisions are made by someone (usually the physician) other than the patient, but this is not to say that the patients have no interest in the process.

Stimson, in a British study, found that patients were not as prescription oriented when visiting the physician as many seem to believe.[6] Rappoport, also in England, found that 56 percent of a sample of patients expected to receive a prescription.[7] Perhaps most interesting was the finding that 24 percent intended to buy an OTC product from a pharmacy after leaving the physician's office. Perhaps most interesting, 50 percent of those who expected a prescription but did not obtain one intended to purchase a product for self-medication. To further confuse the issue, another study reported finding that the patients who did not receive prescriptions reported more satisfaction with the communicative aspects of their visit to physicians than did patients who received prescriptions.[8]

The consumer is, of course, intimately involved in the selection and purchase of nonprescription drugs. That process can also be a complex one. Figure 2.4 provides direction in understanding the process of self-medication on a qualitative level. The timing of the steps in this process and the quantification of the proportions of consumers who proceed through the various steps shown are a continuing challenge to OTC drug marketers.

Patient Compliance

Patient compliance is crucial to successful therapy. It is also important to call attention to certain economic factors—notably, the various cost dimensions related to drugs—that may affect the compliance performance of the patient, either positively or negatively. Aside from the medical implications, it should be clear that this is also ultimately a marketing issue at both the retail and manufacturing levels. More later on this issue.

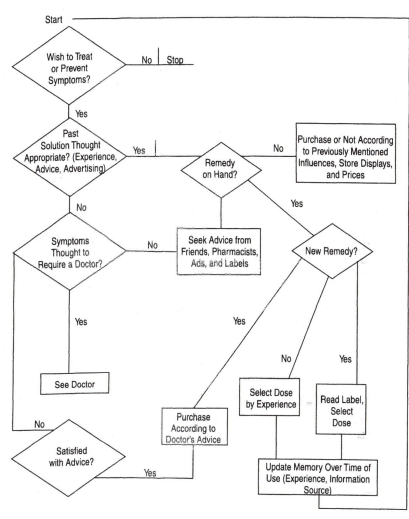

FIGURE 2.4. Self-Medication Model (*Source:* Adapted from T. P. Hustad, A. E. Courtney, and R. M. Heeler. An Emerging Model for Purchase and Consumption of Nonprescription Drugs, *Journal of Consumer Affairs* 13(1):81-85, 1979.)

What Do These People Need?

The difference between demand (want) and need is intuitively easy to understand. One may *want* a new Lexus, but it would be difficult to imagine why one would *need* a new Lexus. In the field of health care this sometimes frivolous difference can, and often does, take on more serious consequences. Here are two possible mismatches between need and demand in the pharmaceutical field:

1. Patient wants for a variety of reasons (direct-to-consumer advertising, word-of-mouth recommendation, addiction/habituation) a medication but does not need it.
2. Patient needs a medication but for a different variety of reasons (ignorance, cost, no diagnosis or misdiagnosis) does not want it.

In many ways, the greatest social contribution of marketing to the field of pharmaceuticals is the efficient and effective matching of needs and wants.

Defining needs among potential customers for pharmaceutical products can be deceptively easy. Morbidity and mortality rates are a logical starting place. If heart attack, cancer, and stroke are the leading causes of death in a society, then there is a clear need for medications to prevent or postpone these deaths. In the words of Tom Lehrer's satirical song "The Old Dope Peddler," it is "doing well by doing good." Dubos quoted Malthus: "I feel not the slightest doubt that, if the introduction of the cow pox should extirpate the small pox we shall find . . . increased mortality of some other disease."[9]

Well, of course! For as long as everyone is destined to die from some cause, a decline in one can only come at the expense of an increase in another. This is an inescapable truth, yet there seems to be some failure to recognize it. What society, and the pharmaceutical industry to some degree, is doing is making conscious or unconscious decisions about "tolerable" causes of death. (Perhaps the ultimate goal is for every death certificate to list "natural causes" as the reason for demise.)

Given the foregoing, it would seem that the pharmaceutical industry will never exhaust the supply of pharmaceutically preventable or postponable mortality. (Indeed, no one does die from smallpox today, but each person still dies.) The same is true for morbidity. In fact, treating, controlling, and preventing illness or the precursors of illness constitute the mission of the pharmaceutical industry as we have known it. One must add, however, given the comments on "lifestyle drugs" mentioned earlier, that this mission has been, and seems likely to continue to be, expanded. The existing and potential technology promises to test the definition of the industry. Theodore Levitt's question "What businesses are you in?" could result in some very interesting and different answers in the near future. In the meantime marketing has much to do just in affecting the proper use of medications. Patient compliance is a fertile field for such activity.*

---

*Material in this section is adapted from the report "Compliance: Rx for Optimal Sales," written by Mickey Smith and copyrighted (1993) by Med Strategy, Inc., a division of the Mattson Jack Group.

Compliance Enhancement: Turning Need into a Want

Consider two short stories. In the first story, John Doe, after several days of worrisome symptoms, makes an appointment with his physician. He takes time off from work, spends more than an hour waiting to see the doctor, fights traffic going and coming, and pays the doctor $40 for a diagnosis. He leaves the doctor's office with a prescription in hand and never gets it filled. How can one explain such apparently irrational behavior?

The second story concerns Jane Brown, Product Manager, who spent $7 million on various kinds of promotions to generate the prescription that John Doe received. Her promotional strategies were brilliant, but the company will never realize a penny from that particular prescription—and Jane does not even know it. Equally irrational behavior?

Fortunately, there are solutions to these behaviors; even more fortunately, these solutions are marketing strategies, too. Some drug manufacturers show a strong awareness of the importance of the compliance issue and of the value of a strong response.

A Glaxo (then) advertisement appearing in the spring of 1992 showed a physician observing, "When my patients don't return, I assume the therapy is working." On the facing page, one of these patients says, "I couldn't tell my doctor his migraine therapy didn't work."

The text of the ad cites data indicating that nearly one-half of all migraine sufferers have given up on their physicians either because of failure to improve or because of side effects of the medication prescribed. This example is illustrative of the complexity, subtlety, and importance of the compliance problem. Among the potential consequences of the situation with migraine are the following:

- Physician misjudgment of the effectiveness of his or her therapy, in this case probably resulting in repetition of this scenario with the next medication prescribed for this patient
- Patient's loss of confidence in the efficacy of medications and perhaps in the skill of the physician
- Continued migraine attacks with continued erosion of the patient's quality of life
- Loss of patient productivity (one estimate, cited in the ad, found that annual lost productivity from migraine attacks was in the $6 billion to $17 billion range.
- Cost of other therapies, including OTC medicines, used by the patient to no avail

We will devote some attention to the marketing consequences of non-compliance. In Figure 2.5 we have created a hypothetical market of a mil-

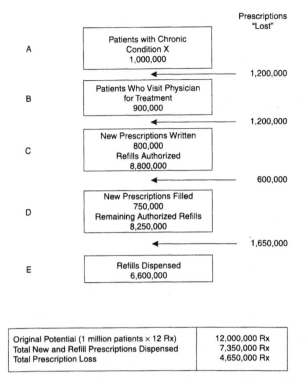

FIGURE 2.5. Decomposition of a Market

lion patients with condition X (A). The initial potential market is 12 million over a year (a new prescription and 11 refills per patient). We postulate that 10 percent do not go to the doctor (B), and that 12 percent of those who do see a doctor do not receive a prescription (C). Consistent with statistics cited earlier, we project that just more than 6 percent will not have their original prescription filled and therefore receive no refills (D). Finally, we project a further loss of 20 percent of refills through either failure at or delays in all. The total loss from the original potential market is nearly 39 percent! Let us carry the example further and assume a revenue of $10 per prescription (for ease of calculation). A company with a 20 percent market share of new prescriptions can use several ways to increase total revenue. The traditional way is to increase a market share of new prescriptions through promotions, price changes, and so forth. Focusing on compliance, however, yields some interesting data. Assuming one could effect full compliance for the company's product, what would happen? The data in Table 2.3 tell us.

TABLE 2.3. Effect of Full Compliance

	Decomposed Market		Fully Compliant Market
New Rx Written	160,000		160,000
New Rx Filled	150,000		160,000
Authorized Refills	1,920,000		1,920,000
Refills Dispensed	1,320,000		1,920,000
Difference (new and refill)	610,000	or	$6,100,000

Of course, full compliance is an unreal expectation, but an improvement of even 50 percent in the compliance statistics could generate an additional $3 million in revenue in this example. It would take a 4 percent increase in market share to match this result. Unfortunately, few data to date focus on the relative cost-effectiveness of expenditures on compliance enhancement versus expenditures on promotion with regard to increased sales.

Knowledge, Beliefs, and Culture

Importance has been attached to the role of the health belief model (HBM) in explaining compliance-related behavior. The model was originally postulated, and has been used, to explain all manners of health-related, especially preventive, behavior. As a marketing model HBM is very helpful in pointing out specific perceptions that may need changing through marketing activities (see Figure 2.6).

Perceptions, in this case, not practically different from beliefs, are amenable to change. Such change can be altered, with varying degrees of success, through education. Real knowledge has as a necessary, though not sufficient, component the possession of the relevant facts. Education is a means of providing those facts, and marketing has the tools to do this. Early direct-to-consumer education had as its goal the simple act of informing potential consumers that an effective treatment for their condition might be available through their physicians.

Knowledge alone is not, of course, a guarantee of rational action on the part of the public. Past and present beliefs (whether based on facts or not) and cultural context have an important and complex influence on consumer behavior. Believing is an important component of successful medical treatment. It is the basis for the placebo response and the reason for double-blind clinical trials. Dubos reminds us that Hippocrates anticipated the need for double-blind studies with this statement: "He doth the best cures in whom we trust."[10]

Culture as a marketing consideration does not often receive a great deal of attention. In this field of medicine, however, it can be a critical factor. The term "drug culture" emerged in the 1960s to describe the phenomenon of

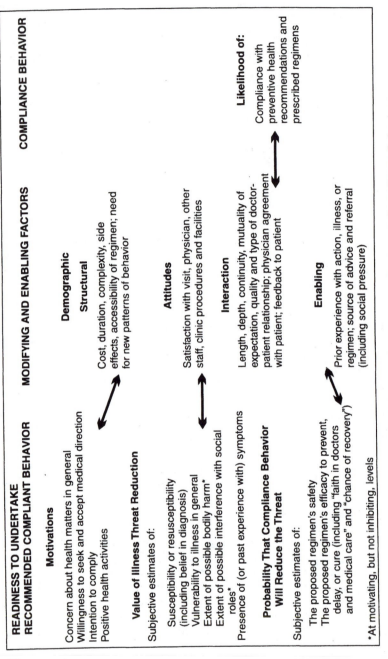

FIGURE 2.6. Health Belief Model for Predicting and Explaining Compliance Behavior

READINESS TO UNDERTAKE RECOMMENDED COMPLIANT BEHAVIOR

Motivations

Concern about health matters in general
Willingness to seek and accept medical direction
Intention to comply
Positive health activities

Value of Illness Threat Reduction

Subjective estimates of:

Susceptibility or resusceptibility (including belief in diagnosis)
Vulnerability to illness in general
Extent of possible bodily harm*
Extent of possible interference with social roles*
Presence of (or past experience with) symptoms

Probability That Compliance Behavior Will Reduce the Threat

Subjective estimates of:

The proposed regimen's safety
The proposed regimen's efficacy to prevent, delay, or cure (including "faith in doctors and medical care" and "chance of recovery")

*At motivating, but not inhibiting, levels

MODIFYING AND ENABLING FACTORS

Demographic

Structural

Cost, duration, complexity, side effects, accessibility of regimen; need for new patterns of behavior

Attitudes

Satisfaction with visit, physician, other staff, clinic procedures and facilities

Interaction

Length, depth, continuity, mutuality of expectation, quality and type of doctor-patient relationship; physician agreement with patient; feedback to patient

Enabling

Prior experience with action, illness, or regimen; source of advice and referral (including social pressure)

COMPLIANCE BEHAVIOR

Likelihood of:

Compliance with preventive health recommendations and prescribed regimens

36

using drugs for nonmedical reasons. Such colloquial use of the term tends to diminish the wider impact of culture as a total way of living, including one's values, beliefs, norms, and traditions. The marketing implications of cultural considerations are real, but not necessarily obvious. "Cultural lag" is a good example.

Physician Paul Stolley described cultural lag as the situation wherein technological advances outstrip the ability of society to adapt to and utilize these advances.[11] An early example was the oral contraceptive. It is highly unlikely that this pharmaceutical discovery could have been introduced if available in the 1930s. Without the so-called sexual revolution in the late 1950s to early 1960s (a cultural phenomenon), could "the Pill" have been accepted? (Some have argued that the first two shots in the sexual revolution—the Pill and *Playboy* magazine—were fired in the drugstore.) At the end of the twentieth century, the future of the oral abortifacient RU-486 was shaped by decisions that are as much cultural as legal and regulatory.

Another cultural change in the United States seems to encompass a switch to a combination of self-care through changes in lifestyle and diet and the use of "natural" remedies. If these changes are as real as the trends suggest, they will represent a real shift in the twenty-first century from patterns of life in the twentieth century.

"To ward off disease," Dubos wrote, "men as a rule find it easier to depend on healers than to attempt the more difficult task of living wisely."[12] He describes a progression in popularity from Hygeia, goddess of health, to her sister, Panakeia, who "became omnipotent as a healing goddess through knowledge of drugs either from plants or from the earth" (if the pharmaceutical industry has a goddess she is certainly the one). Both of these goddesses served the famous physician Asclepius, described by Luther as "God's body patcher."[13]

A final example of cultural impact on the use of medications is the "medicalization of life." In 1971, Lewis reported that nearly two-thirds of his (nonscientific) sample of physician respondents felt that other physicians were prescribing too many tranquilizers. He made clear through the example of a Valium advertisement his belief that a major reason for overprescribing is the "medicalization of human problems," noting that "once daily living is defined as disease, how logical it is for us to attempt to treat that disease."[14]

Again, if one looks to Freidson's exposition on medicine, one finds an explanation, if not an excuse, for the medicalization of human problems. As he observes (and supports by argument), "The medical profession has first claim to jurisdiction over the label of illness and anything to which it may be attached, irrespective of its capacity to deal with it effectively."[15] In fact, people come to physicians because of anxiety in their lives. By the simple act of seeking medical assistance, the patient has medicalized the problem. Of course, by treating the patient, the physician confirms that the medicalization

was appropriate. If the drug works, even if only briefly, the actions of both patient and physician are reinforced, and the drugs have worked—criticism of
the *effectiveness* of the benzodiazepines, at least, has been rare.

One may argue (and many do) that the drugs do not "cure" the anxiety
and do not eliminate the cause. True enough, but the same can be said of
antihypertensive medication, antiarthritics, and even aspirin. Should the patient be denied relief of mental discomfort when it is caused by problems of
daily living?

Unless and until society is provided with an acceptable alternative to the
physician in dealing with personal problems, as long as people continue to
seek relief from this source, it is unrealistic to expect the physician to turn
them away because they have a problem with which he or she should not deal.

Society has medicalized human problems, it appears. Medicine has perhaps been an accessory, and the pharmaceutical industry, certainly, has provided both with the means. To expect either of the latter parties to do, or
have done, otherwise bespeaks a considerable naïveté.

Freidson pointed out that "while medicine is hardly independent of the
society in which it exists, by becoming a vehicle for society's values it came
to play a major role in the forming and shaping of the social meanings im-
bued with such a role."[16] He argued that physicians became "moral entre-
preneurs," seeing "mental illness" where the layperson sees "nervousness"
or "problems." Yet, the same layperson has come to the physician for help.
If the physician eschews treatment (with drugs), the patient is likely to be
disappointed, and the physician becomes equally a moral entrepreneur, saying, in effect, "You were wrong to come to me. Pull yourself together and
get your life in order." However correct that judgment may be, the personal
burden on the physician can be enormous.

The 1971 quotation from Lewis, cited earlier, was revisited in 1997 by international pharmacoepidemiologist Graham Dukes. In an editorial in the
International Journal of Risk and Safety in Medicine, Duke's writings ac-
company an extensive review of the use of selective serotonin reuptake inhibitors and other antidepressant medications.[17]

A concern expressed by Dukes is that

> the medicalization of life—a process which transforms aspects of ev-
> eryday existence into pathological conditions requiring diagnosis,
> medical involvement and treatment [—has] happened to pregnancy
> and the menopause, . . . with unusually active children who were sup-
> posed to require (CNS stimulants), and . . . over the last thirty years
> with the broad spectrum of various depressive states which in part rep-
> resent a normal reaction to the stresses of life.[18]

Two observations before continuing. First, the attention to the "lifestyle
drugs" mentioned earlier in this chapter may presage a major cultural

change. Second, one wonders what our culture would do with the drug developments shown in Table 2.4 that were predicted in 1971 for the year 2000.

System Constraints

It is clear that nothing can happen for the pharmaceutical industry without some initial action by a prospective consumer. But taking action is surely not easy. Assuming a successful, and appropriate, decision that something is wrong and something needs to be done about it, here is just a partial list of the constraints that the various components of the health care system place on even the most sophisticated potential consumer of medication:

- The patient must decide whether to treat the illness with a non-prescription (OTC) medication or try to get a prescription medicine.
- If the OTC decision wins, the medicine is probably not covered for payment by the patient's insurance or other benefit plan.
- If the prescription drug route is taken, there is a good chance that only certain physicians may be approached under a patient's benefit payment program. (Remember, of course, that regulatory constraints already limit access to legend drugs to prescription by a licensed practitioner.) So access to *medications* may be limited by federal regulation and access to that *practitioner* may be limited by the patient's benefit program.
- But the limits go further! The practitioner may be limited in prescribing by the benefit program to a generic equivalent of his or her drug product choice or forced to choose a lower cost or other alternative from the same therapeutic class.
- Limits may also determine the number of refills allowed, the quantity allowed, or the number of prescriptions allowed in a given time period.
- The patient may even be expected to order prescription medications by mail in order to realize the full economic value of a benefit program.

Now we have used the phrase "benefit program" several times already, and we have purposely used it in a generic way. What does it mean? First, we will limit the following discussion to prescription medications. There are effects on OTC reductions—especially those which are being switched to OTC from prescription status—but we will address these later. Also, the benefit program represents yet another intervening variable in an already complicated transaction.

The original (well maybe not original, but first early modern) model for treatment was for the patient to visit the healer/physician and receive treat-

TABLE 2.4. Probable Future Alterations of Life Patterns by Drugs

1. Prolong childhood and (shorten?) adolescence
2. Reduce need for sleep
3. Provide safe, short-acting intoxicants
4. Regulate sexual responses
5. Control affect and aggression
6. Mediate nutrition, metabolism, and physical growth
7. Increase or decrease reactivity (alertness, relaxation)
8. Prolong or shorten memory
9. Induct or prevent learning
   a. experience without reinforcement
   b. vicariously with reinforcement
10. Produce or discontinue transference
11. Provoke or relieve guilt
12. Foster or terminate mothering behavior
13. Shorten or extend experienced time
14. Create conditions of *jamais vu* (novelty) or *déjà vu* (familiarity)
15. Deepen our awareness of beauty and our sense of awe

Source: Adapted from Nathan S. Kline, Probable Future Alterations of Life Patterns by Drugs, in *Psychotropic Drugs in the Year 2000,* eds. William O. Evans and Nathan S. Kline (Springfield, IL: Charles C Thomas, 1971), p. 78.

ment on the spot. When materia medica became somewhat more specific and precise, it became timely to defer to a knowledgeable specialist (pharmacist) to prepare the medications. It was not required, but it was convenient and logical. After World War II real medicines began to be discovered and developed. In the face of these new potent remedies the "legendary," Durham-Humphrey Amendment to the Food, Drug, and Cosmetic Act was enacted requiring a prescription to gain access to certain medications judged by the FDA to be unsafe for use by an unsupervised general public. The term "legend," a designation used in printing, refers to the sentence required, by law, to appear on the packages of these drug products: "Caution: Federal law prohibits dispensing without a prescription." This set up the extraordinary, if not unique, class of goods that one could not necessarily buy, even if one had the money (other such goods include nuclear arms and alcohol and tobacco, if under a certain age). Now, by law, three parties were involved in a prescription drug transaction—patient, prescriber, and pharmacist.

In spite of the three-party relationship just described, the 1950s and beyond saw the invention of the term "third party" to describe yet another—this time a fiscal player. In this case, the *patient* visits the *prescriber,* who issues a prescription to the *pharmacist* and who is, usually, reimbursed for his or her

[handwritten margin note: after WWII needed Rx to gain access to some medications.]

goods and services (see *Section III: Pricing*) by a payer of some kind. Sure, that is a fourth party, but a third party between the pharmacist and the patient. It is probably essential to note that from a pure market perspective it would be difficult to identify another case in which the consumer does not decide which commodity to consume and also pays for none or only a part of it.

Let us return to "pharmacy benefits." It is as good a euphemism as any. The idea of providing needed medicines to various publics goes way back in history—farther back than will we. Perhaps the first serious initiative in the United States was the Kerr-Mills program.

Finally, in response to unremitting pressure for a public drug program, Wilbur Mills (then chairman of the Ways and Means Committee) began to search for some compromise. First, he sounded out colleagues on a plan that would have given Social Security beneficiaries a choice between higher cash benefits or hospitalization benefits. Department of Health, Education and Welfare (HEW) Secretary Flemming rejected this idea and implied that President Eisenhower would veto such legislation. Nor, in all likelihood, were there enough votes for the idea in the committee at that point. In any case, it was quietly dropped. But Chairman Mills moved to break on impasse. With the cooperation of the American Medical Association (AMA), Mills devised a plan to expand greatly the program of medical vendor payments provided under the state-run public assistance programs. This was to be accomplished by creating a new assistance category called "medical indigency," for elderly people who might not otherwise qualify for welfare in their states but who needed help with their medical bills. This plan was the forerunner of what we know today as Medicaid. From the point of view of the members of Congress, the Mills plan had several merits: It was more modest in cost and scope than either a so-called Forand bill or the Republican "subsidy" plan; from a technical standpoint it was a logical first step; it was a "Democratic bill" in a Democratic Congress and was sponsored by the respected Ways and Means Committee chairman; and, not least, it had the backing of the AMA. Therefore, Chairman Mills's proposal proved to be the one upon which a congressional consensus could be reached. The proposal (H.R. 12580) was quickly approved by the Ways and Means Committee, easily won clearance for a floor vote from the House Rule Committee, and whisked through the House of Representatives by a vote of 381 to 23.

The most important public effort to provide medicines to a defined population (the "needy") was the Medicaid legislation enacted during the Kennedy Administration. While a plethora of special interest groups were busy fighting or supporting the *Medicare* legislature, *Medicaid* slipped by nearly unnoticed. Yet its impact on the public and on the pharmaceutical industry has been enormous.

It is interesting that the Medicare program, designed to serve the elderly population who use and need more medications per person as of the year

2000, still lacked an outpatient pharmacy benefits program. The last serious effort to provide such a benefit resulted in the Medicare Catastrophic Coverage Act, which was both passed and repealed by the same Congress because, among other things, the various agencies of the federal government could not agree on how much it would cost and whether the American taxpayers could/would afford it. Such drug benefits were a major point in the presidential election of 2000.

Medicaid, a partnership between state and federal governments, continues today to provide recipients with an assortment of prescription and nonprescription medication, at an assortment of persona costs, and with a bewildering array of individual drug constraints.

In the private sector, some insurance programs have long offered pharmaceutical benefits—for a premium, of course. Union contracts, health maintenance organizations (HMOs), and professional association programs have, together, contrived to make prescription benefits, variously, a bargaining chip, a negotiated fringe, or a prerequisite of membership. Each and all have played a role in the makeup and future development of the industry and influenced the behavior of individual consumers.

A brief analogy might help, although we will revisit pharmacy benefits at other times in this text.

Suppose you are a homeowner belonging to a homeowners improvement association to which you pay an annual premium. The premium is designed to help you handle the things that can go wrong around the house in such a way that you will not be financially devastated by a major disaster but also to help you deal with day-to-day maintenance of a home during the normal aging process. One day you notice a ventilation problem that you believe can be solved fairly easily, but to take care of it, you will need an electric drill.

Now, drills are covered by your homeowner's policy, but to receive the economic benefits of your policy, you are required to visit a "house doctor," describe your problem (he or she will not make house calls), and receive an authorizing note allowing your acquisition of a drill, after assessing your ability to use such a drill in compliance with directions (sure!). You have seen some advertisements and ask if it could be a Black & Decker drill. "Certainly," says the doctor, who specifies that brand on the note. You take the note to the designated hardware store (only certain stores are approved by your hardware benefit plan). You are informed by the hardware dealer that Black & Decker drills are not covered by the plan. Certainly you may buy *that* drill out of your own cash, but the drill that is covered is a Knobstock. That, in a nutshell, and certainly incompletely, is the systems environment in which the consumer often functions.

These influences on the individual have an effect on and are affected by the aggregate. That is what we address in The Outer Ring.

THE OUTER RING: THE AGGREGATE ENVIRONMENT

A convenient segue between the discussions of the inner and outer rings in Figure 2.1 was provided by Figure 2.2.

In addition to our individual characteristics and behavior, each of us has other identities as parts of even larger groups, including family, various formal and informal communities, and finally the total society. There is some value in understanding the parallels illustrated in Figure 2.2, in which is shown the dual position of humans in nature. Just as the entire human organism must often take action to correct disruptions at the lower levels of the mental and physical organization, so the total society must frequently initiate programs to correct health problems among its individual members.

Rene Dubos has found in the earlier writings of famed medical scholar Virchow further justification for studying society in order to study health care:

> In [Virchow's] words, "Epidemics resemble great warnings from which a statesman in the grand style can read that a disturbance has taken place in the development of his people, a disturbance that not even a carefree policy can long overlook." Thus, according to Virchow, the treatment of individual cases is only a small aspect of medicine. More important is the control of crowd disease which demands social and, if need be, political action. In this light medicine is a social science.[19]

As Wilson points out:

> Although it is quite clear that society, like the body, is composed of interdependent systems and that events occurring in any given system reverberate in other subsystems, we must recognize that mutuality among sections of a community (society) is far less thoroughgoing than the pervasive mutuality of body process. Further, we must be aware of imagining that communities possess anything approaching the central nervous system, either in singleness of purpose or unitary mechanisms of control, is foolish.[20]

In spite of these limitations, however, the study of a society and its goals is imperative for anyone who intends to operate in the health system that the society has developed. For, in spite of its failure to reach unanimity of purpose consistently, society does on occasion act as one organism: setting priorities, defining goals, choosing methods. When *society* is the patient, it decides how much health care it will seek and who will provide it.

The social component of medical care includes the goals of the individual patient and the individual health professional as manifested by public action. The products of such action are the various public health programs initiated in response to the demands of society.

In general, the community participates in the medical care complex in order to promote, protect, and restore the health of individuals in its population. It recognizes that expenditures of money, manpower, and material in the field of health represent investments in the total structure of a community and cannot be considered on only the consumption side of the ledger. Ideally, therefore, society's goals are to reduce, as far as possible, mortality and morbidity in all segments of the population; to ensure that everyone has access to personal health services of high quality; and to remove or reduce unnecessary social or economic consequences of dependencies that the population may suffer as the result of disease and disability. In striving to accomplish these goals, different communities and societies may use different means, depending upon the combination of different cultural values, political attitudes, economic circumstances, and technological capacities.

The importance of social forces in accepting responsibility for health care and the tortuous path that the changes in social attitudes may take are illustrated in the example of Medicare, which, "from idea to law," seems to have spanned a period from 1883 to 1965. For this major, and by now seemingly completely acceptable, piece of social legislation to be enacted, almost tangible shifts in public opinion and pressure had to occur. Considering the problems involved in bringing an *insurance* program of this type to law, it seems incredible that, at the same time, without major tumult, a *welfare* health program (Medicaid) was also passed.

Noted medical historian James Harvey Young has described the characteristic pattern of food and drug legislation as consisting of "change, complexity, competition, crusading, compromise, catastrophe." The laws to which he referred were primarily those which regulate practices relating to drugs. In fact, the same pattern, with less obvious "catastrophe," seems to characterize legislation establishing other types of health programs.

It is entirely appropriate that social goals should have become more and more clearly identified and more and more forcefully pursued. The social changes that have been occurring so rapidly have had a serious impact through creation of both psychologic and physical environmental hazards. Individual health needs quickly become community health needs—more numerous, diversified, and complex. More community participation is required to provide the comprehensive services necessary for resolution and/or prevention of the multiplication of problems.

Many of the problems are relatively new: urbanization, increased population density with its pollution of all kinds, automation, industrialization, and depersonalization. Successful functioning in isolation is no longer possible, as the components of this intensely complex society have, of necessity, become interdependent.

This is the social overlay that affects society's views and goals in health. Historically people have tended to be satisfied with medical care of the curative or "crisis" type. Medicine has been importantly affected by major discoveries and changes (including drugs) that have allowed a shift in emphasis from almost exclusive concentration on diagnosis and treatment to a much broader approach that includes the prevention of disease and rehabilitation from its effects.

Our society has become better informed on health matters, and its stated goals reflect a more knowledgeable public. Freedom from disease has been expanded to include the desire to live in a state of well-being. The public no longer regards medical care as only a means of *restoring* health; this care is now considered to include the means for *maintaining* good health. It is now expected that the highest quality of medical protection should be available and accessible to all of the people when they are sick or when they are well.

A further comparison of patients as individuals and in the broader social context is provided by the data in Table 2.5. These data reflect responses of more than 10,000 people regarding what individual patients and their responding health care systems should do in an ideal system. Although the two lists are not incompatible, obviously compromises are needed.

The ultimate test of a business or its industry is its social relevance. Clearly the pharmaceutical industry is socially relevant. The relevance of an individual firm or its individual products is ultimately determined by those in the marketplace.

In the final analysis, it is society itself that controls all marketing activities. The principal means of control resides in the decision to buy or not to buy. This is the most potent form of regulation. Since the people elect the legislators, they do, indirectly, enact the laws as well. In fact control by *regulation* is probably the farthest removed from the people.

The average layperson does not, of course, have sufficient information to decide the merits of all of the controls imposed on marketing. In many cases, he or she does not have even enough knowledge to appraise the value of the products that this marketing activity brings.

Economic Environment

A national health insurance was established in Germany in the 1880s. The motives were previously economic—healthy workers would be more productive workers. The age for retirement—sixty-five—was also selected for economic reasons. Most workers were expected to be dead by that age. Social Security, still saddled with that aged and arbitrary cutoff, is just addressing yet another economic fact of life.

Another economic fact of life is that the demand for health care is nearly inexhaustible, but the funds to pay for such care is exhaustible. For this simple reason, and for many more complicated reasons, economics, in addition to humane and medical concerns, will always be a serious concern for the pharmaceutical industry.

TABLE 2.5. What Patients and the Health Care System Should Do

People believe patients should . . .	People believe the health care system should . . .
Responsibility	
Risk-related behavior: be responsible for the consequences of their own lifestyle	Civic issues: offer support for unexpected crises
Personal responsibility: offer Rx compliance	*Financial obligation:* pay in the event of crisis
Financial obligation: pay for elective care	
Fairness	
Convenience: have health care services close and information readily available	*Universal access:* offer care of equal quality
	Community issues: give sense of caring and support
	Convenience: make services accessible
Affordability and Efficiency	
Cost/benefit/value: have information about the cost and effectiveness of treatment	*Accountability:* identify good performers
	Cost/benefit/value: benefit the whole
Prudence: recognize the limits of their care	*Productivity:* minimize waste
Simplicity: have understandable information	*Prudence:* act intelligently for personal and national interests
	Affordability: price services affordably
	Simplicity: make the system more consumer friendly
Dignity	
Humaneness: have personal choice in death and dying	*Humaneness:* help patients avoid pain and suffering
Caring: receive emotional support from providers	*Caring:* view its caregivers' role as "healers" rather than "doctors"
Compassion: receive understanding and patience	*Compassion:* understand patient etiology
Trust/honesty: be able to cultivate personal relationships with providers	*Trust/honesty:* offer accurate, honest information
Respect: have providers accept wishes	
Choice	
Information: be allowed more individual decision making	*Information:* make decisions in cooperation with patients
Control: have some control over health outcomes	*Control:* cede some control to patients
Informed consent: be given the opportunity to investigate in advance of decisions	*Informed consent:* give patients full information for health care decisions
Personal responsibility: be permitted a choice, such as to accept or reject treatments	*Personal issues:* allow patients to select providers
	Autonomy: allow patients to make decisions
Quality	
Quality of life: maintain their quality of life	*Quality of life:* make quality paramount
Quality of care: receive the best individual care and attention	*Quality of care:* give the best care possible and offer a hospitable environment
Technical excellence: have access to the best and latest technology	*Technical excellence:* adopt techniques that improve
Healing/caring: have providers who are understanding and supportive	*Healing/caring:* make system more approachable

Source: Adapted from Elizabeth Moench, "What Does DM Mean to Patients," *Pharmaceutical Executive,* May 15(5): 52, 53, 56, 1995.

Examples of economic trends and events affecting most businesses include the following possibilities:

- Depression; worldwide economic collapse
- Increasing foreign ownership of U.S. economy
- Increasing regulation and management of national economies
- Several developing nations becoming superpowers
- World food production
- Decline in real world growth, or stable growth
- Collapse of world monetary system
- Increase in inflation
- Significant employee-union ownership of U.S. businesses
- Worldwide free trade
- Significant epidemics threatening patients, as with AIDS in Africa

It is not unrealistic to say that all companies, small or large, engaged in strategic planning examine the economic environment. Relevant published information is usually gathered, analyzed, and interpreted for use in planning. In some corporations the entire process of dealing with economic information may be manual and intuitive. Several pharmaceutical companies, however, have established full-blown pharmaceutical economics study groups. Part of the work of these groups is to access and predict the economic environment. Another part is to explain, for marketing purposes, the economics of medication use.

Dubos anticipated the current emphasis on quality of life and pharmaceutical economic research and application in marketing:

> If one were to use a criteria [sic] the amount of life spoiled by disease, instead of measuring only that destroyed by death; or the number of days lost from pleasure and work because of so-called minor ailments; or merely the sums paid for drugs, hospital, and doctor's bills, the toll exacted by microbial pathogens would seem very large indeed.[21]

Ethical/Cultural Environment

For many years in the third quarter of the twentieth century the prescription pharmaceutical industry styled itself as the "ethical drug industry." Presumably this self-bestowed sobriquet referred to the fact that the industry dealings were mainly with health professionals—primarily physicians—who were themselves "ethical." Although this title has largely disappeared from use, it made a convenient target for those who found plenty of unethical behavior to criticize.

The pharmaceutical industry has received somewhat more than its share of attention from a group of writers aiming at social control and changes *authors to look into* ←

through their activities as "medical muckrakers." As unflattering as the term sounds, "muckraking" has an honorable role in society. The term "muckraker" was originally coined by President Theodore Roosevelt and has come to refer to journalistic reformers. Two of the first to bear the appellation were Upton Sinclair and Samuel Hopkins Adams. Their activities were culminated in published books, *The Jungle* and *The Great American Fraud*, respectively, together, were in large part responsible for passage of the original Food and Drugs Act.

The most widely read among the early medical muckrakers were Martin Gross *(The Doctors)* and Morton Mintz *(The Therapeutic Nightmare,* reissued under the title *By Prescription Only).* The latter author based much of his material on the Kefauver investigations. Gross attacked primarily the "medical establishment," but in his single chapter dealing with the drug industry, he

1. called for elimination of all types of drug promotion to physicians;
2. asked for denial of patients to "molecular or other modification of an existing drug, or combination of two or more existing drugs, unless the Secretary of Health, Education and Welfare determines that the therapeutic effect of the modified drug is significantly greater";
3. asked for compulsory licensing of drug patents after three years; and
4. suggested that patients insist on prescription by generic name.[22]

It is the ethical environment of society as a whole, however, that fits our outer ring. And while the industry must somehow adapt to changes therein, those changes tend to be evolutionary, rather than rapid and responses may be equally slow.

Defining death, determining the terminality of disease, and measuring changes in quality of life are among the social goals to which the industry must be prepared to respond. Dubos introduced the theories of Elle Metchnikoff to illustrate a fascinating concept that is at least indirectly related to the core of pharmaceuticals.[23] Metchnikoff, a Nobel Prize winner in the 1800s, noted that every bodily function calls into play an "instinct of satiety." A satisfying meal leaves us without desire for food; we seek rest after any sort of exercise. Why, then, is there no instinct of satiety for living—an "instinct of death"?

Referring to Metchnikoff's philosophy Dubos notes:

> It is . . . because human life is usually much shorter than the number of years of which he is potentially capable. Human beings who reach a really ripe age—say 100 years or more—do welcome death without regrets even though they are not sick and do not suffer, just as a normal person welcomes sleep at the end of a day.[24]

Measuring changes in quality of life—an exercise that may seem at first to be interesting to only academics and the clergy—has taken on marketing importance, which is discussed elsewhere in the book. For present purposes we will treat the concept as part of the cultural environment.

Quality of life (QOL) is one of those concepts (e.g., positioning) that everyone knows, no one can really define, but of which it is easy to give examples. This is true in large part because QOL measurements, such as side effects, have long been an implicit part of clinical investigations. QOL studies, especially when applied in an economic context as they often are, simply assess the impact of disease and of therapy, directly and explicitly. This is a favorable development in that it is bringing focus and vigor to such investigative considerations.

For the drug industry, QOL issues can range from something as simple as being able to thread a needle to situations as somber as determining the degree and nature of pain relief to provide to the terminally ill cancer patient.

The ability to define QOL, to measure differences in it, and to demonstrate positive effects of medications on it are matters of great potential commercial significance to drug marketers, but they should also understand the deeper philosophical issues. The *commercial* importance of QOL springs from its *human* importance.

Human dimensions of QOL include the following:

- Factors related to physical problems
- Presence or absence of physical symptoms
- Toxicity and side effects of therapy
- Body image and mobility
- Psychological, social, and spiritual dimensions
- Coping abilities
- Quality of interpersonal relations
- "Happiness" or sense of well-being
- Inner peace, not necessarily religious
- Economic costs and effects
- Wider dimensions, such as external effects on others
- Personal preferences, ambitions, priorities
- Cultural variations
- Political and policy considerations
- Philosophical and ethical dimensions
- Value and meaning of time

An example of how this somewhat vague, sometimes difficult-to-measure concept has been applied to real-world health-related social decisions comes from the United Kingdom.

Quality-adjusted life years (QALY) is a synthetic common denominator that attempts to allow comparability of results of differing treatments. To the degree that it is a reliable and valid measure it would allow, for any treatment, determination of lives saved and prolonged. For example, it would yield different cost-effectiveness data for two patients, each of whose life was extended by five years, but one of whom spent the time in a coma and the other in a reasonably functional state.

Cost utility analysis (CUA) is a new label that emphasizes the economic concept of health "utility" as a measure of benefits obtained from an intervention. Utility values are used to express the impairment of health experienced by survivors of a disease. A scale ranging from 0 (death) to 1 (perfect health) reflects the utility value for each health state.* When combined with survival data, utility values allow the researcher to estimate the number of life years gained weighted by their QALY. This has seen very limited application in the United States because of practical difficulties in developing the utility values for difference health states. In the United Kingdom, however, there is significant support for using "cost per QALY" as a measure of value for money in the debate about national health care priorities. Qualms about using the QALY concept and cost utility as a means to allocate health care resources in the United Kingdom are, however, quite abundant. Concerns range from arbitrarily selected values for utility to ethical implications of favoring patients whose age and disease suggest the prospect of longer and better QOL at the expense of the old and very sick.

The QALY concept represents a natural extension of the way medicine has been practiced in the United Kingdom since the introduction of the National Health Service (NHS) in 1947. NHS was originally conceived as an access to high-quality medical care with no charge at the point of use, funded through general taxation. With no or little cost of access, demand rapidly exceeded the ability to supply. Supply and demand were brought into equilibrium by an ad hoc application of the queuing principle.

Access to some form of health care is rarely denied but may be deferred. Individual physicians have to make value judgments about individual patients as to their positions in the queue. The criteria most physicians use are very similar to those involved in calculating QALY; i.e., given a limitation of resources, which patients are likely to receive the greatest benefits for the longest time?

The application of these principles can readily be visualized in a hospital setting; the number of operation theaters and the people to staff them are limited, and the demand for procedures exceeds this supply; a waiting list is formed with those who will benefit most (not necessarily the most needy) at

---

*Some argue that the scale should range from +1 (perfect health) to −1 (better to be dead).

the top of the list. For some patients this does imply that the situation is resolved by an untimely death while waiting for the procedure.

This situation is most dramatically exemplified by the U.K. attitude toward treating end stage renal disease (ESRD). The NHS recognized that treating all patients who could benefit from renal dialysis would rapidly bankrupt the system. Instead, they opted for very limited dialysis facilities and a concentration on organ transplant. The cynical observer might note that this plan puts the blame for the failure to provide adequate therapy on the low supply of organs rather than on the government's unwillingness to fund an adequate number of dialysis centers.

With community care, a slightly different tactic is taken. There is free access to a primary care physician for all, but the primary care physician acts as a gatekeeper for access to specialist care. Physicians have the freedom to prescribe any drug approved by the committee on safety of medicines but their prescribing habits are carefully monitored. In practice, if a physician wishes to use an expensive therapy, he or she may do so but must compensate by reducing the average price of his or her other prescriptions.

Political Environment

The political environment is an obvious but not always accurate reflection of the previously discussed components of the outer ring, although it must be admitted that a reverse influence also exists.

International assessment of the political environment is a daily necessity for the pharmaceutical industry. The framework provided in Table 2.6 is only a partial list of the concerns.

In the United States politics and pharmaceuticals have "enjoyed" a rich history together. Members of both political parties have used the industry, its products, its prices, and its practices as a source of political activity for more than half a century. Some, notably, the late Estes Kefauver, have used congressional investigating powers and the forums associated with them to seek the presidency.

In the 1992 presidential election, health care reform was a central issue for the Democratic Party, with the cost of prescription medications being a frequently cited concern. (Interestingly, considerable reform did follow that election, but it was brought about in large part by private industry and not by career politicians.) Health care for the elderly has been and promises to be a continuing public policy issue, with outpatient drug benefits an elusive goal.

A Political Example

The Medicare outpatient drug benefit moved through Congress in 1987-1988 at the legislative equivalent of the speed of light. As a visible benefit for the elderly in an election year, it quickly got the support of the Democratic leadership. The Republicans, in turn, were not inclined to a protracted fight on the bill, pro-

TABLE 2.6. A Framework for Analyzing the Political Environment

Sources of Political Risk	Groups Through Which Political Risk Can Be Generated	Effects on International Business Operations
Comparing political philosophies (nationalism, socialism, communism) Social unrest and disorder Vested interests of local business groups Recent and impending political independence Armed conflicts and internal rebellions for political power New international alliances	Government in power and its operating agencies Parliamentary opposition groups Nonparliamentary opposition groups (Algerian FLN, guerilla movements working within or outside country) Nonorganized common interest groups: students, workers, peasants, minorities, and so on Foreign governments or intergovernmental agencies such as the EEC Foreign governments willing to enter the armed conflict or to support internal rebellion	Confiscation: loss of assets without compensation Expropriation with compensation: loss of freedom to operate Operational restrictions: market shares, product characteristics, employment policies, locally shared ownership, and so on Loss of transfer freedom: financial (dividends, interest payments, goods, personnel, or ownership rights, for example) Breaches or unilateral revisions in contracts and agreements Discrimination such as taxes or compulsory subcontractings Damage to property or personnel from riots, insurrections, revolutions, and wars

Source: Adapted from Stefan H. Robock and Kenneth Simmonds, *International Business and Multinational Enterprises,* Fourth Edition (Homewood, IL: Richard D. Irwin, Inc., 1989), p. 383.

Note: FLN - Front de Libéracion Nationale (National Liberation Front); EEC = European Economic Community.

viding the Democrats with a ready-made election issue. One of the prime Capitol proponents of the bill, in fact, was a Republican.

Although the ultimate legislative action on Medicare outpatient coverage was rapid, the process leading up to it was much slower. The final act can be viewed as the progeny of previous health care entitlements and prescription drug legislation.

The concept of adding an outpatient prescription drug benefit to the Medicare program goes back to 1967, when the Johnson Administration set up a task force to study the issue. That group issued a report supporting the addition of a drug benefit, a recommendation that was then seconded by a nongovernment commission established to review the task force's work.

In the early 1970s, Congress increased its focus on the drug industry. Senator Kennedy held a series of hearings that focused on drug prices to argue that the price differential between brand-name drugs and generic products was not justified by quality concerns.

In this atmosphere, the Department of Health and Human Services began to look at ways to reduce costs, and the prescription drug reimbursement system was one area singled out for reform. The result was the Maximum Allowable Cost/Estimated Acquisition Cost (MAC) program, which incorporated the basic ideas contained in the task force report prepared for HEW in the late 1960s. The basic cost control element of the program was reimbursement limits for individual drugs, encouraging the dispensing of lower-cost generic equivalents in place of brand-name products.

A major change in the pharmaceutical environment since the advent of MAC in 1977 has been the explosive growth in the availability of generic products. That change was brought about legislatively in 1984 with the enactment of the Drug Price Competition and Patent Term Restoration Act of 1984 (discussed in later chapters).

The Waxman-Hatch Act, as it is known in recognition of the two principle sponsors, contained two major sections that together represented the most significant piece of legislation affecting the drug industry since the 1962 effectiveness amendments were added to the Food, Drug, and Cosmetic Act.

Under Title I of the Waxman-Hatch Act, Congress established a procedure to extend the patent terms for pharmaceutical products meeting specified eligibility criteria. The purpose of extending the patents of some new pharmaceutical products beyond the standard seventeen-year period was to compensate research-based firms for patent time lost during the premarket approval process at the FDA.

The second section of the Waxman-Hatch Act is more significant in relation to the coverage of outpatient drugs under Medicare. In Title II of the Waxman-Hatch Act, Congress authorized procedures for the first time for the FDA to review and approve generic versions of prescription drugs first approved after 1962 when the effectiveness amendments were added to the Food, Drug, and Cosmetic Act.

Title II of the Waxman-Hatch Act immediately and dramatically expanded the multisource drug marketplace so that it now includes many of the most commonly prescribed drugs. In some ways, the inclusion of a Medicare outpatient drug reimbursement system is merely an extension of the Waxman-Hatch Act. Federal reimbursement of outpatient drugs on a scale proposed by the Medicare Catastrophic Coverage Act would simply be unaffordable without the existence of the large pool of multisource drugs that developed as a result of the Waxman-Hatch Act.

By early 1989, only a few months after the election, many members of Congress were "discovering" that they had voted for the bill without a full appreciation of its potential cost.

The case just related is a prime example of the nature of the influence of the political environment on the pharmaceutical industry. It is also a good example of a good political "horse trade"—the generic components of the industry get easier access to the market, the brand-name components get the potential for patent life extension, and the government gets a promise of lower drug costs. By the end of the twentieth century, there was still no Medicare outpatient drug benefit.

Legal/Regulatory Environment

In his treatise *Medizinische Polizei*, Johann Peter Frank proposed that the State was responsible for people's health.[25] This concept seems to be mentioned today in various ways from providing health care to protecting the people from harm. Most of the activity of the state in this regard finds form in laws and regulations.

No business can operate without considering a myriad of government restrictions and regulations. Costs and profits can be affected as much by a regulation written by a government official as by their own management decisions or their customers' changing preferences. The types of management decisions that increasingly are subject to governmental influence, review, or control are fundamental to the business system:

- What lines of business should be explored?
- What products can be produced?
- Which investments can be financed?
- Under what conditions can products be produced?
- Where can products be made?
- How can products be marketed?
- What prices can be charged?
- What profits can be kept?

Virtually every major department of every corporation in the industry has one or more counterparts in a federal and/or state agency that controls or strongly influences its internal decision making. Many feel, with considerable justification, that the pharmaceutical industry, from manufacturer to practicing pharmacist, is the most highly regulated of all. Why would that be the case?

An imperfect model to explain the development of legal controls in the pharmaceutical industry would look like this:

Individuals Express Needs and Concerns
↓
Individuals As a Society Express Collective Needs and Concerns
Through Election of
↓
"Politicians" Who Have Identified Social Needs and Concerns and Who
↓
Enact Laws to Fulfill the Needs and Address the Concerns,
Leaving the Actual Implementation of Such Laws to
↓
Regulations, Promulgated Usually by Nonelected Officials
of State and Federal Agencies

This progression is fraught with the opportunity for error, both in sensing the will and needs of those in the previous step and in their implementation even if properly identified. Nevertheless, that is how it works, and the good news is that opportunity exists at each step.

In this section we briefly examine laws, regulations, and judicial controls at both the federal and state levels. We will return to many of these at appropriate parts in the text.

Federal Laws

Laws at the federal level include those which affect business generally and those which have specific importance to the pharmaceutical industry.

Laws of general industry application include the following:

- Sherman Antitrust Act, 1890
- Federal Trade Commission Act, 1914
- Clayton Antitrust Act, 1914
- Robinson-Patman Act, 1936
- Wheeler-Lea Act, 1938
- Lanham Trademark Act, 1946
- Fair Packaging and Labeling Act, 1966
- Consumer Product Safety Act, 1972

It is neither practical nor necessary to review the provisions of each of these laws here. It should be noted, however, that each of these laws has had important specific effects on the pharmaceutical industry despite their general applicability. They have affected pricing, promotion, distribution, and product development (the four Ps that are the focus of much of this book).

Laws specific to the pharmaceutical industry are as follows:

- Food and Drugs Act, 1906 ("the original")
- Harrison Narcotic Act, 1914
- Food, Drug, and Cosmetic Act, 1938
- Durham-Humphrey Amendment, 1951
- Kefauver-Harris Drug Amendments, 1962
- Drug Abuse Control Amendments, 1965
- Comprehensive Drug Abuse Prevention and Control Act, 1970
- Drug Price Competition and Patent Term Restoration Act, 1984

Other laws are specific to the pharmaceutical industry but this list should provide an appreciation of the industry's legislative controls. Again, it is impractical here to discuss details of each, but two of the laws and their histories are so important to marketing that we attend to them in some detail, particularly as they also illustrate the interaction between the general and the specific laws.

The well-known sulfanilamide disaster in which a toxic agent was used as a solvent occurred in 1937. More than 100 people died from ingestion of this elixir of sulfanilamide.

It is interesting to note that the court order for seizure of the substance was not founded on allegations that the drug was adulterated or unsafe. Rather, the product was labeled as an "elixir," which necessarily implies an alcoholic solution. The product contained no alcohol and was therefore misbranded. Accordingly, if it had been properly labeled as a solution rather than as an elixir, no violation would have occurred.*

This tragedy, coupled with books such as *200,000,000 Guinea Pigs,* by John Grant, and *American Chamber of Horrors,* by Ruth Lamb, detailing hazards caused by current manufacturing practices of the food, drug, and cosmetic industry, aroused public pressure and overcame government inertia. As a result, the Federal Food, Drug, and Cosmetic Act was passed in 1938. The act identified certain prohibited practices, including introduction into interstate commerce of any food, drug, or cosmetic that is adulterated or misbranded.

Provisions regarding the advertising of drugs were of critical significance to the marketing of pharmaceuticals. At issue was enforcement jurisdiction for false advertising. Should the Federal Trade Commission (FTC) or the FDA assume responsibility for these provisions in the new bill? The FTC actively lobbied against jurisdiction with the FDA. The Proprietary Association (now the nonprescription Drug Manufacturers Association), the United Medicine Manufacturers of America, and the Institute of the Medicine Manufacturers supported the FTC.

The central objection against assigning drug advertising responsibilities to the FTC was the restriction imposed by the Supreme Court in *Federal Trade Commission v. Raladam Co.* This decision limited FTC authority to only false advertising in which an injury to competition could be shown. Pharmacist-legislators Wheeler and Lea sought to overrule the Raladam decision and give the FTC responsibility for advertising by congressional enactment. They drafted the Wheeler-Lea Amendments to the Federal Trade Commission Act.

The Wheeler-Lea Amendments prohibited dissemination of any false advertising for the purpose of inducing, directly or indirectly, the purchase of food, drugs, devices, or cosmetics. Such actions constitute unfair or deceptive practices under the Federal Trade Commission Act. An advertisement

---

*This subsection is adapted from Chapter 21, "External Controls," in Mickey Smith (Ed.), *Principles of Pharmaceutical Marketing,* Third Edition (Binghamton, NY: The Haworth Press, 1988), pp. 485-513. Original material written by Gary C. Wilkerson and Michael Pietrangelo.

is false when misleading in any material respect. Furthermore, omission of any material fact may result in a misleading advertisement. The Wheeler-Lea Act abolished the rule of caveat emptor. The consumer has a right to rely upon statements contained in advertising, and if the advertisement has the capacity or tendency to deceive, its language contravenes the law.

Passage of the Wheeler-Lea Amendments resolved the issue of regulation of drug advertising. The FDA still retained jurisdiction over labels and labeling.

The 1938 Food, Drug, and Cosmetic Act required drug packages to be labeled with adequate warnings and directions for use. Drugs not labeled were deemed misbranded. However, an exemption from the "directions" requirement existed for medications not necessary for protection of public health. After World War II many pharmaceutical companies that had previously restricted marketing of their products through professional channels began labeling all packages for prescription sale. This created a problem because the statute required adequate directions for use unless otherwise exempted.

Then, in 1948, the Supreme Court handed down its landmark decision in *U.S. v. Sullivan.* In this case, a pharmacist, who purchased properly labeled sulfathiazole from a wholesaler, removed twelve tablets from the bulk container, placed them in a pill box, labeled it "sulfathiazole," and sold it to a patient. The court held that the pharmacist violated the misbranding provision of the act by not providing adequate directions and warnings for use to the customer.

Following this decision, Congress passed the Miller Amendment, which clearly extended to wholesale and retail establishments for violation of the act. Pharmacists consequently became concerned over possible prosecution for selling prescription drugs over the counter, even though such actions were not expressly prohibited by the Food, Drug, and Cosmetic Act. Obviously a need existed for a statutory definition of prescription drugs. Two pharmacist-legislators, Representative Carl Durham (North Carolina) and Senator Hubert Humphrey (Minnesota), sponsored such legislation. Supported by the National Association of Retail Druggists and by the FDA, the Durham-Humphrey Amendment to the Food, Drug, and Cosmetic Act became law in 1951. In effect, this measure provided for the existence of two classes of drugs, those dispensed pursuant to a prescription and those sold over the counter.

Three general categories of prescription drugs were defined in the amendment:

1. Hypnotic or habit-forming drugs that are specifically named in the law, and their derivatives, unless specifically exempted by a regulation
2. A drug that is not safe for self-medication "because of its toxicity or other potentiality for harmful effect, or the method of its use, or the collateral measures necessary to its use"

3. A "new drug" that has not been shown to be safe for use in self-medication, and that, under the terms of an effective new drug application, is limited to prescription dispensing

Additionally, it amended the act by (1) restricting the dispensing of legend drugs pursuant only to prescription, oral or written (with certain exemptions), and (2) prohibiting the refilling of such prescriptions without the expressed authorization of the prescriber (oral or written in appropriate circumstances).

It further required that all prescription medications, prior to dispensing to the patient, bear the following statement: "Caution: Federal law prohibits dispensing without a prescription" (see System Constraints). This measure directly affected the marketing of prescription pharmaceuticals. Drug firms discovered the need for and benefit of physician advertising by the use of detail people (salespeople), medical journals, and direct mail. However, the companies tended to describe the therapeutic *advantages* of their drugs, neglecting to identify side effects and contraindications. Consequently, the drug manufacturers were to some extent replacing medical schools as principal sources of drug information.

The FDA recognized the need for physicians to have at their disposal all necessary information for each medication prescribed. Accordingly, the "full disclosure" regulations were promulgated. These regulations required that the label specify, among other things, the format for full disclosure, including the kind and amount of active ingredient and the dosage.

The most significant amendments to the 1938 Food, Drug, and Cosmetic Act were the Kefauver-Harris Drug Amendments of 1962. Senator Estes Kefauver (Tennessee) held a series of hearings in the late 1950s and 1960s that questioned the marketing and pricing methods of the pharmaceutical industry. Then, in late 1961, the thalidomide tragedy unfolded.

Thalidomide was a tranquilizer/sedative marketed by Chemie Grunenthal in West Germany as an OTC. The product was distributed for approximately three years before Dr. Leng, a pediatrician a the University of Hamburg, discovered and reported to the company that it caused phocomelia, a birth defect in infants. By this time several thousand infants had been affected.

The European experience was reported in early 1962, at which time all U.S. clinical trials on thalidomide were terminated. All new drug applications were either rejected or withdrawn—public condemnation and legislative reaction were swift. Another tragedy, therefore, provided impetus for congressional activity, and in 1962 the Kefauver-Harris Amendments were passed unanimously.

These amendments have significantly affected the marketing of pharmaceuticals in the United States by requiring substantial evidence of efficacy for drugs approved between 1938, the enactment date of the Food, Drug, and Cosmetic Act, and 1962. Of course, "new" drugs introduced after 1962 must also comply with this standard. Consequently, introduction of new drugs was necessarily delayed for several years because of the extensive testing required. Target dates for the products, ordering, receipt of labels and packaging, and shipment of the finished product required new time schedules, causing considerable increases in premarket expenditures. Also, the effective patent life of new chemical entities consequently decreased.

Federal Regulations

It is nearly impossible for legislators to write laws that cover every specific and detailed aspect of the enforcement of that law. Such specificity comes through regulations. Thus, the 1962 drug amendments had as their primary purpose to ensure both the safety and effectiveness of medications. To make that happen, Congress, in its law, delegated to the FDA the power to promulgate regulations designed to enforce the intent of the law. The regulations are thus backed by the law and have the force of law. At the national level, FDA regulations are, in effect, the "rule book" for pharmaceutical research, development, and marketing.

Specifics of FDA regulations will be covered at appropriate places in this book, but a few comments are necessary here. First, although the FDA regulators are paid and not elected government employees, the commissioner of the FDA is appointed by the president of the United States. Thus, politics *do* have a potential role in the operation of the regulatory agency, often making it a target for criticism by the opposing political party. (An editorial in *The Wall Street Journal,* for example, suggested that a contribution by the manufacturer of Premarin may have been a factor in an FDA decision to delay approval of a generic counterpart.[26])

Some evidence suggests that FDA regulators are also not immune to *social* pressures. Scheduled meetings to discuss OTC status for oral contraceptives were postponed following some public protests. A "fast track" has been developed for review of applications for some classes of drugs—notably AIDS and cancer treatments. Also, it is well-known, if not found in the official regulations, that "me too" drugs may not flow through the review process as quickly as do those with some acknowledged potential advantage over existing therapies.

In an industry dependent to such a great extent on innovation, the agency with the authority to regulate all innovation is powerful indeed. The FDA is such an agency.

State Laws

With fifty states to consider, it will not be possible to go into the specifics of their laws, but the states can, and sometimes do, enact laws affecting pharmaceutical products and practices within their states. (For a long time most states had laws prohibiting generic substitution, and some still have statutes providing the prescriber with the opportunity to do so.)

Generally speaking, the most important law regarding the pharmaceutical industry in any state is the pharmacy practice act. Known under various official names, these acts typically (but not always) boil down to authorizing a state board of pharmacy to regulate pharmaceutical products in order to protect the public.

State Regulations

The regulatory effect of state boards of pharmacy on marketing practice is substantial, as they, in effect, grant monopolies at the retail (including hospitals) level in the pharmaceutical industry. The license to practice pharmacy or to operate a pharmacy is by regulation limited to certain individuals and under certain conditions. One of these has had interesting marketing implications.

All state boards of pharmacy now require proof of a certain number of hours of continuing professional education in order to renew the license to practice. The number of hours required varies and the content of the education is sometimes, but not always, restricted. Many manufacturers and wholesalers have developed programs to provide directly to pharmacists or sponsor financially such education programs as a promotional device.

The Human Medical Condition

Ultimately and obviously, the pharmaceutical industry is affected by health and illness in the population to a greater extent than by any of the other environmental factors displayed in Figure 2.1. Eventually each of us will die, and each death will be a consequence of one or more pathological conditions. Thus, this industry will be busiest because it has predicted needs and succeeded in filling them.

Most of what is described in this book relates to the environment in industrialized nations, with the United States most often used as an example. In that context it is comparatively easy to explain trends and developments in morbidity and mortality in the twentieth century. In a nutshell:

- People are living longer because they are not dying younger from some of the scourges of childhood common earlier in the century (diphtheria, small pox, etc.). This is the good news and it *is* good news. Declines in infant mortality, more than any other factor, account for the continuing increase in life expectancy. (This is not the place to explain it, but saving the life of a single one-year-old to reach "old age"

has the effect of adding a year to the life of more than sixty septua-
genarians.)

- The bad news, depending on one's point of view, is that a population
consisting of one-sixth to one-fifth "old people" will also include
great numbers of "old, sick people."
- In effect, the success achieved in extending the average length of life
has also made it possible for people to live long enough to have all manner of ailments. Many, if not most, may be treated with pharmaceuticals. Few may be cured.

In addition to these obvious changes over the past century are new problems
as well. The most obvious and overwhelming example is AIDS. Totally unexpected, the AIDS epidemic has perhaps served to remind us that nature
has ways of keeping us on our collective toes (which reminds us that television advertisements in the late 1990s suggest an epidemic of toe fungus).
And AIDS may be just a beginning.

In her book *The Coming Plague,* Laurie Garrett describes "The Revenge
of the Germs" as a constantly evolving evolutionary resistance by bacteria
to scientists' best efforts to eradicate or control them.[27] The battle between
science and nature can be expected to continue unabated with one or the
other having the upper hand at any point in time. Successes and failures in
the battles against AIDS, various kinds of cancers, and other plagues attest
to the continued efforts by the industry to fight morbidity, affect mortality,
and make a profit.

Dubos reminds us that these battles are not new: "The paleopathological
records leave no doubt—that most of the known organic and microbial disorders of man and animals are extremely ancient."[28] The prevalence, incidence, and consequences have been altered over time, of course. Not that
new diseases do not exist. Male pattern baldness comes to mind.

Technical Environment

A final environment component of the Outer Circle is the technical one.
Here we refer to not only technical changes developed by and in the pharmaceutical industry but also those developed for other purposes but adapted
by clever, imaginative people to applications in health care. Two examples
should support this:

- The microencapsulation techniques used by the National Cash Register company were originally designed to produce carbon-paper-free
copy capabilities. They were eventually adapted to prolonged active
medications.

- The microscope sprang from interests in nonpharmaceutical applications, yet its invention was a necessity for the entire field of antibiotic therapy.

The "germ theory" of disease changed medical treatment dramatically, holding that each disease had a well-defined cause and that treatment should be focused specifically on that causative agent or at least on the affected part of the body. (It is notable that this therapeutic breakthrough almost certainly prevented others.) The search for the "germ" that causes heart attacks, arthritis, and stomach ulcers, e.g., was doomed to failure—or was it? It seems likely that such little germs may in fact play a significant role in development of ulcers. See how medical technological developments can affect this industry, sometimes in contradictory ways?

With Koch's discovery of the specific microbial agents of disease (made possible by that microscope—"Thank you, Antony van Leeuwenhoek") the hope for "magic bullets" in the form of specific drugs did not seem unrealistic. And indeed many such magic bullets have been, and continue to be, discovered. As Paul Erlich described it, "Antibacterial substances are, so to speak, charmed bullets which strike only those objects for whose destruction they have been produced."[29]

The pharmaceutical industry lives and thrives because of technological advances in therapy. That is well understood. What should also be understood is that changes in technology outside the industry can and often do have significant impact on pharmaceutical marketing practices. An example is the Medicare outpatient drug program in the United States, which, when proposed, would have been impossible without the computer technology to allow immediate verification of eligibility, deductible status, etc. The success of cable television made it possible to utilize a new sales/education tool by bringing pharmaceutical programs into the physician's office or home (and also the homes of consumers).

Sometimes with and sometimes without the contributions of an industry, technology evolves that at least influences, and at times transforms, the character of that industry. Clearly, the pharmaceutical industry is technology based, and it would be folly to attempt future planning without careful scanning of the environment to identify incipient technological developments.

THE MIDDLE RING

The Four Ps

Included as environment items in this circle are the classic four Ps: product, price, place, and promotion. Each of these receives separate and extensive treatment in the chapters that follow and therefore will not be addressed now.

The Competitive Environment

To outperform competitors and to grow despite them, a company must understand why competition prevails, why firms attack, and how firms respond. Insights into competitors' perspectives can be gained by undertaking two types of analysis: industry and competitive. Industry analysis assesses the attractiveness of a market based on its economic structure. Competitive analysis indicates how every firm in a particular market is likely to perform given the structure of the industry.

Every industry has a few peculiar characteristics. These characteristics are bound by time and thus are subject to change. We may call them the dynamics of the industry. No matter how hard a company tries, if it fails to fit into the dynamics of the industry, ultimate success may be difficult to achieve.

To formulate marketing strategy, a company should determine the relevance of each of the competitive factors in its industry and the position it occupies with respect to competitors. An attempt should be made to highlight the dynamics of the company in the industry environment.

There are many approaches to the analysis of an industry. One is Porter's "five-factor" model.[30] Although this model is not perfectly adaptable to the pharmaceutical industry, it does provide a convenient framework for a discussion of several pharmaceutical industry institutions and characteristics.

As shown in this model (see Figure 2.7), the degree of rivalry among different firms is a function of the number of competitors, industry growth, product differentiation, and exit barriers. Among these variables, the number of competitors and industry growth are the most influential. Further, industries with high fixed costs tend to be more competitive, since the competing firms are forced to cut prices to enable them to operate at capacity. Differentiation, both real and perceived, among the competing offerings, however, lessens rivalry. Finally, difficulty of exit from an industry intensifies competition.

Threat of entry into the industry by new firms is likely to enhance competition. However, several barriers make it difficult to enter an industry. The three-cost-related entry barriers are economies of scale, absolute cost advantage, and research and development costs. Economies of scale require potential entrants either to establish high levels of production or to accept a cost disadvantage. Absolute cost advantage is enjoyed by firms with proprietary technology or favorable access to raw materials and by firms with production experience. In addition, high capital requirements, limited access to distribution channels, and government policy can act as entry barriers.

Substitute products that serve essentially the same function as the industry products are another source of competition. Since substitute products place a ceiling on the prices the firms can charge, they affect the industry po-

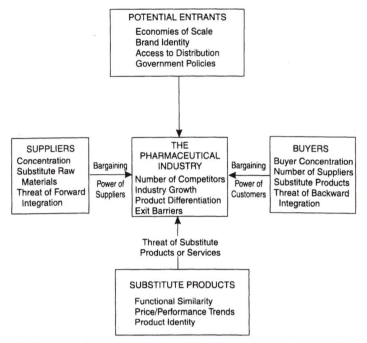

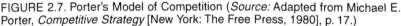

FIGURE 2.7. Porter's Model of Competition (*Source:* Adapted from Michael E. Porter, *Competitive Strategy* [New York: The Free Press, 1980], p. 17.)

tential. The threat posed by a substitute also depends on its long-term price and performance trends relative to the industry's product.

Bargaining power of buyers refers to the ability of the industry's customers to force the industry to reduce prices or increase features, thus bidding away profits. Buyers gain power when they have choices—when their needs can be met by a substitute product or the same product offered by another supplier. In addition, high buyer concentration, the threat of backward integration, and low switching costs add to buyer power.

Bargaining power of suppliers is the degree to which suppliers of the industry's raw materials have the ability to force the industry to accept higher prices or reduced services, thus affecting the profits. The factors influencing supplier power are the same as those influencing buyer power. In this case, however, industry members act as buyers.

These five forces of competition interact to determine the characteristics and the attractiveness of an industry. The strongest forces become dominant in determining profitability and become the focal points of strategy formulation.

A firm should first diagnose the forces affecting competition in the industry and their underlying causes and then identify its own strengths and weaknesses relative to the industry. Finally, the firm should formulate its strategy, which amounts to taking offensive or defensive action in order to achieve a secure position against the five competitive forces. According to Porter, this involves

- positioning the firm so that its capabilities provide the best defense against the existing array of competitive forces;
- influencing the balance of forces through strategic moves, thereby improving the firm's relative position; or
- anticipating shifts in the factors underlying the forces and responding to them, exploiting change by choosing a strategy appropriate to the new competitive balance before rivals recognize it.

The Internal Environment

In some ways this is the most difficult environmental element of all. Even if one were clever enough to recognize and utilize all of the other environmental elements mentioned previously, it is still possible—maybe likely?—that the plans, strategies, and tactics so carefully prepared will be ruined by factors in the environment within the company. An extraordinary range of possibilities exists. The monthly cover stories on corporate chief executive officers (CEOs) in *Pharmaceutical Executive* provide an interesting array of corporate philosophies. A similar series on middle management (with identities protected) would, perhaps, be even more illuminating.

The great marketing theorist Wroe Alderson defined an industry as consisting of "all the firms producing products which the market accepts as identical or all firms making products which the individual producers are deliberately trying to differentiate from each other."[31]

How do they go about this differentiation, and why? John T. Conner, former Secretary of Commerce, described the marketing responsibilities of the pharmaceutical industry a long time ago:

> . . . the chief objective in a revolutionary industry such as pharmaceuticals or computers is to get wide-spread acceptance and skilled use of new products as quickly as possible. This means, in our case, that the rate at which the medical profession and the public are able and willing to accept innovation must equal the rate at which new products are coming out of our laboratories. It is not the goal of our society to produce idle discoveries.

He described a remarkable contract.

> . . . the case of chlorothiazide, which took our laboratories twelve years of a renal research program to discover, plus another year of animal tests and fourteen months of clinical trials to get on the market. Within three months after it was introduced as a product, physicians were administering it to half of the patients requiring diuretic therapy in the country.[32]

Not every pharmaceutical firm sees its goals clearly, however. In carving a niche for itself in the market, each firm must employ its resources in such a way as to develop a total "personality," for competitive purposes, which gives it the greatest economic power and which rivals will find hardest to duplicate.

The ability of executives in the pharmaceutical industry to achieve the goal just suggested would seem to depend upon their abilities of definition and implementation. This "personality" includes engineering skills, production efficiency, research and development talents, and the effectiveness of the marketing organization.

The activities necessary to achieve competitive superiority would seem to depend upon the goal of the firm. Although maximum profit is most often cited as the ultimate goal, alternate goals do *exist,* and the importance of profit as the ultimate goal of the firm is often questioned.

It is a practical fact that the goals of firms (or of individuals) are usually expressed in optimal terms. One does not desire simply "a car," but the best car possible. If profit is a desirable target, it stands to reason, under most circumstances, that a firm will attempt to achieve maximum profit, not just "a profit." The same will be true of sales volume and savings in production costs.

Different types of goals have been postulated for the business firm. One is the marketing, or sales, goal. Beginning with the assumption that the firm is able to maintain its present position, it follows that it will be expected to better this position. Although profits cannot be ignored in achieving maximum sales goals, they may be relegated to a secondary position.

The problem of creation of corporate image is one that has created jobs for psychologists, sociologists, and advertising executives—jobs that might not otherwise exist. Although creation of an image would hardly be expected to serve as the primary goal for a company, the important long-term effects on the profit motive cannot be overlooked. Creation of an image costs money, which reduces profits.

The goal of power is another important one with an appreciable effect on the profit goal. Whether the power is exercised or not, large corporate size is probably the most effective measure of all types of corporate power—at any rate, this is the view taken by the Federal Trade Commission in the area of regulation. Power may result in profits, but profits also may constitute a source of power.

The ultimate internal goal, the financial one, may be defined in general terms by stating that the financial requirements of all possible future conditions of the firm should be adequately met. This is particularly true for such short-run circumstances as might exist if the firm suddenly found it crucial to maintain liquidity.

Most certainly the pursuit of alternate goals affects the "competitive personality," which in turn radically alters the effectiveness of the pharmaceutical company's pursuit of these goals.

Perhaps the hardest facets of the competitive "personality" to develop and evaluate are those which actually resemble personality as it is usually defined. These are such things as company image and quality of management.

A public relations director for a large pharmaceutical company has listed six questions that he believes the corporate executives should consider before attempting to establish a good image:

1. Has your management agreed on the corporate image your organization hopes to achieve?
2. In addition to the general long-range objectives you want to accomplish, do you also have specific short-term objectives for your program?
3. Do you do enough listening and research to find out what your different "publics" think of your organization?
4. Do you look to case histories of firms in fields other than your own for ideas you could borrow and improve?
5. Do you hold necessary periodic reviews of your program to consider what clicked, what failed, etc.?
6. Do you identify yourself closely with the "publics" you are trying to reach?

The marketing environment holds both threat and promise for the pharmaceutical industry. However, important obstacles may lie in the path to the exploitation of areas of attractive market opportunity. Indeed, it has been suggested that marketing as a separate discipline grew out of the attempt to evaluate the positive and negative factors in the business environment.

Any forward-looking business firm allots considerable time and effort to planning, implementation, and control. All of the activities of planning and implementation may be wasted without an adequate system of controls. Business controls, in their purpose and complexity, are not unlike the controls in the cockpit of a jet plane. Long before the jetliner taxis down the runway, the pilots, the navigator, and their supervisors have carefully plotted the course over which the plane is to fly to reach a preselected destination (this is equivalent to the planning function). In the course of planning the flight, fuel supplies, passenger capacities, crew needs, and air fares have all been determined. Following the planning phase, the resources of the airline are mobilized to start the plane on its way (implementation). All has been carefully planned and implemented. The function of the controls is to keep the plan (or business) "on course" regardless of unexpected or unforeseen events.

Keeping business on course requires that the enterprise not only functions as expected when the environment is unchanged but also has the ability to adapt when it does change. Using the airplane analogy again, we might say that marketing controls for the firm would include a sort of complex "automatic pilot" for use during normal marketing conditions, as well as a series of sensing devices—marketing radar, altimeter, and air speed indicator, if you will—ready for any change in conditions.

Unfortunately, for those whose job it is to plan for control within the marketing function, the problems are infinitely more complex than those of control for the plane. The environments within which the system operates are dynamic, requiring continuous adjustment of this system. In fact, the firm may have multiple objectives from subsystems within the general system. Further, the objectives of the subsystems may be at least partially in conflict. (For example, production desires a uniform product, while marketing desires a variety of products.) The variations within which the airplane's system of control must operate are finite (temperature, pressure, weather, etc.). The changes in the marketing environment are so varied and so dynamic that sensing devices may not be equally effective in forecasting all types of change.

The problem of instituting and maintaining marketing controls is both crucial and difficult. It is biphasic, both in definition and in fact. The dominant dictionary meaning given for "control" when used as a verb is "to restrain, govern, regulate." Indeed, this is an important aspect of the control function. The original French word from which the English term is derived, however, means "to verify by comparison." This, too, is an integral part of the control process. Control, then, is a combination of surveillance, appropriate regulation, and both internal and external controls, if needed.

In some, if not most, ways the internal environments of pharmaceutical companies shape their collective future. As Levitt noted, "Good work in the pursuit of wrong purposes is more damaging than bad work in the pursuit of right purposes. In business, the marketing imagination is the central tool for deciding on what the purposes are to be."[33]

CONCLUSION

In this (very long) chapter we have identified some, but certainly not all, of the environmental factors that have an impact on marketing decisions and practices in the pharmaceutical industry. In the next chapter we will use a similarly broad approach to describe some of the activities used by that industry to identify and deal with these environmental challenges.

Chapter 3

General Practices

Mickey Smith

INTRODUCTION

In the previous chapter we discussed a wide range of general environmental factors that affect the practice of pharmaceutical marketing. In this chapter, we will examine some of the practices of pharmaceutical marketers in anticipating and dealing with their current and expected environmental influences.

In that previous chapter we covered many environmental issues, but certainly not all of them. In addition, the environment does change—sometimes without any warning, but often without warning for the unprepared. Being prepared for environmental change, as well as being able accurately to assess the current environment are two of the many challenges facing marketing professionals. *—2 main mkt. challenge*

Jain described the "environmental approach" as one of several philosophical directions from which to address markets and marketing plans. This approach, he wrote, "portrays the marketing decision maker as the focal point of numerous environments within which the firm operates and that affect the success of the firm's marketing programs."[1] Other approaches exist, of course, but, as we have obviously chosen this one, let us see what we can do with it.

Levitt quoted Henry Kissinger's assessment of the then continued Japanese economic successes: "What could be more effective than a society voracious in its collection of information, impervious to pressure, and implacable in execution?"[2] Strong words, indeed, and when written in the 1980s, they seemed to presage a virtual takeover of American enterprise via successes in the fields of automobiles and electronics. Some believed that similar dramatic successes lay ahead in pharmaceuticals. That has not happened, certainly. Although the Japanese presence in the U.S. market is significant, there is, so far at least, nothing to rival the successes of other, equally foreign, companies such as . . . well, by the time this is read the names will have changed, but I was thinking of Roche, Hoechst, Ciba-Geigy, Glaxo, and others.

At any rate, environmental assessment is a necessary, but not sufficient, activity for any pharmaceutical company hoping for long-term success. It is not suggested that the Japanese lacked the will to do such assessment, but rather the ability to interpret the data. American (and other non-Japanese) firms seem to have gotten one environmental factor right—if you want to do business in Japan, you better have a Japanese partner.

Environmental assessment, for our purposes, may take two general forms: a broad assessment of the total environment and the much more specific assessment usually known as market and/or marketing research.

The broad assessment can include steps described by Jain and listed, with examples, here:

1. Watch for broad trends appearing in the environments. Such things as self-care, preventive practices, expansion of personal use of computers would fit here.
2. Evaluate each trend for relevance. Use of the personal computer extended to the cyberspace that now exists would show obvious relevance. Indeed, it would be difficult, but not impossible, to find an environmental trend with *no* possible relevance to pharmaceuticals.
3. Estimate the impact of the trend on your market or even an individual product. A facetious example might be a trend toward "fashionable baldness." Even if short-lived (but not necessarily, or perhaps head shapeliness could become important), such a trend would have an obvious impact on both topical and systemic hair growers.
4. Forecast the direction and potential longevity of the trend. "Hairlessness" has, of course, other sites of potential influence with regard to the human body. Is that a real possibility, and how long might it last? (This is especially important in colder areas.)
5. What is the momentum? Is this a gradual change, but a strong one? Is the change rapid, but with considerable potential to "fizzle"?
6. Does a trend provide an opportunity? Would, using this example, a systemic, whole-body depilatory make sense (especially if reversible)?
7. What does it mean for corporate strategy? Should the company "fight 'em" or "join 'em"? Each of those decisions leads to more strategy decisions.[3]

A bit later we will devote considerable attention to market and marketing research as the major focus of the pharmaceutical industry in environmental scanning, but first a brief look at other scanning techniques. (As is the case with many topics mentioned in this book, other books have been written solely on the subject.) Jain is used as the basis for this.

- *Extrapolation techniques:* Essentially these involve using past trends to predict the future. Plenty of room for surprises here, but if the trend is stable, such tools as regression analysis are helpful.
- *Historical analogy:* This involves a look at what happened in the past when certain events have occurred. An example is downsizing of sales personnel in response to a variety of external forces. This has *always* been followed by "upsizing" at a later date.
- *Intuitive reasoning:* What does intuition, "unconstrained by past experience and personal bias," suggest? This is the sort of thing that keeps consultants in business.
- *Scenario building:* A series of "what ifs" or "if this, then what." Probabilities should be an important part of this process.
- *Cross-impact matrices:* This technique allows the scanner to analyze the simultaneous study of two conflicting futures.
- *Morphological analysis:* In this case, all (identifiable) ways to achieve an objective are used, with the goal of developing the optimal approach.
- *Network methods:* Contingency trees and relevance trees are used here. The former uses logic to display graphically environmental trends with the alternative outcomes. The relevance tree assigns degrees of importance to the branches.
- *Model building:* Widely used, especially by consulting firms skilled in the process, this technique uses deductive and inductive procedures to identify multivariate possible responses to strategic decisions.
- *Delphi techniques:* As is true of the previous technique, Delphi methods are not unique to pharmaceutical applications but are rather broadly used to "forecast" the future. Generally, they require selection of a group of "experts" to assess the likelihood of the occurrence of specified events. Sometimes, but not always, the experts also tell how confident (how "expert") they feel about their ability to make the prediction. Reiteration and feedback are used to fine-tune the results.[4]
- *Content analysis* (not in the Jain list): This procedure uses systematic analysis of printed materials to detect trends. The best-selling book *Megatrends* was based on this technique. The assumption is that the printed materials (e.g., newspapers) reflect and/or influence future events.

Market and Marketing Research As Environmental Scanning

For the pharmaceutical industry, environmental scanning can range from the macro level (movements toward self-care, political trends) to the micro level (activities and trends within a given market). It is at the micro level that the industry is "data rich." One would be hard-pressed to name an industry with as much information about its own markets (the inner circle in Figure 2.1, Chapter 2) as the pharmaceutical industry.*

Whatever the term "market" may imply in a given situation, its size and growth patterns are a fundamental requirement of business. Management needs to know the characteristics of the market they are in, or which they may plan to enter.

Historically, this application has always been the first demand of a business that finds itself becoming concerned with its progress in the marketing area. This is why, also, the term "market research" is usually the forerunner to the broader "marketing research." Once markets have been defined and characterized by market research, the need for marketing research quickly manifests itself. Although the two terms are often used interchangeably, it is useful to distinguish market research—determination and assessment of the qualitative and quantitative dimensions of a market (however defined)—from marketing research—analysis of the effects of the various marketing activities of a firm and its competitors.

Another useful distinction is that between primary and secondary research and/or data sources. That distinction is shown in Figure 3.1.

It has often been stated that, with regard to the marketplace in which it operates, the pharmaceutical industry is perhaps the most "data rich" of all industries. As a result, it is one of the most, if not the most, sophisticated users of market and marketing research information. To a large degree, this wealth of data regarding the pharmaceutical marketplace is a function of the many inherently unique aspects of the pharmaceutical marketing process as described in Chapter 1.

Remember that pharmaceutical companies produce and market two types of products. One type is the prescription product that may be obtained by consumers only upon the presentation of authorization by a licensed prescriber. The other is the over-the-counter product that may be purchased without a prescription. The primary target of the marketing effort for prescription products is the population of licensed prescribers in the country, rather than the consumers of the products. Another target of the marketing effort for prescription pharmaceuticals is the population of licensed pharmacists in the country, this group having assumed more importance because of their increased role as decision makers with regard to the specific brand of drug to be dispensed to the patient. Here, too, however, the focus is on an intermediary rather than on the ultimate consumer, although that has been changing, as later discussion of promotion will illustrate.

---

*This section draws freely from the writings of Stephen C. Chappell in Mickey Smith (Ed.), *Principles of Pharmaceutical Marketing,* Third Edition (Binghamton, NY: The Haworth Press, 1988), pp. 115-138, and in Mickey C. Smith, *Pharmaceutical Marketing: Strategy and Cases* (Binghamton, NY: The Haworth Press, 1991), pp. 110-150.

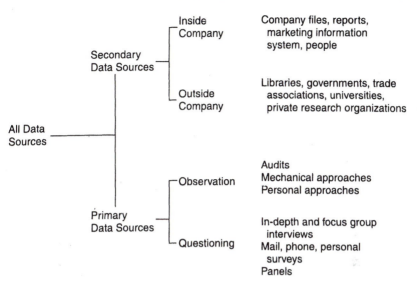

FIGURE 3.1. Types of Market Data Sources

The selling of prescription pharmaceuticals to the public also involves some atypical characteristics. Professional licensure is required for an establishment to stock and sell prescription products. Further, the seller (or dispenser) of these products must be licensed to do so. The selling of prescription pharmaceuticals to the public is thus restricted to the comparatively small numbers of pharmacists and pharmacies in the country, rather than to the substantially larger number of retailers and retail outlets, which would normally be the case for a consumer product.

Uniqueness also characterizes prescription products in the sense that, as mentioned previously, purchase of these products by consumers requires the presentation of authorization by a licensed prescriber in the form of a written prescription. A record of every transaction involving the sale or dispensing of a prescription drug to the consumer is therefore created and maintained, with these records being specific to the patient, physician, pharmacy, and product. As the majority of the population becomes covered by one of many public and private prescription payment plans, these data can also be found in their records. Indeed, the sale of such information has become a major source of revenue for payers.

In effect, product choice decisions and product movement in the multi-billion-dollar prescription drug industry are accounted for or represented by what basically amounts to a relative handful of the population. The number of licensed prescribers of medication in the United States is probably about

500,000, and the number of registered pharmacists is roughly 150,000. There are approximately 55,000 retail pharmacies in the country and slightly more than 7,000 hospitals. Contrast these numbers, for example, with the potential hundred million decision makers who might be involved in a consumer product, and the many hundreds of thousands of outlets that might sell a consumer product, with few, if any, records maintained regarding these decisions or sales. (We should note, however, that the use of bar code scanning and consumer credit cards at the checkout counter make it *electronically* feasible to identify buyers of, say, Preparation H, at least if they do so on credit. Issues of confidentiality do exist, of course, but the technology is in place.)

These examples, along with other unique aspects of prescription marketing, are of considerable importance in the gathering of data regarding the marketplace. In one sense, there is virtually no difficulty in finding physicians, pharmacists, pharmacies, or hospitals. Primarily because of professional licensure requirements, all are on continually maintained lists of one type or another. Additionally, the number of members in each of these groups is known to within a very small degree of error. The person who wants to know the number of physicians in the country does not have to initiate a study to find this information. Consider this as compared to the problems that would be encountered by the researcher who wanted to know the number of coffee drinkers in the United States and wanted to conduct research among them—no definitive list of coffee drinkers exists.

Relatively little is required of the researcher in the pharmaceutical marketplace in terms of characterizing potential research subjects. Information is available, for example, on the physician's type of practice, specialty, year graduated from medical school, medical school attended, and location of practice. Information is also available on retail pharmacies in terms of their type, size, and location. Hospitals are identified by type, bed size, affiliation with learning institutions, presence of a formulary, and whether certain types of equipment are available. This precharacterizing of research subjects is generally not available to the researcher in the consumer marketplace.

Another element that facilitates the conduct of market research in the pharmaceutical marketplace is the fair amount of homogeneity that is found within and among the various groups of participants in the marketplace. Physicians and pharmacists, for example, have received the same basic education as other physicians or pharmacists. As with most purchasers of consumer products, no wide variations from physician to physician are found in terms of socioeconomic considerations. Most participants in the health care area are professionals and tend to communicate on an inter- and intragroup basis better than the average consumer does with other consumers. Similarity in thinking and activity among the members of a particular group generally tends to facilitate researching of the group.

The conduct of market research in the prescription product area is also made somewhat easier than doing the same in the consumer sector because most of the decisions made by principals in the market are presumed to be based on knowledge, rather than on emotion.

Finally, in many segments of pharmaceutical market research, the researcher does not have to create or search extensively for records of fact regarding decision or activity. As pointed out earlier, for instance, records are required to exist for every transaction regarding the sale of a prescription product to a consumer.

In summary, many of the unique characteristics of prescription product marketing have the effect, in one fashion or another, of eliminating or minimizing many of the requirements and effort associated with market research in the general sense. This is certainly a major reason for the enormous amount of data available regarding the prescription product marketplace.

Of course, one should not carry away the impression that market research in the pharmaceutical industry is an effortless undertaking. Although many areas of advantage exist relative to other industries, many of the peculiar aspects found in pharmaceutical marketing create complications with which the researcher has to deal. As one illustration, the construction of a sample of retail pharmacies has to take into consideration the fact that pharmacies vary a great deal in the composition of their sales volume. Some may fill only a few prescriptions yet have an extremely high volume of business overall. Others may do a negligible business in items other than prescriptions from several hundred physicians. The customary probability or random statistical sample of the drugstores in the country may not necessarily constitute a representative sample of the prescription market in the country.

The difficulties of market research have resulted in opportunities. Responding to these have been scores of companies who specialize in or devote at least a part of a larger business to pharmaceutical market and marketing research. In practice, much of the data gathering in the drug industry is done by such firms. The interpretation of these data, especially when coupled with internal company records, occupies much of the time and creativity of the market research personnel of pharmaceutical companies. This is not to say that they never design and execute their own data collection projects, but rather that the integration of company records, available data services, and custom-designed studies is a challenge to the marketing strategist.

Secondary Data from Commercial Suppliers

A large number of market and marketing research services have been developed for the pharmaceutical industry by independent research companies, sometimes referred to as service agencies or suppliers. Many of these services have been in continuous operation since the 1950s; others were initiated over the years in response to changes in the marketplace and to concomitant changes in the information needs of the industry. A service offered to the pharmaceutical marketer that depicts the frequency and characteristics of substitution in retail pharmacies is important in today's market, but it was obviously of no relevance prior to the repeal of antisubstitution legislation. Advances in technology have also been responsible for the development of new services by facilitating the collection and processing of information that either was not available previously or was too difficult to collect and process. As an illustration, the advent of pharmacy service systems has provided as a by-product millions of records of prescription-dispensing information stored on computers, easily accessible for very detailed analyses.

The services provided by independent research companies are generally classified into two major categories: syndicated or custom. A syndicated service is defined here as one in which all subscribers receive identical information. These services are generally supported by a large number of subscribers. The custom service, on the other hand, is supported by only one client to whose specific needs the service or project is tailored. Only the contracting client receives the information in a custom project. Another categorization of these services is based on their periodicity or continuity. They may be periodic, continuing (and periodic), or ad hoc in nature.

Periodic and Continuing Audits and Surveys

The following are seven general types of continuing audits or surveys of the pharmaceutical marketplace:

1. Retail pharmacy purchase audit
2. Hospital purchase audit
3. Warehouse withdrawal audit
4. Retail pharmacy prescription audit
5. Physician panels
6. Promotional media audits
7. Retail sales audit

Broadly defined, these services are nationwide in scope, each covering one aspect of the pharmaceutical marketplace on a regular, periodic basis—monthly, quarterly, etc. With some exceptions, which will be noted, these audits present national estimates of activity—dollars, prescriptions, detail calls. These estimates represent projections of data collected from samples constructed to be representative of the population, or universe—physicians, hospitals, pharmacies—being studied. Again, in general, data are presented at the product level. Product level data are then summarized to therapeutic category or to manufacturer level, and these ultimately to a total marketplace figure. In addition to absolute volume estimates, market share and trend information are customarily provided.

Retail Pharmacy Purchase Audit

This is designed to provide a measurement of pharmaceutical product purchases by retail pharmacies. A purchase audit is, in effect, an "inflow" audit, measuring the flow of product (either directly from a manufacturer or from a wholesaler) into retail pharmacies. This is in contrast to an "outflow" audit, such as the prescription audit, which monitors the flow of a product out of the pharmacy into the hands of the consumer. In theory, at any one point in time, the difference between an inflow audit and an outflow audit is represented by inventory on the shelf. The scope of the retail pharmacy purchase audit is not limited to prescription, or legend, pharmaceuticals but includes over-the-counter medications as well.

Hospital Purchase Audit

In general methodology, style, and form, this is a replica of the retail pharmacy purchase audit. The obvious difference is that this audit focuses on hospital purchases of pharmaceutical products. The hospital sector has increased substantially as a market for pharmaceutical products. The growth in purchases of pharmaceuticals by hospitals has on a relative basis far exceeded that of the retail pharmacy segment. There are a number of reasons for this, but of probably prime importance to the pharmaceutical marketer is the fact that in many communities around the country the hospital has become more of a factor in routine patient care. The increase in the number of patient visits to hospital *out*patient facilities has been remarkable, as has been the growth in the filling of prescriptions by hospital pharmacies for these outpatients.

Warehouse Withdrawal Audit

This service measures the withdrawal of pharmaceutical products from the pharmaceutical wholesaler and from major drug chain warehouses. Although this audit monitors withdrawal or outflow from warehouses, note that this is basically the same as measuring inflow to the pharmacy or hospital. Because it is, this service is actually similar to the purchase audits described previously, and one may question the need for both types of services. Major differences, however, do exist. The purchase audits reflect all purchases by a pharmacy or hospital, whether or not they were purchased directly from a manufacturer or from a wholesaler. Given the focus of the warehouse withdrawal audit on the warehouse segment only, purchases directly from the manufacturer are not represented in the auditing process.

On the other hand, although the purchase audits are based on samples of hospitals and pharmacies, the warehouse withdrawal study is, for all intents and purposes, a census of warehouse withdrawal activity for pharmaceutical products. The amount of data available from such a census is enormous as compared to that developed with the purchase audit. This mass of data provides the capability to isolate and analyze small segments of the marketplace, such as zip code or specific sales territories. This capability is quite valuable in dealing with questions of individual territory potential and performance needs for territorial realignment, or differential selling techniques.

Retail Pharmacy Prescription Audit

This is designed to measure the outflow of prescription drugs from the pharmacy into the hands of the consumer. In many ways, it may be logically argued that prescription audit data are the most sensitive indicators of prescription product performance in the marketplace. The prescription is not an expression of opinion, attitude, or speculation on the part of the prescriber but is a matter of record. As prescribers collectively change their minds about individual drugs or areas of therapy, these changes are, in essence, automatically recorded in the prescription files of pharmacies. Prescriptions, further, are indicators of what is presently occurring in terms of demand. Purchase data, for example, may record a pharmacy's purchase of antibiotics in the month of August in anticipation of the antibiotic "season." That purchase record, however, does not signify current physician demand for antibiotics.

Prescription data are also viewed by most pharmaceutical marketers as the best indicators of the results of marketing or promotional efforts to create new business. If one looks at purchase data for an antihypertensive product, it is impossible to sort out that portion of dollars representative of new business as opposed to that portion reflective of patients who are already using the product. New prescription volume for the same product, however, is a reasonably good indicator of the trend in generating new patient business for the product.

There are presently two primary methods of collecting data for continuing syndicated prescription audits. One method relies on a sample of retail pharmacies, with pharmacists in each of these pharmacies recording information regarding prescriptions filled by the pharmacy. The other method takes advantage of pharmacy service system-generated prescription records and extracts required information from records stored on computers. Each method has inherent advantages and disadvantages. Pharmacy service system data are voluminous and easily and quickly collected and processed. These data, however, represent information on only what is dispensed by the pharmacy. The method that relies on pharmacist reporting of information produces a smaller volume of data and takes more time to collect and process but yields information on what was prescribed by the physician as well as on what was dispensed by the pharmacist. Prescription data are available at national and subnational levels, the latter allowing prescription generation analysis at more discrete geographic levels.

Physician Panels

These represent research services of a somewhat different type. One physician panel is a study of medical practice in the United States. Although most of the services discussed thus far are oriented toward the depiction of product movement in one way or another, this physician panel goes somewhat further in that it portrays usage of pharmaceutical products along a number of variables.

A sample of physicians is utilized. Each physician in the sample is asked to provide specific information regarding each patient seen during an assigned reporting period. Information requested includes diagnosis; patient characteristics; location of visit; drugs, if any, used to treat the condition; and action desired from these drugs. Beyond simple estimates of volume and trend of drug usage, data resulting from this study are used to determine such considerations as which conditions a drug is used for, by what specialty of physician, in what frequency, and for what patient type.

Another type of physician panel is designed to collect the daily new prescription output of individual physicians. Followed over time, data from this panel can demonstrate changes in prescribing habits by a physician or groups of physicians based on specialty, age, location of practice, and prescribing volume. These data are often used to track new products, whereby physicians are identified as to certain characteristics and monitored as to if and when they began to prescribe a new product, in what volume, for how long, and how, if at all, previous prescribing patterns were altered.

Still other physician panels are maintained which are narrower in scope in terms of drug use or diagnosis areas but which are more detailed in the information provided within these more limited parameters.

Promotional Media Audits

Three segments of promotional activity in the pharmaceutical marketplace are monitored by continuing audits: detailing, journal advertising, and direct mail advertising. Projections of detailing effort as perceived by physicians in office-based practice, and the receipt of direct mail advertisements by this group of physicians, are made from information provided by samples of physicians who report on these respective promotional approaches. An audit that depicts the detailing of pharmacists is also available. The amount of dollars spent by pharmaceutical companies for the placement of advertising in professional journals is monitored for the industry, with the dollar estimate based on a census of all publications that carry ethical pharmaceutical product advertising. This audit has declined in use.

Retail Sales Audit

This has historically been used primarily for nonprescription pharmaceuticals. One type of retail sales audit may be described as "opening inventory plus delivered purchases minus ending inventory." Mainly because of time and cost considerations, this type of audit is conducted for selected products of interest to the subscriber as opposed to the "all products, all categories" approach of most of the audit services already described.

These descriptions are of the general types of continuing audits and surveys offered to the pharmaceutical marketer. Although each has one major objective, you will readily understand that each of these provides data or information ancillary to the main objective but still of considerable use. Because the purchase audits, for example, collect unit and dollar information at the package size level, the opportunity exists for performing pricing analysis. The main use of prescription audits is to provide prescription counts by product, but information may also be collected on daily dosage, patient price, and number of units of a drug prescribed. An analysis of dosage is, therefore, capable of being done.

It should also be pointed out that a great deal of work is done using segments of a particular study. Prescription data, for example, are studied to obtain both prescribing and dispensing information.

Finally, in recent years, much progress has been made in combining the information available in the individual audits into one general database that offers the potential for an almost unlimited number of cross tabulations and interrelating exercises.

Other Commercial Research Services

A wide variety of custom and syndicated research services are available to pharmaceutical marketers. The Pharmaceutical Marketing Research Group, an organization of professional researchers working for drug firms, refers to those who provide such services as "vendors."

The variety of research services provided by these vendors is extraordinary. The following is a partial list of words used by the vendors themselves to describe their services. It is obvious that the market research departments who require outside services have an extensive (perhaps bewildering) array from which to choose.

Ad Layout Testing
Ad Recall Studies
Attitude Measures
Audits
Brand Awareness
Brand Imagery
Concept Testing
Convention Surveys
Copy Testing
Corporate Image Studies
Distribution Analysis
Focus Panels/Groups
Mail Surveys
Mall Intercept
Market Segmentation
Market Share
Media Research

Medication Histories
Multivariate Statistics
Name Tests
Packaging Studies
Panel Studies
Penetration Studies
Personal Interviews
Prescription Audits
Product Positioning
Questionnaire Design
Readership Studies
Sales Force Effectiveness
 Studies
Sample Evaluations
Shelf Life Audits
Telephone Interviews
Tracking Studies

In addition to market research offerings, various other sources of information regarding pharmaceuticals, the pharmaceutical marketplace, and the population in general are available to the pharmaceutical marketer or market researcher. These usually provide background information or intelligence or are reference works. *The Pink Sheet* and *Scrip* are examples of publications that provide news or intelligence regarding the industry. Publications such as the *Merck Manual, Merck Index, AMA Drug Evaluations, Facts and Comparisons,* and *Remington's Practice of Pharmacy* are excellent for obtaining background information on diseases and drugs. *The Journal of the American Hospital Association* and its *Annual Guide* issue provide a wealth of demographic information on the hospital universe in the United States. Many government agencies publish a variety of reports and studies of potential interest, such as *United States Census Data, the Statistical Abstract of the United States,* and, of more specific interest to the pharmaceutical market researcher, studies such as those on specific diseases and health care financing.

The industry trade and professional presses also offer an array of valuable statistics. *MedAd News, Medical Marketing and Media, Pharmaceutical Executive,* and a number of retail-oriented magazines provide regular special statistical reports. Research media, such as *The Journal of Pharmaceutical Marketing and Management, The Journal of Research in Pharmaceutical Economics,* and *Pharmacoeconomics* also publish the results of original, primary research.

"In House" Market and Marketing Research Activities

Because of the abundance of market and marketing research services offered to the pharmaceutical industry, one may be left with the impression that these offerings satisfy all the needs of companies, and that the function of the market research department within the company is simply to analyze the data provided. This is not the case; many research studies are initiated, carried out, and analyzed by in-house personnel. In some cases this is due to requirements of confidentiality. In others, company personnel may have more knowledge of a particular subject area. Third, there may be a need for correlation of the market research study with other company data, and this is often more easily accomplished by in-house staff. Finally, a company may view the use of its own staff as being less costly than contracting out a project. Analyses of internal company data, such as factory sales, promotional spending, and detailing call reports, also generally fall within the market research department's area of responsibility. A third major segment of activity is the analysis of data provided by independent research companies who work with these outside suppliers on particular projects.

Applications and Uses

The services and data that have been discussed have been labeled as market research, marketing research, or marketing services and data. Although these data are designed to measure or portray the marketplace in one way or another and are perhaps of special importance to the marketer, their utility and application extend well beyond the sector of the marketing department. Probably few areas in any pharmaceutical company do not, at one time or another, have use for these services and data.

As an example, a major strategic question that companies have to deal with is research and development planning. What disease or product appears to warrant long-term research and development investment? Which seems to suggest the plausibility of short-term involvement? Marketing data can aid in this planning process in such areas as identifying market size and potential, whether a therapy is available, where therapy is available but not used, and what is to be the next logical step in therapy. Short-term focus is illustrated by analyzing the data to help identify areas that may be available for subdivision. The analgesic market, for example, is a broad one. Some companies have been successful in orienting their development efforts toward a segment of that market, such as migraine headache analgesia. Similarly, companies have had success in segmenting the respiratory condition area by offering products specifically for sinusitis. Data analysis may help identify product sectors in which more convenient dosing of a drug would be beneficial to the patient and to marketing.

These data may be useful with regard to the serendipitous research and development discovery. Should the company that finds itself with a compound that appears effective in the treatment of a particular disorder pursue the study of the compound? Available data can help in this decision by delineating such parameters as the prevalence of this disorder, the potential market size, or drugs presently employed. It should be pointed out here that for neither directed nor serendipitous research results is market size or potential necessarily the key determinant in deciding whether to continue studying a product. Many companies have marketed drugs for treating minuscule patient populations.

It should also be noted that real market potential is affected by many variables. As Figure 3.2 shows, the theoretical market potential may be considerably different from that which is ultimately realized.

Other segments of the broadly defined development process benefit from the use of marketing data. Diverse conditions, such as osteoarthritis and hypertension, are often found in the same patients. If an antiarthritic compound has a blood pressure-elevating property, this compound would not be used to treat arthritic patients who are also hypertensive. Data from physician panels on medical practice can quantify how frequently these condi-

Demographics

↓   Incidence/Prevalence

Potential Patients

↓   Diagnosis

Diagnosed Patients

↓   Limiting Factors

Achievable Patients

↓   Prescribing/Ordering

Treated Patients

↓   Compliance

Patient Days of Drug Therapy

FIGURE 3.2. From Theoretical to Real Market Potential

tions exist together and thus suggest the minimization of usage potential that would be caused by this property of the compound. Questions on the need for specific dosage forms required for a product may be answered by reviewing the marketing data. Diagnosis data, for instance, would indicate that otitis media is mainly a disorder of pediatric patients. If an anti-infective with efficacy in otitis media cannot be formulated in liquid form, it would be used infrequently.

Data are useful in planning clinical trials. If a product demonstrates activity in more than one condition, data showing the relative importance of the various conditions might be used to determine for which condition clinical testing should be performed. Seasonality, regionality, and specialty data are also of interest in planning clinical trials. Companies may determine the combination of region, season, and specialty that are most likely to produce large numbers of patients with a specific condition.

Assuming that a product is to be marketed or is already on the market, the manufacturing area of a company needs direction in regard to how much of the product is required. Marketing data can be used to assist in these determinations. The need for samples, for instance, in terms of such factors as overall quantity or package size, is often decided by analysis of competitive sampling, as shown by audits of promotional activity.

Corporate development departments rely on marketing data in many cases to analyze potential company or product acquisitions and licensing opportunities. Financial and legal personnel also have occasion to view market data as an aid in their activities.

The most frequent use of market data occurs, of course, in the marketing area of the company. One major use is for premarketing planning. Much of this use is involved with analysis of the market that the drug is to enter. A marketer needs to know various pieces of information to ensure successful marketing of a product. What physician specialties are important in a given therapy or diagnosis category? Is the hospital an important sector? What patient characteristics are apparent? What is the present state of the market in terms of competition? How do competitors promote their products? Are there presently unsatisfied portions of the market? Attitudinal research is generally carried out to determine how physicians perceive a proposed product or the advantages and disadvantages of currently available products. Advertising personnel study data to depict in print media a patient type that the physician finds relevant to the condition for which a drug is to be used.

Once a product is on the market, the main use of marketing data is to monitor the performance of a product across all the various aspects of the marketplace. Product sales, prescriptions, overall physician usage or by specialty or high prescribers, diagnosis, and location, for example, are all analyzed continuously to monitor progress of a product by itself as well as in relation to the market in which it competes. Invariably, this monitoring process reveals information that suggests the need for additional information or action, and the market or marketing research process takes another turn.

As the late Raymond Gosselin, one of the fathers of pharmaceutical market research, has so aptly stated, the task of market and marketing research is to keep those who need to be kept informed supplied with all the facts possible to amass. The extraordinarily dynamic nature of the pharmaceutical industry coupled with the ever-increasing ability to collect facts suggest the need for an ability of the market research function to contribute even more significantly in the future. Although the pharmaceutical industry is, in fact, a data-rich industry, and much is presently known, much more needs to be known.

WHO ARE WE? WHO ARE THOSE OTHER PEOPLE? WHAT CAN WE DO ABOUT THEM?

In this section we will consider industry practices regarding the internal environment and the competitive environment (see Figure 2.1, Chapter 2).

Who Are We?

There is no shortage of information on how pharmaceutical companies (or at least their CEOs) answer the question just posed. For a number of years, *Pharmaceutical Executive* has published cover stories in which industry leaders describe corporate philosophies and plans in broad, but sometimes surprisingly specific, terms. From these and other sources, such as corporate annual reports, it is possible to gain considerable insight into the process of analysis of the internal environment.

Analysis of the internal environment of the firm can range from the often chatty comments by executives in magazine stories, to investment analysts, to more formal study such as SWOT and portfolio analysis.

SWOT is an acronym signifying a systematic review of a company's *S*trengths, *W*eaknesses, *O*pportunities, and *T*hreats. This analysis can, and *should,* be conducted regularly by staff of the company itself, but similar analyses by (presumably) objective outsiders are valuable as well.

O.T.C. Update, a publication of Nicholas Hall and Company, regularly publishes SWOT analyses of companies in the nonprescription drug business. Table 3.1 is an example. As Table 3.1 indicates, Procter & Gamble had, in 1997 and by the publisher's accounting, considerable assets in the areas of strengths and opportunities, but some significant weaknesses and threats as well. Such SWOT analyses can be elaborated to include priority ratings for action, but their basic value is in providing structure for planning.

TABLE 3.1. SWOT Analysis, Procter & Gamble

Strengths	Powerful global brands
	Critical mass in United States, Germany, and United Kingdom
	Participation in emerging markets
	Consumer marketing expertise
	Ambition to be a health care player
Weaknesses	Lack of organic Rx-to-OTC switch pipeline
	Does not have an analgesic or dietary supplement lineup
	Market heavily weighted toward mature United States and European markets
Opportunities	License or acquire new OTCs, or Rx drugs with switch potential, in the United States
	Penetrate emerging markets
	Step up research and development
	Streamline existing OTC portfolio to enhance focus on core brands
Threats	Failure to retain partner with an Rx-to-OTC switch pipeline
	Paired brands lose shelf space to competitors
	Rx drugs become main focus, diverting investment from OTCs

Similar to SWOT analysis in its function is "portfolio analysis." The most prominent conceptual framework for this technique is the portfolio matrix, usually attributed to the Boston Consulting Group (BCG). As originally formulated, this matrix consisted of four categories of business or products based on a combination of sales growth rate and relative market share.

- *Stars* are high-growth market leaders. The large amounts of cash that they generate are often offset by heavy reinvestment. They do, nevertheless, represent considerable profit opportunity.
- *Cash cows* attract money because of a high market share and a limited need for cash outflow. Low market growth, although true, is not an issue. As Jain puts it, they are the foundation on which everything else depends (e.g., McDonald's Big Mac).[5] They must be protected. Premarin comes to mind as the "poster child" for cash cows.
- *Question marks* exist in growth markets with a low market share. The strategy is obvious: increase market share. But how, and how much to spend? This category is the true test of market strategists.
- *Dogs* show low market share and low growth. What to do? Kill them? Sell them to someone who might change their status? This category,

too, is a marketing challenge, but not one that generates much excitement.

A new approach of BCG and detailed descriptions of how to use portfolio analysis in strategy formulation are available in basic marketing texts, such as in Jain's chapter on strategy formulation.

Who Are Those Other People?

They are our competitors! They threaten our sales and our profits, sometimes without intention or knowledge, but usually because they are very much aware of our company as *their* competition.

In a free-market economy, each company tries to exceed its competitors in performance. A competitor is like an enemy. To outperform its competitors, a company must know how it stands against each one of them with regard to "arms and ammunition"—skill in maneuvering opportunities, preparedness in reacting to threats, and so on. To get adequate knowledge about the competition it faces, the company needs an excellent intelligence network.

Typically, whenever one talks in terms of competition, emphasis is placed on price, quality of products, distribution, and other marketing variables. For the purposes of strategy development, however, one needs to go far beyond these marketing tactics employed by a competitor. Simply knowing that a competitor has been lowering prices, for example, is not sufficient. Over and above that, we must know how much flexibility the competitor has in further reducing prices. Implicit here is the need for information about the competitor's cost structure.

Perhaps the best way to define competition is to differentiate between natural and strategic competition. Natural competition refers to the survival of the fittest in a given environment. It is an evolutionary process that weeds out the weaker of the two rivals. Applied to the business world, it means that no two firms doing business across the board the same way in the same market can coexist forever. To survive, each firm must define how it is uniquely superior to other competitors.

Strategic competition, in contrast, relies on leaving nothing to chance. Bruce Henderson has defined it as the "studied deployment of resources based on a high degree of insight into the systematic cause and effect in the business ecological system."[6] Strategic competition requires

1. an adequate amount of information surrounding the situation;
2. development of a framework to understand the dynamic interactive system;
3. postponement of current consumption to provide investment capital;
4. commitment to invest major resources to an irreversible outcome; and

5. ability to predict the output consequences, even with incomplete knowledge of inputs.

The degree of competition in a market depends on the moves and countermoves of the various firms that are active in the market. Usually it starts with one firm trying to achieve a favorable position by pursuing appropriate strategies. Since what is good for one firm may be harmful to the rival firms, however, the latter then respond with counterstrategies to protect their own interests.

Competitive intelligence is the publicly available information on competitors, current and potential, that serves as an important input in formulating marketing strategy. No general orders an army to march without first fully knowing about the enemy's position and intentions. Likewise, before deciding on the competitive moves to make, a firm must be aware of the perspectives of its competitors. There are many sources of competitive intelligence in the drug industry. Promotional activities may be monitored through promotional audits. Pricing practices are easily monitored from the field. Even drugs in research are easily identified well before they reach the marketplace. This is both a blessing and a curse of a highly regulated industry.

Industry economist Thi Dao has described the evolution of competition in the pharmaceutical industry as progressing from almost total emphasis on product differentiation to a current spectrum of competitive issues ranging from pure price competition to product innovation. For the future, it seems obvious that competition will have a strong economic component. Dao notes:

> To compete effectively in the future marketplace, pharmaceutical companies need more than just new medicines—they need new medicines that are cost-effective. Product competition based on cost-effectiveness will have a significant impact on the way companies do business and their collective and individual public image. At the industry level, the cost-effectiveness standard will preempt any need for governments to institute new price controls. For, as a mechanism by which medicines can be differentiated (by therapeutic benefits and/or quantified economic values), cost-effectiveness is, in effect, a form of economic regulation.
>
> And with this mechanism, product competition can take only one of the two following forms: first, if a new medicine is found to be more cost-effective than its competitors, the marketer can justify a higher price. Further, the medicine is likely to enjoy a leading market position because its cost-effectiveness will induce decision makers to grant it "medicine-of-choice" status. Second, if the therapeutic and safety benefits offered by the medicine are not sufficient to make it more cost-effective than existing competitors, its marketer will be forced to accept a lower price.[7]

Analysis of the competition should proceed along lines similar to those used in self-analysis—and on a product-by-product basis. Once this has been accomplished, one will have a clearer idea of where and how to compete and on what strategic basis, i.e., the changes in the marketing mix that are possible given the corporate strengths and weaknesses as well as those of the competition.

What Can Be Done About Those Other People?

The annual issues of *MedAd News* provide a review of activities of the top fifty pharmaceutical firms based on past, present, and future proposals. Each issue includes for each company some identifiable strategies from the previous year. Examples included are well worth careful study.

It would seem reasonable to conclude that this industry is in the process of consolidation on all fronts. With that as an assumption, Editor Wayne Koberstein, in *Pharmaceutical Executive*, proposed a typology of pharmaceutical companies as follows:[8]

Type	Characteristics	Examples (in 1998)
Behemoths	*Merger Bent*	Glaxo Wellcome
	Global/constant integration	Novartis
	Market share/board portfolio	
	Vertical strategies/multifront marketing	
	Dominate by size/resources	
	Acquisition over alliances	
Performers	*Merger Averse*	Pfizer
	Highly organized/centralized	Lilly
	Traditional sales/marketing	
	Internal hedging, e.g., disease management	
	Managed care units, regional business units (RBUs), globalization	
	External hedging, e.g., research/marketing alliances	
Contenders	*Focused*	Warner Lambert
	Merger resistant	Searle
	Development specialties/speed	
	Comarketing/copromotion	
	Therapeutic focus, e.g., opportunity seeking	
	Outsourcing	

Challengers	*Partner/Niche Player*	Amgen
	Research intensive	Genzyme
	Extensively outsourced, e.g., virtual company	
	Low or no profit	
	Licensed or "networked"	

So, Who Are "They"?

Chances are they may be you! Consider as a not atypical example the case of Astra, a company with roots in Sweden, but with a worldwide future. Astra and Merck, after a period of joint venture (fifty-fifty) agreed in 1998 to restructuring, resulting in a new Astra. Merck did not go away—revenue and income from then current and pipeline products would be slowed. In late 1998 Astra and Zeneca, in a "merger of equals," created a new company, Astra Zeneca, resulting in a company on equivalent footing with Merck, Glaxo Wellcome, Pfizer, and Novartis (and these have changed as well).

At this rate, the possibility, as cited by a representative of Pricewaterhouse Coopers, that "by the year 2000 there may be as few as thirteen industry giants" seems credible. So what does this mean for the marketing executive? Not only does one need to know the competition as competitors, but also as possible partners. Integrating the marketing plans for products of newly merged partners is yet another challenge.

WHAT BUSINESS ARE WE IN?
HOW DOES THIS GUIDE US?

Definition of business mission has an intimate, chicken-and-egg relationship to market boundary definition. On the one hand, business mission must be defined, at least in part, in terms of market scope. On the other hand, the market scope should emerge from the business mission. Mission is a broad term that refers to the total perspectives or purpose of a business. Traditionally, the mission of a business corporation was framed around its product line and expressed in mottoes such as "Our business is textiles," "We manufacture cameras," and so on.

The mission of a business is neither a statement of current business nor a random extension of current involvements. It signifies the scope and nature of business, not just as it is today, but as it could be in the future. The mission plays an important role in designating opportunities for diversification either through research and development or acquisitions. To be meaningful, the mission should be based on a comprehensive analysis of the business's technology and customer mission. Examples of companies with technology-based definitions are computer companies and aerospace companies. Customer mission refers to the fulfillment of a particular type of customer need, such as the need for basic nutrition, health care, or entertainment.

An adequate business definition requires proper consideration of the strategic three Cs: customer (e.g., buying behavior), competition (e.g., competitive definitions of the business), and company (e.g., cost behavior such as efficiencies via economies of scale, resources/skills such as financial strength, managerial talent, engineering/manufacturing capability, physical distribution system, etc., and differences in marketing, manufacturing, research and development requirements, and so on, resulting from marketing segmentation).

The mission deals with these questions: What type of business do we want to be in at some future time? What do we want to become? At any given point in time, most of the resources of a business are frozen or locked into their current uses, and the outputs in services and/or products are for the most part defined by current operations. Over an interval of a few years, however, environmental changes place demands on the business for new types of resources. Management has the option of choosing the environment in which the company will operate and acquiring commensurate new resources, rather than replacing the old ones in kind. This explains the importance of defining the business's mission. The mission should be so defined that it has a bearing on the business's strengths and weaknesses. The corporate mission of Eli Lilly and Company, reprinted here, reflects some of these:

> Eli Lilly and Company is a research-based corporation that develops, manufactures, and markets human medicines, medical instrument systems, diagnostic products, agricultural products, and cosmetics.

> To guide its affairs, the company follows certain fundamental principles. These principles, which we believe are in the best long-term interests of all shareholders, are the following:

> The company is committed to the discovery and marketing of innovative products of the highest quality that offer benefits to customers in all of our markets.

> The company is dedicated to the highest levels of ethics, integrity, and excellence in research, manufacturing, marketing, and all other phases of its operations.

> The company recognizes a primary responsibility to its employees because of the key role employees play in the achievement of corporate goals. The company's objective is to attract and retain outstanding people at all levels and in all parts of the organization. It is committed to fair and equitable treatment of all employees and to policies and

programs that offer the opportunity for employees to develop meaningful and rewarding careers.

The company feels an obligation to be a good corporate citizen wherever it operates.

Marketing Goals and Objectives

Goals and objectives flow from and must be consistent with the company mission. There are differences of opinion about the definition of each. Goals are often described as long-term (five to fifteen years) accomplishments consistent with the mission. Objectives are often shorter term and should always be measurable. These terms are used interchangeably in practice, but within a company a commonly understood definition of both is essential.

Objectives form a specific expression of purpose, thus helping to remove any uncertainty about the company's policy or about the intended purpose of effort. If properly designed, objectives permit measurement of progress. Without some form of progress measurement, it may not be possible to know whether adequate resources are being applied or whether these resources are being managed effectively. Finally, objectives facilitate the relationships between units, especially in a diversified corporation, where the separate goals of different units may not be consistent with some higher corporate purpose.

Despite their overriding importance, defining objectives is far from easy. Defining goals as the future becomes the present is a long, time-consuming, and continuous process. In practice, many businesses are run either without any commonly accepted objectives and goals or with conflicting objectives and goals, which, in some cases, are different in such general terms that their significance for the job is not understood.

Setting Goals and Objectives

The first step in the process of setting goals and objectives should probably be an inventory of objectives, as they are currently understood. For example, senior executives may state what the current goals are and what type of company they want it to be in the future. Various executives will perceive current goals differently; of course they will have varying ambitions for the future. It will take several top-level meetings and a good deal of effort on the part of the CEO to settle on the final goals.

Each executive may be asked to make a presentation on the goals and objectives in the future. The executives should be asked to justify the significance of each goal in terms of measuring performance, satisfying environmental conditions, and achieving growth. Foreseeably, the executives will have different goals or may express the same goals in terms that make them appear different, but there should emerge, on analysis, a desire for a common destiny. Sometimes disharmony of goals may be based on diverse perceptions of a business's resource potential and corporate strategy. Thus, before embarking on setting goals, it is helpful if information on the resource potential and corporate strategy is circulated among the executives.

Before finalizing the goal, it is necessary that the executive team show a consensus; that is, each one of them should believe in the viability of the set goals and willingly agree to work toward their achievement. A way must be found to persuade a dissenting executive to cooperate. For example, if a very ambitious executive works with stability-oriented people, in the absence of an opportunity to be creative, the executive may fail to perform adequately even on routine matters, thus becoming a liability to the organization.

Once broad goals have been worked out, they should be translated into specific objectives. This is an equally challenging task. Should the objectives be set so high that only an outstanding manager can achieve them, or should they be set so that they are attainable by the average manager? At what level does frustration inhibit a manager's best efforts? Does an attainable budget lead to complacency? A company might start with three levels of objectives: (1) easily attainable, (2) most desirable, and (3) optimistic. Thereafter, the company may choose a position somewhere between the most desirable and the optimistic objectives, depending on the organization's resources and the value orientation of the management. In no case, however, should the performance fall below the easily attainable level, even if everything goes wrong.

The Concept of Strategic Planning

Strategy in a firm is concerned with the basic goals and objectives of the business, the product-market matches chosen on which to compete, the major patterns of resource allocations, and the major operating policies used to relate the firm to its environment.

Each functional area (e.g., marketing) makes its own unique contribution to strategy formulation at different levels. In a great many firms, the marketing function represents the greatest degree of contact with the external environment—the environment least controllable by the firm. In such firms, marketing plays a pivotal role in strategy development. (A Searle advertisement stated, "Marketing is the force that drives our business.")

In its strategic role, marketing consists of establishing a match between the firm and its environment to seek solutions to problems of deciding how the chosen field(s) of endeavor may be successfully run in a competitive environment by pursuing product, price, promotion, and distribution perspectives to serve target markets. Marketing provides the core element for future relationships between the firm and its environment. It specifies inputs for defining objectives and helps in formulating plans to achieve them. Strategy specifies the direction. Its intent is to influence the behavior of competitors and the evolution of the market to the advantage of the strategist. It seeks to change the competitive environment. Thus, a strategy statement includes a description of the new competitive equilibrium to be created, the cause-and-effect relationships that will bring it about, and the logic to support the course of action.

Planning articulates the means of implementing strategy. A strategic plan specifies the sequence and timing that will alter competitive relationships.

Marketing strategies should devise ways in which the corporation can differentiate itself effectively from its competitors, capitalizing on its distinctive strengths to deliver better value to its customers. A good marketing strategy should be characterized by

1. a clear market definition;
2. a good match between corporate strengths and the needs of the market; and
3. superior performance, relative to the competition, in the key success factors of the business.

Such a strategy assumes development of an effective marketing mix—the four Ps—which are discussed in Sections II through V of this book. Matching the needs of the marketplace with corporate strengths requires a thorough knowledge of both. We have seen how market research can help with the former. Only objective, honest introspection can supply the latter.

INTERNAL REVIEW—
ANOTHER LOOK AT THE CORPORATE NAVEL

In the prescription drug industry, much is usually made of the relative potential of drugs in the companies' various pipelines. Indeed, imminent blockbusters are desirable, but a company cannot simply wait around for its scientists to pull a rabbit out of the laboratory hat. The research-intensive nature of this industry tends to overshadow the importance of marketing savvy and strategy.

In the same sense that a company may be known for its eminence in the field of, say, cardiovascular research, it may also be noted for various areas of strength in marketing. A regular, systematic audit of marketing strengths and weaknesses is essential to strategy development. A nonexhaustive list of potential strengths would include the following:

- Customer service/channel relationships
- Corporate image
- Capital availability
- Quality of sales force

- Effectiveness of promotion in print media
- Pricing knowledge and skills
- Product distribution efficiency
- Exclusivity in markets, even in "niche" markets
- Dominant market share position
- Morale and commitment of marketing personnel
- Expertise in market research

A short list of potential weaknesses could include these factors:

- Lack of coordination between sales and marketing
- Lack of clear understanding of corporate marketing strategies by those who must implement them
- Ambiguity in identities of differing divisions of the marketing effort
- Uncertainty regarding job security, especially in a time of mergers and acquisitions

Regular *internal* environmental scanning is essential to exploitation of strengths and correction of weaknesses. This is difficult to do efficiently and effectively for at least two reasons:

1. It is tempting to lose one's objectivity when studying one's own performance.
2. There is some risk of engendering fear among employees while getting information.

These difficulties do not excuse failure to make such assessments on a regular basis. Table 3.2 provides an overview of some of the steps that can be taken, while Table 3.3 delineates some of the challenges and opportunities. The ability to meet the challenges and exploit the opportunities is the mark of a successful marketer.

TABLE 3.2. Steps in the Process of Assessing Strengths and Weaknesses

Which attributes can be examined?	What types of measurements can a manager make?	What criteria are applicable to judge a strength or a weakness?	How can the manager get the information to make these assessments?
Organization structure	Measure the existence of an attribute	Historical experience of the company	Personal observation
Major stated policies		Intracompany competition	Customer contacts
Top manager's skills	Measure an attribute's efficiency		Experience
Information systems		Direct competitors	Exit interviews

TABLE 3.2 (continued)

Which attributes can be examined?	What types of measurements can a manager make?	What criteria are applicable to judge a strength or a weakness?	How can the manager get the information to make these assessments?
Planning system	Measure an attribute's effectiveness	Consultant's opinions	Control system documents
Employee attitudes			
Technical skills		Normative judgments based on management's understanding of literature	Meetings
Research skills			Planning system documents
New product pipeline			Employees
Demographic characteristics of personnel		Personal opinions	Subordinate managers
Channel relations		Specific targets of accomplishment, such as sales quotas	Superordinate managers
Sales force skills			Peers
Breadth of product line		Employee turnover	Published documents
Stock market performance			Competitive intelligence
Knowledge of customers' needs			Consultants
Market domination			Published materials
			Professional meetings

Source: Adapted and expanded from Howard H. Stevenson, Defining Corporate Strengths, and Weaknesses, Sloan Management Review, 17(spring):54, 1976.

TABLE 3.3. Challenges and Opportunities in the Marketing Mix

Product	Price	Promotion	Place
Less differentiation	Less pricing flexibility	Greater competitive "noise" levels	More customers
More R&D risk			Changing demographics of U.S. population
Shorter life cycles	Commodity pricing of patented products	New message including economics	
More generics		Greater message	Greater centralization of purchasing and treatment decisions
More emphasis on outcomes	Harmonization of worldwide prices	Requirement for more efficient media	
Entry of brand manufacturers into generics business	Decreased profits	Subject to new public values	More emphasis on self-care
Greater demand to prove value	Greater justification	Greater regulation	Greater cost control efforts
	Possible controls		

TABLE 3.3 *(continued)*

Product	Price	Promotion	Place
	Entry of economics into sale dialogue	Greater copromotional/comarketing with "customer" to drive market share	Decreased economic growth
	Lower prices, increased units	Growing importance of patient	Health care reform efforts
	Limited awareness of price among doctors		Greater governmental intervention

SECTION II:
PRODUCT

Chapter 4

Principles of Product Research and Development

Greg Perkins

The accepted definition of "product" is "the benefits or positive results that markets derive out of doing business with the company using the products you offer in the way you offer them."

People do not buy drills, it is said, they buy holes. Similarly, patients do not want medication—they want relief from pain, a longer life, or better function. Those who prescribe or dispense to those patients want those things as well as their own professional needs to be satisfied.

It is the product strategies that eventually come to dominate the overall market strategy of the company. In this chapter we will discuss the following several aspects of product strategy. The new product strategy will receive the most attention—as it does in the pharmaceutical industry.

- Product scope strategy
- New product strategy
- Product positioning strategy
- Product repositioning strategy
- Product elimination strategy
- Diversification strategy

PRODUCT SCOPE STRATEGY

The product scope strategy deals with the perspectives of the product mix of a company (i.e., the number of product lines and items in each line that the company may offer). The product scope strategy is determined by making a reference to the business mission. Presumably, the mission defines what sort of business it is going to be, which helps in selecting the products and services that are to become a part of the product mix.

The product scope strategy must be finalized after a careful review of all facets of the business, since it involves a long-term commitment. Additionally, the strategy must be reviewed from time to time to make any changes called for because of shifts in the environment. Product scope strategy is also related to market scope strategy. The strategy alternatives discussed briefly here are as follows:

- Single market
- Single product
- Multimarket
- Multiple products
- Total market
- System of products

Single Market

A variety of reasons may lead a company to concentrate its efforts on a single segment of the market. For example, a small company, to avoid confrontation with large competitors, may find a unique niche in the market and devote its energies to serving this market. The single-market or niche strategy is often born of necessity. Lacking the resources to fight head-to-head battles across the board with larger, entrenched competitors, the winners typically seek out niches that are too small to interest the giants or can be captured and protected by sheer perseverance and by serving customers surprisingly well.

Single Product

A business may have just one product in its line and try to live on the success of this one product. This strategy has several advantages. First, concentration on a single product leads to specialization, which helps in scale and productivity gains. Second, management of operations is much more efficient when a single product is the focus. Third, a single-product company may become so specialized in its field that it can withstand virtually any competition. Fleets Enema is an acceptable example.

Innovative imitation may not only gain a foothold into a fruitful market, but go a long way toward preventing a decline. Ortho-McNeil Pharmaceuticals, for example, might have been content to remain in the "prophylactics and diaphragm" business. Instead, defining their "market province" to be control of conception, they were ready with their own version of the oral contraceptive early in the development of this market. Since then, of course, they have diversified.

Despite its obvious advantages, the single-product company has one drawback: if changes in the environment make the product obsolete, the single-product company can be in deep trouble.

The single-product strategy has an additional drawback. It is not co
cive to seeking growth or market share. Its main advantage is profitability
a company with a single-product focus is not able to earn higher margins,
is better to seek a new posture. Companies interested in growth and/or market share will find the single-product strategy to be of limited, but real,
value.

Multimarket

Instead of limiting business to one segment and thus putting all its eggs in
one basket, a company may opt to serve several distinct segments. To successfully implement the multimarket strategy, it is necessary to choose those segments with which the company feels most comfortable and in which the company is able to avoid confronting companies that serve the entire market. This
strategy accepts the premise that it is possible to differentiate between such
markets as prescription and OTC, hospital and drugstore, brand name and generic, and so forth. Strategy is then formulated accordingly.

Multiple Products

The multiple-products strategy amounts to offering two or more products. A variety of factors leads companies to choose this strategic posture. A
company having a single product has nowhere to go if that product gets into
trouble; with multiple products, however, poor performance by one product
often can be balanced out. In addition, it is essential for a company seeking
growth to have multiple product offerings.

While not all products may be fast-moving items, they must complement
each other in a portfolio of products. The multiple-products strategy is directed toward achieving growth, market share, and profitability. Not all
companies will prosper simply by having multiple products. This is because
growth, market share, and profitability are the functions of a large number
of variables, only one of which is having multiple products. Most of the major drug companies have some sort of multiple-products strategy.

Total Market

A company using the total-market strategy serves the entire spectrum
of the market by selling different products directed toward different segments in the market. The strategy evolves over a great number of years
of operation. As the market grows and different segments emerge, leading
competitors may attempt to compete in all of the segments. This may be
done by employing different combinations of product, price, promotion,
and distribution strategies. These dominant companies may also attempt to
enter new segments as they emerge.

et strategy is risky. For this reason, only a very small num-
n an industry may follow this strategy. It requires a top
tment to embracing the entire market. Additionally, a
ple amount of resources to implement this strategy.
in a strong financial position may find this strategy
panies in the drug industry seem to flirt with this strat-
through mergers and acquisitions, especially in recent years.

...a of Products

The word "system" as applied to products is a post–World War II phenomenon. Two related forces have been responsible for the emergence of
this phenomenon. These are the popularity of the marketing concept that
businesses do not sell products but customer satisfaction, and the complexi-
ties of the product itself, which call for the use of complementary products
and after-sales services.

Offering a *system* of products rather than a single product is a viable
strategy in a number of ways. It makes the customer fully dependent on the
company, which in turn gains monopolistic control over the market. Additionally, the system-of-products strategy blocks the way for the competition
to move in. With such benefits, this strategy is extremely useful in seeking
growth, profitability, and market share.

The successful implementation of this strategy requires a thorough understanding of customer requirements—the processes and functions the
consumer must perform when using the product. Effective implementation
of this strategy broadens both the company's concept of its product and the
market opportunities for it, which in turn helps meet the product and market
objectives of growth, profitability, and market share.

The system strategy is unlikely to occur in this industry unless there are
even more mergers. It is, however, the approach attempted by wholesalers
(see Section IV).

NEW PRODUCT STRATEGY

New products continue to be the lifeblood of the research-intensive pharmaceutical industry. They may be new in the sense of new chemical entities,
new to an individual firm's product line, or a new name for an existing (especially OTC) product. However, new products are usually necessary for
sustained profitability and growth.

Top management can affect the implementation of new product strategy:
first, by establishing policies and broad strategic directions for the kinds of
new products the company should seek; second, by providing the kind of
leadership that will create the environmental climate needed to stimulate in-

novative drive in the organization; and, third, by instituting review ana
itoring procedures so that the manager is involved at the right deci.
points and can know whether work schedules are being met in ways that a
consistent with the broad policy direction.

New product strategies can focus on imitation of existing products, modification and improvement of existing products, or truly new products. The
latter will receive the most attention here, but all of these are widely employed in the drug industry.

Product Imitation

Exact product imitation is, of course, the heart of the generic drug industry. Indeed, the FDA requires the imitation to be identical, at least insofar as
its bioequivalence is concerned. A sort of quasi-imitation exists in the form
of new, patented drug products which are molecular analogues of existing
products but which offer little or no therapeutic advantage. (The FDA, in
fact, makes such a judgment on each new product.)

This strategy particularly suits companies with limited resources. Many
companies, as a matter of fact, develop such talent that they can imitate any
product, no matter how complicated. With a limited investment in research
and development, the imitator may sometimes have a lower cost, which
gives it a pricing advantage in the market over the leader.

The imitation strategy may also be adopted on defensive grounds. Being
sure of its existing product(s), a company may initially ignore new developments in the field. If the new developments *gain a foothold in the marketplace,* however, they may cut into the ground held by the existing prod-
uct(s). In such a situation, a company may be forced into imitating the new
developments as a matter of survival.

It should be noted that truly innovative imitation attempts to improve
upon the original article and, as such, tends to lend its own contribution to
better pharmaceuticals. On balance, the gains to be realized by this type of
competitive activity seem to outweigh the problems created by the numbers
of available drugs.

Any pioneer in the field has a strong talking point when referring to the
need to recover research and development costs plus a fair profit in a short
period. All of the advertising, no matter how actively oriented toward promotion of the brand name, tends to contribute to the primary demand for the
product type and, thus, aids competitors. Further, simply by being first, a
company must take a stand as to products and policies. The followers, then,
are free to deviate from this stand and, if these deviations are good from a
marketing point of view, to profit by it.

nent/Modification

...ct of a company may reach a stage at which something
...it viable. The product may have reached the maturity
...cycle because of shifts in environment, thus ceasing
...turn, or new product, pricing, distribution, and pro-
...ployed by competitors may have reduced the status of
...a "me too" category. At that stage, management has two op-
...er eliminate the product or revitalize it by making improvements or
...ifications. Improvements or modifications are achieved by redesigning, remodeling, or reformulating so that the product satisfies customer needs more fully. This strategy, commonly known as *life cycle management,* seeks not only to restore the health of the product but also sometimes to help distinguish it from those of competitors.

There are a number of reasons for "molecule manipulation" within a firm's product line. Sometimes an expiring patent may move a firm to search for a slight but patentable modification of a successful product. Sometimes, as noted earlier, slight modifications bring about completely new uses for the compound. Often, efforts are made to provide a full spectrum of analogues active in different types of conditions, or at least sufficiently different to be promoted for these differing conditions. Tranquilizers in a series are often handled in this manner. Further, it has been shown that the introduction of a new product by a firm having an older one already a success usually exerts an incremental effect on sales, rather than cutting into the market share of the established product. Finally, in the understandable rush to be first, some firms may market the first product possible, with the acknowledged aim of replacing it with another at a later time.

Structural modifications are not, of course, the only means of changing the character of existing products. Another method is finding new uses for them.

The following excerpt from a National Pharmaceutical Council publication provides the industry's position.[1]

Pharmaceutical Research and Innovation

The vast majority of clinically important drugs developed over the last 50 years have resulted from an evolutionary process, involving multiple, small, successive improvements within a pharmacological class. This should come as no surprise, since the process of repeated incremental improvement is the predominant mechanism of innovation and product development within many industries.

"Small Wins" and Incremental Improvement: The Basic Mechanism of Technological Innovation

Most technological advances are built from bits and pieces rather than from large leaps or breakthroughs in discovery or technology. This means that the products of technology-driven industries improve as a result of a series of small steps forward. Over time, succession of "small wins" adds up to a big advance in technology. The importance of small wins in the success of most enterprises is often underestimated:

> "It is by no means certain that the increase in productivity over a longer period of time is chiefly due to the great inventors and their inventions. It may well be the case that the sum total of all minor improvements, each too small to be called an invention, has contributed to the increase in productivity more than the great inventions themselves."[1]

Small wins and incremental innovation have played a major role in product development in the computer, automobile, and aviation industries.

> "In the last 20 years the number of bits on a [computer] chip has gone from one to one million. Incremental improvement has also given us better resolution screens and quieter, better quality printers, . . . jet engines with double the thrust per unit weight of two decades ago, plastics that can be used at temperatures twice as high as a decade ago, and incandescent light bulbs that are 15 times as efficient as Edison's; in short, an array of products across the entire spectrum of modern industry that are much better, and often less costly, than those of an earlier era."[2]

Further, most competition is between variants of the same product, for example, automobile vs. automobile, not automobile vs. helicopter, and "where the United States has not been competitive, we have lost, usually not to radical new technology, but to better refinements . . ."[2]

The old Bell Telephone System, with its research-oriented subsidiary of Western Electric, was the inventor and most consistent practitioner of incremental innovation.[3] And that is why we have the best telephone system in the world. America's pharmaceutical industry is the best in the world for the same reason.

Incremental Advances Characterize the History of Pharmaceutical Innovation

Great strides in pharmacology and therapeutics have resulted from very small variations in the chemistry of active molecules.[4] In fact, the history of pharmacology is characterized by incremental improvements in the safety, efficacy, selectivity, and utility of drugs within a given class. As a result, many pharmacological classes now contain numerous agents. Although these agents are molecularly similar, their therapeutic properties are often significantly different. The public benefits are striking because a broad class of drugs enables physicians to treat with precision the individual needs of diverse patients.

Examples of Small Changes Resulting in Important Progress

Minor alternations in the chemical structure of a drug can make a vast difference in biologic activity, as illustrated by the following examples:

- In 1989, the FDA approved a new drug, clozapine, a modification of the dibenzodiazepine class of tricyclic drugs. This new agent promises relief for thousands of schizophrenics who have not responded to prior treatment with available antipsychotic agents.
- Efforts to improve the antibiotic sulfanilamide unexpectedly brought forth potent new diuretics, improved antibacterials, and the first oral antidiabetic agents.
- Addition of two carbon atoms to morphine resulted in nalorphine, a morphine antagonist used to treat narcotic overdose. A minor modifcation of nalorphine gave naltrexone, a narcotic antagonist with long duration of action, enabling its use as an oral formulation in the treatment of narcotic addiction.
- A small change in dehydrocorticosterone, a virtually inactive compound, produced cortisone, which has a great range of biological effects. Other modifications of steroid drugs separate their anti-inflammatory activities from their glucocorticoid and mineralocorticoid activities.
- Minor modifications in cephaloridine, a cephalosporin antibiotic effective only by injection, produced cephaloglycin and cephalexin which have the advantage of being effective by oral administration.
- Vincristine and vinblastine are nearly identical compounds that attack different forms of cancer. Vincristine is effective against actue leukemia, while vinblastine is not.

These examples illustrate the fact that incremental advances, providing a succession of small improvements, have historically been the most common pattern for the development of medicines.[5] *Only recently has the introduction of "biotech" drugs such as recombinant proteins and monoclonal antibodies significantly begun to impact the picture.[6]*

The Drug Class Is the Fundamental Therapeutic Unit

Although "breakthrough" therapies such as the beta-blocker propranolol and the ulcer drug cimetidine attract public attention, it is the small, successive developments that generally make the difference to the majority of patients. The breakthroughs, which are usually the first of a class, inevitably display deficiencies after they are widely distributed. Pharmaceutical companies use these revealed deficiencies as opportunities to develop related compounds that are more effective, more selective, and less toxic. The drugs of choice in a well-developed class are almost never the ones that were marketed first.

A pioneer or breakthrough drug, representing a novel therapeutic entity, is best seen as the organizing principle for the eventual evolution of a new class of agents. In time, other agents with similar properties are discovered and developed. The drug class as a whole eventually becomes the fundamental therapeutic unit. The therapeutic power, stability, and utility of a class are defined through the contributions of its multiple agents.

Classes of drugs have important properties that are not possessed by individual agents. Features which emerge only at the class level include:

- variability in pharmacological properties to fit the needs of individual patients;
- cumulative improvements in efficacy, selectivity, and reduced toxicity;
- comprehensive knowledge of the extent and limits of pharmacological action, derived from research and clinical experience with multiple chemically related agents; and
- the availability of a "tool chest" for further research on basic disease mechanisms.

Because of these attributes, the collective therapeutic advantage of the class as a whole may be of greater clinical significance than the original advantage of the pioneer compound.

1 Weick KE. Small wins. Redefining the scale of social problems. Am Psychol. 1984; 39:40-49.
2 Gomory RE, Schmitt RW. Science and product. Science. 1988; 240:1131-2/1203-4.
3 Drucker PF. The 10 rules of effective research. Wall Street Journal. May 30, 1989.
4 Maxwell RA. The state of the art of the science of drug discovery—an opinion. Drug Dev Res. 1984; 4:375-89.
5 Snell ES. Postmarketing development of medicines. Pharm Int. 1989; 7(2):33-7.
6 Drews. Drug discovery: A historical perspective. Science. 2000; 1960-64.

New Product Development

New product development* and marketing in the pharmaceutical industry, perhaps as in no other industry, requires the close and efficient cooperation of the research and marketing functions in the firm: The interface between basic research that produces (one hopes) the breakthrough chemical compounds and marketing, charged with the creation of a successful promotion, price, and distribution plan, is the site of action of drug development. Drug development is the process by which a chemical entity is transformed into a drug product.

The success of a pharmaceutical firm is the result of more than just the efficiency of its R&D laboratories, however, because the input of research is essentially information that is used by manufacturing and marketing to make and sell products. For the pharmaceutical firm to be successful, these three key functions must operate in an integrated and productive manner.

All regulatory and pricing policies that make it difficult for marketing to compete successfully will also affect the research process indirectly. Consequently, the technoscientific success of the pharmaceutical company is de-

---

*Much of the material in this section was adapted from Chapter 7, by Richard E. Faust, in Mickey Smith (Ed.), *Principles of Pharmaceutical Marketing*, Third Edition (Binghamton, NY: The Haworth Press, 1988), pp. 141-171.

pendent upon the integration of key functions and the proficiency of research to create, manufacturing to make, and marketing to sell new and improved products. More attention is being given to the development of the total corporation through managed creativity applied to every business function. In addition to new and improved products and processes, corporations may seek growth and efficiency through new distribution channels and customers, new financial and administrative practices, and new marketing strategies. Close interaction with and collaboration between R&D and marketing is therefore needed to support various corporate development plans and objectives.

Unquestionably, investing in long-range R&D requires an act of faith by top management. In spite of all the elaborate models available for identifying market opportunities, establishing research priorities, and forecasting return on investment, research investment still requires the judgment of top-level managers. There is little doubt, however, that the success of a major new drug product can have a profound impact on a firm's sales and profit profile, and it is this possibility that often encourages continued investments in R&D in many firms.

The nature of the "research planning" function varies considerably within pharmaceutical firms, but, in general, it focuses on the allocation of research resources involving project selection and monitoring. It may also encompass such activities as those associated with generating R&D budgets and forecasting output, personnel administration, and organizational development.

Research functional or operational plans are often designed to convey the status of research activities and commitments, to present a profile of the use of research resources, and to generate a picture of outputs both in the near and long term. Most research plans seek to create a balance between programs yielding near-term results (one to five years) and those providing rewards further along (five to ten years). In addition, the major research-oriented firms invest in more exploratory or basic programs that may be termed "new horizon research," in which the payback may not occur for at least fifteen to twenty years. The contents of a typical strategic or functional research plan may be outlined as follows:

1. *Introduction:* a statement of the orientation of the plan, its relationship to previous and related plans, and current information being developed in research
2. *Objectives:* a statement of research objectives and their relationship to corporate and business objectives
3. *Research environment:* an overview of research and how it is affected by competitive R&D trends, political/legislative pressures, various major scientific and technological factors, and socioeconomic forces, as well as the presentation of strategies to respond to these dynamic environmental elements

4. *Research resource analysis:* an analysis of research personnel, expenses, and facilities, including recent growth patterns, current allocations, and present needs
5. *Drug development project analysis:*
   a. Drug development projects (years one to five)
   b. Drug development projects (years five to ten): analysis of compounds projected in the pharmaceutical business plan using a "one-pager" format that encompasses such information as the project objective, sales projections, patient status, development timetable, and competitive products
6. *Exploratory research activities:*
   a. Overview of exploratory effort: perspectives on magnitude of the effort, emerging trends and changing patterns, and commentary on research activities that have an impact on broad areas, such as aging
   b. Important research areas and activities: a review of current important and emerging research efforts and integrated programs aimed at generating significant new products and product leads beyond those of the current project planning period
7. *Support for marketed products:* a summary of research efforts aimed at developing new dosage forms and indications, as well as special clinical and other studies that support current products
8. *Research operational improvement strategies and goals:* an elaboration of research actions, plans, and strategies aimed at improving operations and the probability of success over the planning board; an assessment of broad trends, patterns, and considerations to aid in evaluating research output and contributions to corporate success
9. *Research requirements and resource projections:* a profile of personnel, funding, and facility needs during the next five years, including perspectives on alternative output patterns influenced by the magnitude of budget and personnel increases
10. *Planning highlights and summary:* an overview and summary of planning goals, operating strategies, and projections for near-, mid-, and long-term achievements

A strategic business plan is designed to convey the thrust of the business operation. The areas covered usually include an analysis of environmental forces and other factors that influence the success of the enterprise and indirectly impact R&D. The contents of a typical pharmaceutical strategic business plan may be outlined as follows:

1. *Description and purpose of the business:* A statement of the basic business growth strategy and goals of the marketing area presents a

picture of the business and its general plans for the planning period, usually five to ten years.

2. *Environmental analysis:* This provides an overview of the environmental forces affecting the business, such as increased substitution, more generic prescribing, efforts to reduce health care costs, inflation, patent expirations, concern for "orphan" drugs, increased competition, and various governmental regulations.

3. *Critical issues:* Many plans contain a description of important issues that will affect the success of the business over the planning period. These issues and concerns will vary with the firm, but they might include such topics as

   a. the impact of various special regulations,
   b. the patent status of marketed products,
   c. an inventory of current research programs and commitments to improve allocation of resources, and
   d. establishment of mechanisms for research program review to ensure consistency with business objectives and goals.

4. *Strategies and programs:* Once critical operational areas have been identified, strategic plans usually describe how the business intends to meet these challenges and to ensure growth and profits. Because one critical issue usually centers on the flow of new products from research over the planning period, various strategies are often mentioned that are designed to improve research productivity and to enhance the functional interface between research and marketing groups. Under a plan to "improve research productivity," one might find such action strategies as the following:

   a. Improve criteria for product candidate selection for development and evaluate compliance to criteria throughout development
   b. Improve the priority-setting process and communication of priorities for research and product development programs
   c. Inventory current research programs and commitments to improve allocation of resources
   d. Establish mechanisms for research program review to ensure consistency with business objectives and goals

5. *Resource requirements:* This section of the planning document presents a detailed analysis of the projected output over the planning period, including sales from existing and new products and dosage forms. The resources needed (e.g., facilities, capital, and personnel) for this are also projected over the planning period. Often probabilities are used to forecast output, and in some cases, "optimistic," "pessimistic," and "most likely" forecasts are presented that are also closely connected to research productivity.

It is obvious that the impact of marketing on the R&D process varies with the stage of the process (see Table 4.1). As we move from the exploratory

TABLE 4.1. Parallel Courses in New Product Development: Bridging the Gap Between Basic Science and Marketing Research

Stage	Basic Science	Marketing Research
Idea generation	Component synthesis New dosage forms New delivery systems	New product/service ideas
Screening	Animal studies of pharmacology, thera-peutic activity, and toxicology	Ratings of product potential and company strengths Market profile of disease prevalence, population/epidemiological trends, and competition Competitive strategies Product life cycles
Business and medical analysis	Added animal studies and phase I, II, and III human studies	Decision makers' reactions to the product concept and suggestions for product development Quantification of market potential to the product concept, and marketing strategies Positioning studies, evaluation of promotion themes, segmentation analysis Sales force training and deployment studies Subjective patient evaluations and preferences
Development	Completion of clinical studies Dosage form, delivery system research	Naming studies Packaging studies Marketing tactics research—ad copy testing, pricing studies
Test marketing		Experimental evaluation of product performance and marketing strategies/tactics
Commerciali-zation	Phase IV studies	Evaluation of marketing tactics implemented, progress toward sales goals, model validation Documentation of product life cycles Development of strategies for later stages of the product life cycles and competitive counter-strategies

Source: Robert N. Zelnio and Juliet G. Zimmerman, "Parallel Courses in New Product Development," *Pharmaceutical Executive,* July 4(7): 25-27, 1984. Reprinted with permission from *Pharmaceutical Executive,* July 1984, pp. 25-27. Copyright 2001 Advanstar Communications Inc. Advanstar Communications Inc. retains all rights to this material.

end of the R&D spectrum to the point at which leads are identified and a decision is made to pursue an IND and an NDA, the goals of projects become better defined and the role of marketing increases. At any point, either inadequate marketing inputs or attempts to exert excessive control over the research process can create major problems. Difficulties may also arise when research programs are too unstructured and are not in tune with marketing strategies and the near-term concern for increased revenues and profits. Once projects are formalized, marketing needs to monitor progress and to provide important insights concerning

1. the nature of the clinical studies to be undertaken and the desired claim structure for the product,
2. dosage forms to be developed and their characteristics, and
3. the timing of the NDA submission.

Marketing should also exert considerable influence on research activities in support of existing products, including broadened claims, new dosage forms, and overall defensive efforts. More emphasis has been placed on projects aimed at prolonging the life cycles of currently marketed products. Even in the large research-based firms, as much as 20 to 25 percent of the R&D budget may be directed to such defensive activities.

In some firms a formal statement of marketing interests and opportunities in various therapeutic categories is developed by marketing specialists and presented to research scientists as a guide to research decision making in the selection of R&D programs and projects. The marketing overview usually includes such information as market definition and potential, patient prevalence, current sales data and projections, leading marketed products, prescribing patterns, and competitive trends. In some cases, marketing experts may provide specific suggestions to research such potential sales for products that might be developed.

Project selection decisions are often influenced by a number of important considerations in addition to the size of the research budget. It should be noted that many research, manufacturing, and marketing concerns must be considered that influence project selection decisions. Consider, for example, the following factors for a firm wishing to develop a market position in antibiotics, essentially a new area for the firm, which has a couple of exciting research leads.

1. Do we have specific objectives in the antibiotic field with regard to market position by a targeted date? Can we obtain commitment of resources (e.g., people, funds, facilities) to obtain these objectives? Should our emphasis be near-term (two to three years) or long-term (five to ten years)?

2. What are the risks and uncertainties associated with the effort? What are the financial implications of these uncertainties?

3. What is the nature of the competition in terms of marketed products and current development efforts? What are their strengths, weaknesses, and abilities?

4. What other known antibiotics are actively being developed? What are their potential market advantages and disadvantages?

5. What are the competitive advantages of the products we are considering to develop? What is the expected market life cycle? Are there possible follow-up products?

6. What are the pricing structure and profit trend with antibiotics?

7. Who are the customers (e.g., physicians, third-party payers, government), and what value is each looking for? How will value differences affect our market positioning and opportunities?

8. Can we market antibiotics more successfully with a dedicated sales group or through our existing field force? Are special promotional efforts needed?

9. How will products be produced? If agents are manufactured by us, where? How much investment is needed? Do we have adequate in-house technical expertise to manufacture? What are the new material requirements? Do we need specialized facilities?

10. What is the patent position for each of our potential market entities? Are areas of litigation of concern?

11. What is the R&D cost to support our strategy? Do we have the internal technical and scientific expertise to support the needed research effort? How will a move to antibiotic research impact other research projects and programs?

12. If we accomplish our objectives, what is the likely response of our competitors? How will we respond to them, and what will be the impact on our market share and profitability?

In addition to the interactions between marketing and research that occur during the drug development stage in the category of project management, most firms have new product coordinators in marketing who are concerned with developing market plans for existing products and who have, in addition, a vital interest in new products moving toward NDA approval. Because these products, when approved, are assigned to the product-planning function, personnel in this area seek to become involved during the latter stages of the drug development cycle.

The basic function of a product director is to plan for and manage the development of assigned, existing, and new pharmaceutical products as individual businesses by assessing marketing needs and opportunities, developing marketing strategies and responsibility, and directing the application of marketing resources in an optimal manner consistent with the goals of the firm. In this capacity the director is responsible for the product- or project-related activities of each member of the marketing teams, composed of the following personnel:

- Advertising manager
- Product sales manager
- Sales planning manager
- Professional services physician
- Professional services writer
- Professional services manager
- Medical affairs physician
- Proofreader
- Marketing research analyst
- Copywriter
- Career development associate
- Other specific team members (as appropriate)

The principal functional responsibilities of the product director are the following:

- Develop annual, intermediate, and long-range marketing and business strategies and plans for the business
- Manage and recommend to the marketing board strategies and plans relative to pricing, distribution, labeling, trademarking, and packaging associated with assigned products
- Establish and achieve all quantifiable product, project, and personnel objectives
- Develop unit and dollar sales projections to ensure appropriate planning to meet the anticipated needs of the marketplace and achievement of profit plans
- Recommend and develop appropriate new dosage forms strategy and plans for assigned products to maximize opportunities
- Conduct team meetings, foster communication among team members and departments, and issue appropriate and timely minutes
- Work with sales management to achieve national and regional sales strategies and plans

- Direct selected projects that will impact across product lines and influence future business policies of the firm
- Ensure, through leadership and direction, that the planning, developing, implementation, and monitoring of marketing programs conform with and fully support the product plan
- Initiate and maintain appropriate linkage between the product and project teams and other functional resources, such as distribution, drug regulatory affairs, finance, law, materials management, product development, packaging development, production, manufacturing, facilities planning, research, public relations, public policy, business development, and strategic planning
- Communicate and actively participate with research and project management to ensure that product R&D plans are implemented that fulfill agreed-to strategies for assigned products and therapeutic areas
- Coordinate to achieve mutually satisfactory resolution of any actual or potential conflicts identified between assigned product marketing strategies or programs and existing local, state, or federal laws and regulations
- Monitor social, political, economic, regulatory, and legal trends affecting the pharmaceutical industry and assigned markets and react with recommendations
- Consult with and engage outside support, consultants, and agencies to ensure the continuous generation of new, innovative, and creative ideas for product and project objectives
- Establish budgets and budget mix and monitor expenditures by specific media and target audiences for products or projects
- Anticipate and apprise management of changes in the marketplace and initiate modifications to the marketing plan based on evolving market dynamics
- Exercise final team approval on promotional copy and field communications related to assigned products
- Assume responsibility in concert with appropriate department heads to assist team members in the informal training process relative to team interactions and activities
- Participate and interact with broad chartered committees, such as the FDA production committee, product coordinating committee, project teams, and product management review committee
- Coordinate the response to the FDA relative to assigned marketed products with drug regulatory affairs and others
- Provide input into project management to maximize potential marketing opportunities prior to issuance of the transfer document
- Review and comment on selling emphasis programs

- Recommend appropriate allocation of sales efforts for the pharmaceutical line to the sales department and marketing board for the current planning period
- Launch new products

PRODUCT POSITIONING STRATEGY

The term "positioning" refers to placing a brand in that part of the market where it will have a favorable reception compared to competing products. Since the market is heterogeneous, one brand cannot make an impact on the entire market. As a matter of strategy, therefore, the product should be matched with that segment of the market where it is most likely to succeed. The product should be so positioned that it stands apart from competing brands. Positioning tells what the product stands for, what it is, and how the customers should evaluate it.

Positioning helps in differentiating the product from competitive offerings. Positioning is achieved by using marketing-mix variables, especially through design and communication efforts. Although differentiation through positioning is more visible in OTC products, it is equally useful with prescription drugs. With some products, positioning can be achieved on the basis of tangible differences (e.g., product features); with many others, intangibles are used to differentiate and position products.

The desired position for a product may be determined by use of the following procedure:

1. Analyze product attributes that are salient to consumers
2. Examine the distribution of these attributes among different market segments
3. Determine the optimal position for the product in regard to each attribute, taking into consideration the positions occupied by existing brands
4. Choose an overall position for the product (based on the overall match between product attributes and their distribution in the population and the positions of existing brands)

Approaches to a positioning strategy take many forms. Among these are

- attribute positioning,
- price/quality positioning,
- use/application positioning,
- user positioning,
- product class positioning, and
- competition positioning.

PRODUCT REPOSITIONING STRATEGY

Often a product may require repositioning. This can happen if

1. a competitive entry has been positioned next to the brand with an adverse effect on its share of the market,
2. preferences have undergone a change,
3. new preference clusters have been discovered with promising opportunities, or
4. a mistake has been made in the original positioning.

Costs and risks of repositioning are high. The technique of perceptual mapping is one that may be gainfully used to reduce substantially those risks. Perceptual mapping helps in examining the position of a product relative to competing products. It helps in

- understanding how competing products or services are perceived by various groups in terms of strengths and weaknesses;
- understanding the similarities and dissimilarities between competing products and services;
- repositioning a current product in the perceptual space of decision-maker segments;
- positioning a new product or service in an established marketplace; and
- tracking the progress of a promotional or marketing campaign on the perceptions of target segments.

PRODUCT ELIMINATION STRATEGY

Marketers have believed for a long time that sick products should be eliminated. It is only in recent years that this belief has become a matter of strategy. It is believed that a business unit's various products represent a portfolio and that each of these products has a unique role to play in making the portfolio viable. If a product's role diminishes or if it does not fit into the portfolio, it ceases to be important.

When a product reaches the stage at which continued support can no longer be justified because its performance falls short of expectations, it is desirable to pull the product out of the market. Poor performance may be characterized by any of the following:

1. Low profitability
2. Stagnant or declining sales volume or market share that would be too costly to build up
3. Risk of technological obsolescence
4. Entry into a mature or declining phase of the product life cycle
5. Poor fit with the business unit's strengths or declared mission

Products that are not able to limp along must be eliminated. They are a drain on a business unit's financial and managerial resources, which can be used more profitably elsewhere. Three alternatives in the product elimination strategy are harvesting, line simplification, and total-line divestment.

Harvesting

Harvesting refers to getting the most from the product while it lasts. It may be considered as controlled divestment, whereby the business unit seeks to get the most cash flow it can from the business. Usually, harvesting strategy is applied to a product or business whose sales volume and market share are slowly declining. An effort is made to cut the costs associated with such a business to help improve the cash flow. Alternatively, prices are increased without a simultaneous increase in costs. Harvesting leads to a slow decline in sales. When the business ceases to provide positive cash flow, it is divested.

Ideally, harvesting strategy should be pursued when the following conditions are present:

1. The product is in a stable or declining market.
2. The product has a small market share and building it up would be too costly, or it has a respectable market share that is becoming increasingly costly to defend or maintain.
3. The product is not producing especially good profits or may even be producing losses.
4. Sales would not decline too rapidly as a result of reduced investment.
5. The company has better uses for the freed-up resources.
6. The product is not a major component of the company's business portfolio.
7. The product does not contribute other desired features, such as sales stability or prestige, to the business portfolio.

Line Simplification

Line simplification strategy refers to a situation in which a product line is trimmed to a manageable size by pruning the number and variety of products or services being offered. This is a defensive strategy, which is adopted to keep the falling line stable. It is hoped that the simplification effort will help to restore the health of the line. This strategy becomes especially relevant during times of rising costs and resource shortages.

The implementation of line simplification strategy can lead to a variety of benefits: potential cost savings from longer production runs; reduced inventories; and a more forceful concentration of marketing, R&D, and other efforts behind a shorter list of products.

Despite the obvious merits, simplification efforts may sometimes be sabotaged. Those who have been closely involved with a product may sincerely feel either that the line as it is will revive when appropriate changes are made in the marketing mix or that the sales and profits will rebound once temporary conditions in the marketplace turn around.

Divestment

Divestment is a situation of reverse acquisition. It may also be a dimension of market strategy. But to the extent that the decision is approached from the product's perspective (i.e., to get rid of the product that is not doing well even in a growing market), it is an aspect of product strategy. Traditionally, companies resisted divestment for the following reasons, which are principally economic or psychological in nature:

1. Divestment means negative growth in sales and assets, which runs counter to the business ethic of expansion.
2. It suggests defeat.
3. It requires changes in personnel, which can be painful and which can result in perceived or real changes in status or have an adverse effect on the entire organization.
4. The candidate for divestment may be carrying overhead, buying from other business units of the company, or contributing earnings.

With the advent of strategic planning, divestment became an accepted option for seeking faster growth. More and more companies are now willing to sell a business if the company will be better off strategically. These companies feel that divestment should not be regarded solely as a means of ridding the company of an unprofitable division or plan; rather, some persuasive reasons support the divestment of even a profitable and growing business.

Divestment of businesses that no longer fit the corporate strategic plan can occur for a number of reasons. For example:

- A strategic connection no longer exists between the base business and the part to be divested.

"Merck said sales growth for the year (1998) was affected by the formation of the Merial joint venture and the divestiture of the crop protection business in the third quarter of 1997."[2]

- The business experiences a permanent downturn, resulting in excess capacity for which no profitable alternative use can be identified.

"In the United States, sales [for 3M]—adjusting for the third-quarter, 1997 divestiture of the company's outdoor advertising business—rose about 2 percent. This followed a 12 percent volume gain in the first quarter last year."[3]

- Inadequate capital may be available to support the natural growth and development of the business.

"Monsanto Co. (U.S.) will spin off Sept. 1 (1997), its chemicals business into an independent entity. Monsanto will retain its life sciences business but form a new company called Solutia, Inc. to take over the chemicals division. Solutia's stock shares will be listed on the New York Stock Exchange."[4]

- It may be dictated in the estate planning of the owner that a business is not to remain in the family.

"In the first quarter of 1997, global Life Sciences leader Novartis achieved sales of 8.2 billion Swiss francs. The increase, 8 percent in local currencies, represents a 22 percent growth in Swiss francs owing to the strong positive currency effect. Growth was particularly strong in Pharmaceuticals, thanks to a good start in the key U.S. market. . . . The divestiture of non-core businesses was completed with the successful spin-off of Ciba Specialty Chemicals."[5]

- Selling a part of the business may release assets for use in other parts of the business where opportunities are growing.

"In the pharmaceutical segment, first quarter (1997) worldwide sales increased 4 percent to $686 million. At constant foreign exchange rates and after adjusting for the sale of the company's Warner Chilcott generic drug business, sales increased 10 percent. In the U.S., segment sales, as reported, rose 13 percent to $367 million. Excluding the impact of the Warner Chilcott divestiture, U.S. segment sales advanced 19 percent."[6]

- Divestment can improve the return on investment and growth rate both by ridding the company of units that are growing more slowly than the basic business and by providing cash for investment in faster-growing, higher-return operations.

"The divestiture of Eli Lilly's medical devices and diagnostics subsidiaries added $910M to its net earnings; discounting this, the figure was 5 percent up on last year."[7]

DIVERSIFICATION STRATEGY

Diversification refers to seeking unfamiliar products or markets, or both, in pursuing growth. Every company is best at certain products; diversification requires substantially different knowledge, thinking, skills, and processes. Thus, diversification is at best a risky strategy, and a company should choose this path only when current product or market orientation does not seem to provide better opportunities for growth.

The term "diversification" must be distinguished from integration and merger. Integration refers to accumulation of additional business in a field through participation in more of the stages between raw materials and ultimate market, or through more intensive coverage of a single stage. Merger implies a combination of corporate entities, which may or may not result in integration. Diversification is a strategic alternative that implies deriving revenues and profits from different products and markets.

Diversification strategies might include internal development of new products or markets (including development of international markets for current products); acquisition of an appropriate firm or firms; a joint venture with a complementary organization; licensing of new product technologies; and importing or distributing a line of products manufactured by another company. The final choice of an entry strategy in most cases involves a combination of the aforementioned alternatives. This combination is determined on the basis of available opportunities and consistency with the company's objectives and available resources.

There are various modes of diversification. We examine concentric diversification and use it as an admittedly imperfect lead to discussion of switching products from prescription to nonprescription status.

Concentric diversification bears a close synergistic relationship to either the company's marketing or its technology. Thus, new products that are introduced share a common thread with the firm's existing products either through marketing or production. Usually, the new products are directed to a new group of customers.

Although a diversification move per se is risky, concentric diversification does not lead a company into an entirely new world, since in one of the two major fields (technology or marketing), the company will operate in familiar territory. When a firm enters the OTC market for the first time, the technology should be familiar if the consumer marketing strategies are not.

Figure 4.1 shows, in very general steps, the development of a marketing plan for the launch of a new OTC product.

It is beyond the scope of this book to discuss in detail the marketing of OTC drugs. Because of the *continuing* interest in the switch of substantial numbers of drugs from prescription to nonprescription status, that phenomenon will be addressed briefly, from the company strategy perspective.*

On the prescription side, the feelings are liable to be primarily negative. That division loses a product and it risks the alienation of physicians who are thought likely to resent the reclassification of former prescription drugs to wider availability.

A potential positive aspect on the prescription side of the pharmaceutical house is that a long-standing successful prescription item can be gracefully pushed aside to make way for a product of new research developed in the laboratories. If it were not for the availability of the OTC outlet, the product manager for the previous prescription (Rx) item or the marketing director might oppose the introduction of a new drug thought likely to cannibalize a successful old one.

On the OTC side, the situation will be reversed, with more pluses than minuses. The marketing department on the OTC side will welcome the possibility of building a product with brand-name loyalty, recognition, and longevity. The patent runs out on new drugs after a finite period of time, but successful brand names can go on forever, frequently with a new formula. Coca-Cola is an example of this, but other well-known brand-name OTC drugs have long outlived a variety of prescription items that have come and gone during their stay on the market.

Also, the move toward OTC means a considerably wider market for the drug than did the prescription limitation. In 1983, Micatin was available only by prescription. In that year, combined hospital and drugstore sales were $1.25 million. In 1984, Micatin was available for the first time as an OTC agent and sales increased 172 percent to $3.4 million. During that same time, sales of the comparable Lotrimin and Mycelex were still prescription only and remained flat. That Johnson & Johnson had econazole for a backup drug as a prescription-only antifungal while Schering-Plough and Miles had nothing with which to replace clotrimazole may have been at least partly responsible for the difference in these two decisions. In an analogous manner, Actifed, introduced by Burroughs Wellcome, was one of the most successful OTC switches in the early 1980s. By the third year after the conversion, sales had increased fivefold ($62.5 million compared to $11.4 million).[8,9]

---

*This section draws heavily from the work of Dr. William Rosenberg.

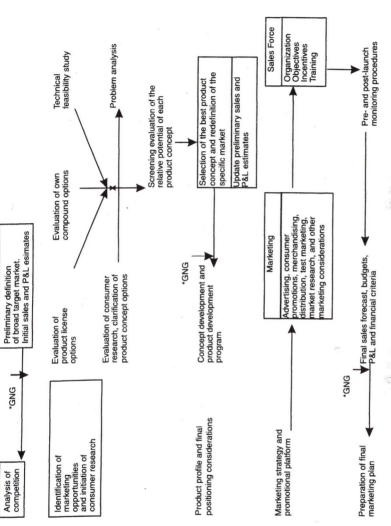

FIGURE 4.1. Development of OTC Marketing Plan (*Source*: Promotional brochure, IMS America, System. GNG = go/no-go decision; P&L = profit and loss.)

127

There is not universal acceptance of former Rx drugs on the OTC side of a pharmaceutical company, either. The change in type of agent means a considerably different way of doing business for many of the participants there. For instance, the research laboratories on the OTC side are frequently composed primarily of formulators and not pharmacologists. They may feel uneasy with the new agents with which they have to deal.

Likewise, the consumer research and marketing forces will find that new agents present both opportunities and challenges. The remarkable success of Actifed illustrates that a significant number of informed consumers are able and willing to purchase a new group of agents that they recognize as different and possibly more effective than those which have had the major push of prior OTC promotion. The same can be said for the initial success of ibuprofen in an intensely competitive analgesic market.

The result of all of this may well mean the emergence of new factors as important in the strategy of marketing OTC drugs. For one thing, it seems that companies which were formerly not considered important factors in the OTC market now are.

Upjohn is a company, for example, with good name recognition among an educated consumer class. They have the added benefit of prior use of the name Motrin in years of televison commercials. Thus, the shift of Motrin, finally, to OTC was a natural phenomenon.

The question of provider recognition is an important one. The nature of the OTC drug market is such that frequently the consumer is surprised to find out that a number of favorite items all come from the same company. He or she frequently does not associate an entire stable of home health remedies as coming from, for example, American Home Products or SmithKline Beecham. The nature of those corporations is such that many of them have acquired their lines through purchase of formerly independent single-product companies. It is not surprising that the name of the product is pushed ahead of the name of the provider.

It may well be, however, that some company will find an advantage in promoting its own corporate identity or perhaps an identifiable kind of brand name that could carry over from one product to another. For instance, a consumer who recognized some brand of nutritional supplement, laxative, analgesic, product for dry skin, or the like might well look with favor on a recognizable sister product for one of the other indications.

That sort of advertising was common in the days before prescription and OTC were so sharply separated in 1938 by the Food, Drug, and Cosmetic Act. For example, the Squibb ads in the 1930s *Saturday Evening Post* tried to convince consumers who were going out to purchase aspirin, mineral oil, boric acid, or whatever else was the OTC agent of the time that they could buy with confidence if it bore the familiar three Squibb columns. It might well be that the time is ready for a return to that type of image. (The red "Lilly" would once have been an ideal candidate for such a campaign.)

A further prospect for the future is the possibility of the innovative coordination of advertising of prescription and related nonprescription drugs. Thus, if related items differ in strength or form or even indication, it may be perhaps possible to pick up some positive associations at the prescription side of the consumers' experience with the expectation that this would carry over further to the OTC side.

Switching prescription drugs to OTC status has evolved since the early 1980s to a point at which the process itself has become increasingly difficult.[10] During this time frame, the trade association dealing with nonprescription drugs has undergone transformation as well, from the Proprietary Association in the late 1980s, to the Non-Prescription Drug Manufacturing Association, to the present-day Consumers Healthcare Products Association.

In 1987, H. I. Silverman delivered a speech to the Proprietary Association in which he forecast a number of developments at the prescription-OTC interface. The following provides a summary of how his predictions have become fact:

1. *Switch continues:* From 1984 to 1999—one switch per year increased to six or seven from 1995 through 1997;[11] no new molecules switched in 1998.[12]
2. *Line extension work:* New products are introduced—Imodium AD (1988) and Imodium Advanced (1997); Rogaine (1996) and Rogaine Extra Strength (1997); Advil (1984) and Children's Advil (1996); Nicorette (1996) and NicoDerm CQ (1998).[13]
3. *Development of certain exceptional ethical OTCs (nonlegend, but promoted to the consumer):* Many current OTCs had ethical OTC histories, e.g., Tagamet, Zantac, and Rogaine.[14]
4. *New delivery systems:* Edible whips, patches, once-a-week controlled release medications, pumps—all have offered exceptional scope in designing OTC products.
5. *New packaging:* Such packages include compliance aids, easy-open tops, and unit-dose packs.
6. *New dosage concepts and combination products:* These should appear and result in market expansion, e.g., Imodium Advanced in 1997 (combination of loperamide and simethicone).
7. *Diagnostics:* This is already a factor in home testing, as demonstrated by a number of pregnancy, glucose monitoring, drug screening, and ovulation detectors.[15]

IBUPROFEN—FROM DRUG TO DRUG PRODUCTS: A CASE

Ibuprofen is, in many ways, the most interesting drug in the modern history of pharmaceutical marketing.* The process by which this new chemical entity became an entire family of drug products offers a smorgasbord of issues: licensing, patent fights, Rx to OTC switch, pricing, promotion, and positioning.

Only brief consideration can be given here to ibuprofen. It is loosely based on Porter's five-factor model as described in Chapter 2 (see Figure 4.2).

Prescription Ibuprofen

The FDA approved ibuprofen to be marketed by its originator, Boots, as a prescription drug (see Figure 4.3). Because Boots lacked the marketing experience in the U.S. market, it sold Upjohn nonexclusive marketing rights to manufacture and sell ibuprofen in 1974. Marketing the drug as Motrin, Upjohn built it into the fifth-largest-selling prescription drug in the United States. In 1985, sales of the nonsteroidal anti-inflammatory agent Motrin were strong from 1984; it contributed to the firm's 7.6 percent sales gain during the second quarter to $543.3 million. In 1986, the sales of Motrin continued to be strong.

In 1981, Boots, which had established a U.S. presence by the acquisition of Rucker Pharmaceuticals in Shreveport, launched its own version of ibuprofen under the brand name Rufen. Competition was keen between Upjohn's Motrin and Boots's Rufen. Both of the companies tried to grasp a bigger market share for their single product, which was the 400 mg tablets. Boots challenged the leader Upjohn by offering buyers a similar product but at a lower price. In its advertisement, Boots focused on the price differential between the two drugs. Rufen, in 1983, achieved sales of $35 million. They also startled the industry by offering consumer rebates.

On the other hand, Motrin was backed and supported by Upjohn and became well-known in the U.S. analgesic market. In its first year of introduction, Motrin was heavily advertised in the medical journals. Motrin targeted the analgesic market, where the competition was very tough among available brands. Upjohn followed two consecutive marketing strategies. The first was the segmentation of the analgesic market to focus on osteoarthritis and rheumatoid arthritis patients (which was the first indication for which they had approval). The second marketing strategy was to differentiate the drug by showing different and better characteristics of the drug than

---

*This case was originally published in an earlier text by Mickey C. Smith, *Pharmaceutical Marketing: Strategy and Cases* (Binghamton, NY: The Haworth Press, 1991), pp. 314-325.

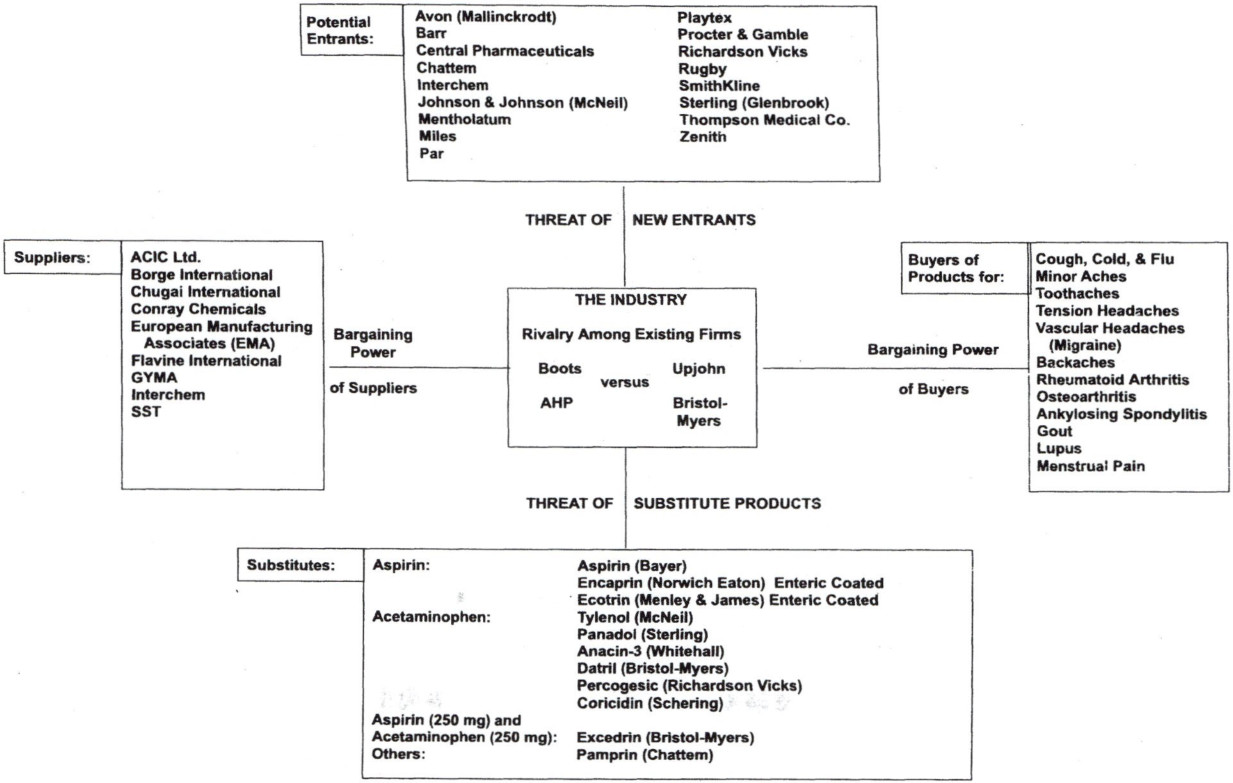

Suppliers: ACIC Ltd.
Borge International
Chugai International
Conray Chemicals
European Manufacturing
Associates (EMA)
Flavine International
GYMA
Interchem
SST

Potential Entrants:
Avon (Mallinckrodt)
Barr
Central Pharmaceuticals
Chattem
Interchem
Johnson & Johnson (McNeil)
Mentholatum
Par
Playtex
Procter & Gamble
Richardson Vicks
Rugby
SmithKline
Sterling (Glenbrook)
Thompson Medical Co.
Zenith

Buyers of Products for:
Cough, Cold, & Flu
Minor Aches
Toothaches
Tension Headaches
Vascular Headaches
(Migraine)
Backaches
Rheumatoid Arthritis
Osteoarthritis
Ankylosing Spondylitis
Gout
Lupus
Menstrual Pain

THREAT OF NEW ENTRANTS

THE INDUSTRY

Rivalry Among Existing Firms

Boots   versus   Upjohn

AHP   Bristol-Myers

Bargaining Power of Suppliers

Bargaining Power of Buyers

THREAT OF SUBSTITUTE PRODUCTS

Substitutes:

Aspirin: Aspirin (Bayer)
Encaprin (Norwich Eaton) Enteric Coated
Ecotrin (Menley & James) Enteric Coated

Acetaminophen: Tylenol (McNeil)
Panadol (Sterling)
Anacin-3 (Whitehall)
Datril (Bristol-Myers)
Percogesic (Richardson Vicks)
Coricidin (Schering)

Aspirin (250 mg) and Acetaminophen (250 mg): Excedrin (Bristol-Myers)
Others: Pamprin (Chattem)

FIGURE 4.2. Selected Components of the Ibuprofen Environment

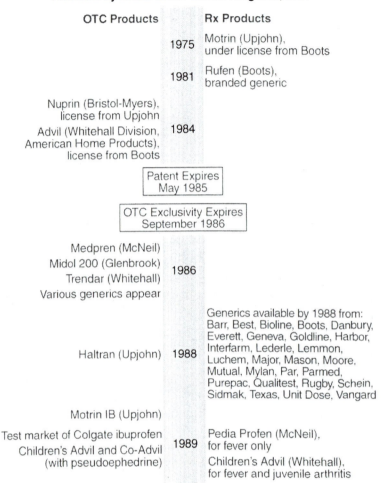

FIGURE 4.3. Ibuprofen from Drug to Drug Products

possessed by other drugs available in the analgesic market. The differentiation techniques were shown in 1974 ads as follows:

- Motrin is chemically unique—unrelated to indomethacin, phenylbutazone, corticosteroids, or salicylate.

- Motrin has better gastrointestinal tolerance than aspirin.
- Motrin is suitable for long-term management.

In 1980, and six years after the introduction of Motrin, Upjohn announced tests proving the effectiveness of the drug in analgesia: "Motrin now proved an effective analgesic for mild to moderate pain." Moreover, Upjohn was providing new features to add to Motrin, thus using new characteristics as a competitive tool for differentiating Motrin from competitors' drugs: "Motrin is not a narcotic, not addictive, and not habit forming."

In 1983, Boots again emphasized in its ads the substantial savings of Rufen over the price of Motrin. For the first time, in TV ads, Boots claimed that Motrin and Rufen were interchangeable and had the same uses, side effects, and contraindications, but the important difference is that Boots's brand of ibuprofen can cost considerably less.

Upjohn provided new services to consumers. They made a brochure available to physicians for distribution to their patients, which was intended to reinforce information presented by the patients' physicians, enhance patient-physician communication, and improve compliance by clarifying medication instructions.

Subsequently, Upjohn introduced 300 mg and 600 mg tablets. On the other hand, Boots, with Rufen 400 mg, extended its line to only 600 mg. However, both companies were considering the extension of ibuprofen to include the 200 mg category and to be targeted to the OTC analgesic market as a pain reliever. Both were also well aware of looming competition once patent protection was lost.

Going OTC

Both Upjohn and Boots decided to enter the OTC market with a partner experienced in selling to consumers. Upjohn chose Bristol-Myers and Boots picked American Home Products (AHP), Whitehall Division. The strategic maneuvers that followed continue today. Only a few can be mentioned.

Both Upjohn and Whitehall presented safety and efficacy data from clinical studies before an August 1983 meeting of the FDA's Arthritis Advisory Committee. The Whitehall NDA reportedly included worldwide data from three clinical studies of the efficacy and safety of the 200 mg dosage form. However, Upjohn produced its own U.S. data for approval and formally objected to Boots's application on the basis that a full NDA was required and, as such, Boots would have to cross-reference confidential data that Upjohn was unwilling to provide. In the meantime, while Upjohn and Whitehall were trying to get an FDA approval to market OTC ibuprofen, several companies tried to break the barriers around the patent holder, Boots, and its licensees, Upjohn and Whitehall. Those companies felt the pressure of introducing OTC ibuprofen into the analgesic market and saw the opportunity to improve their position. Chattem and McNeil were the major potential entrant companies, among others, trying to break the ibuprofen patent.

Chattem sought to head off FDA approval of a recommendation by its Arthritis Advisory Committee to permit the OTC marketing of the Rx analgesic ibuprofen by Upjohn and AHP. The grounds of Chattem's argument were that the pharmaceutical industry is a concentrated one, with relatively few companies possessing enormous economic leverage. In addition, only the largest and most heavily resourced companies were able to maintain NDAs as a routine course of business. Thus, whenever the FDA restricts the introduction of new OTC products to the best financial companies in the industry, inevitably further concentration and monopoly would occur.

Thus, Chattem, a small company engaged in the marketing of OTC drugs in the analgesic market, would be irreparably harmed by the creation of a monopoly in the use of a new OTC analgesic. This injury would occur both because of the direct competition with Chattem's current products, such as Pamprin, and because Chattem would be hindered from marketing a competitive ibuprofen product by the NDA system.

Instead of the NDA system, Chattem urged that the FDA include ibuprofen in its OTC monograph for analgesic drugs. This would mean a determination that the drug is "generally recognized as safe and effective," as it has been marketed to a material extent and time, for the same conditions of general analgesic and menstrual pain and would open up the OTC marketing of ibuprofen to any manufacturer meeting monograph standards.

Moreover, Chattem pointed out that if Upjohn and AHP obtained FDA approval, they would have a great advantage over later competitors, particularly where they have enjoyed a monopoly and have the financial strength to exploit that monopoly. Under these circumstances, Chattem and other small companies would never be able to compete effectively with the large, early marketers of ibuprofen.

Upjohn contended that the apparent but unstated motive for Chattem's petition was to protect its Pamprin menstrual drug product from competition in the OTC marketplace because ibuprofen was being touted as especially effective for menstrual pain. In addition, Upjohn stated that even if ibuprofen were generally recognized as safe and effective for OTC use, it has not been used for a material time under the proposed conditions of use, and a careful evaluation of the published studies would reveal the absence of critical data on the effectiveness of the 200 mg dose, which provides evidence that ibuprofen is a new drug.

AHP contended that "the true purpose of Chattem's request is simply to prevent AHP and Upjohn from marketing [OTC ibuprofen] before the patent expires."

McNeil sought to limit ibuprofen's impact on the OTC analgesic market by saddling the 200 mg dosage with the Rx label warnings. In a petition submitted to the FDA in March 1984, McNeil asked for a series of restrictions, including a contraindication for the OTC product in persons allergic to aspirin. McNeil noted that many patients with known hypersensitivity to aspirin may well select ibuprofen as an alternative "nonaspirin" analgesic, which would create the potential for severe and even fatal reactions due to cross-reactivity of ibuprofen with aspirin.

Neither of these efforts was successful.

On May 18, 1984, the FDA approved OTC 200 mg ibuprofen to be marketed by Bristol-Myers and Whitehall under the brand names Nuprin and Advil, respectively. One of the most important aspects of the original ibuprofen switch was that the patent was to have run out on May 28, 1985, thereby opening up the marketplace for a host of other products. However, under the Drug Price Competition and Patent Term Restoration Act of 1984, exclusivity was granted for an extended period on the OTC version.

Advil and Nuprin were promoted as general pain relievers for headaches, dental pain, muscular aches and pains, reduction of fever, and dysmenorrhea. However, neither drug was labeled for arthritis, as Motrin and Rufen were. Such indications would place Upjohn and Whitehall head-to-head against competitive products or substitutes from aspirin and acetaminophen manufacturers.

Aspirin products were still the cheapest of the over-the-counter painkillers, with generic or house-brand aspirin cheaper than brand names. Thirty Bayer could cost $1.25; 100 Bayer, $1.99; and 100 of a generic brand, $.79. Acetaminophen products were about twice the price of aspirin, with fifty Tylenol costing about $3.99 or sixty Datril, $2.79, but 100 generic, $1.99. As the newest product, ibuprofen was the most expensive. Fifty tablets of Advil were about $4.19 and fifty Nuprin, $3.79.

AHP and Bristol-Myers were blitzing consumers with coupons and spending at least $35 million each on introductory advertising that made essentially the same pitch—"Ibuprofen, once available only by prescription, can now be bought in nonprescription strength"—which might make some consumers think that ibuprofen is better for aches and pains than substitutes such as aspirin or Tylenol.

In response to the appearance of Advil and Nuprin, Johnson & Johnson (Tylenol) announced a program of heavy investment spending to increase Tylenol's massive $50 million advertising budget. Moreover, Johnson & Johnson planned to introduce its own ibuprofen—a one-a-day dose—after the patent expired.

By the end of 1986, Advil and Nuprin had combined for about 15 percent of the market, taking share this time primarily from aspirin. Aspirin had 40 percent of the analgesic market, and acetaminophen, 45 percent.

AHP beat Bristol-Myers to market in 1984 and spent more on advertising. In 1986, Advil outsold Nuprin by about three to one. In 1985, about $35 million in Advil advertising produced retail sales of more than $85 million; Bristol-Myers estimated $25 million brought sales of about only $35 million for Nuprin. Just two months before the patent expiration date of OTC ibuprofen on September 26, 1986, Upjohn decided to introduce its own brand of OTC ibuprofen under the brand name Haltran. Upjohn positioned Haltran in the menstrual pain market in which the company's supplemental approval was exclusively for the dysmenorrhea indication. Thus, Haltran had a two-month advantage over the next wave of OTC ibuprofen introductions.

Next, and upon the expiration of the exclusive marketing period of OTC ibuprofen, several drug companies were ready to jump on the bandwagon. They provided new substitutes and a major challenge to Advil and Nuprin. However, they avoided going head-to-head with them. Instead, they advertised their products as menstrual pain relievers, a $65 million market.

McNeil introduced Medipren; Par and Barr launched a generic ibuprofen; Chattem, Glenbrook Laboratories, Danbury, Chelsea, and many others joined the battle to have a slice of the menstrual pain market.

Whereas most of the later entrants positioned their OTC ibuprofen in the menstrual pain market, the initial OTC ibuprofen products were positioned as painkillers with a reference to menstrual pain. On the other hand, prescription ibuprofen drugs of 400 and 600 mg were positioned in the arthritis market. Thus, ibuprofen has been positioned throughout its life in different markets.

One consideration in the positioning strategies of OTC ibuprofen is whether consumers would perceive OTC ibuprofen as a new brand or a new product. One manufacturer attempted to position its OTC ibuprofen as a new product, as evidenced by its TV ad: "First there was aspirin, then there was Tylenol, and today there is ibuprofen." Another used the following:

> In the fifties menstrual pain meant Midol.
> In the seventies it also meant Pamprin.
> Now there's Trendar. Today's choice for menstrual pain.

Motrin and Rufen chose arthritis as their core segment and hoped to reap the fringe benefits from the menstrual pain and body aches and strains segments. Advil's and Nuprin's core positioning strategies were for headaches, fever, aches, and pains, while Haltran, Midol-200, and Trendar favored positions for relief of menstrual cramps. Medipren positioned itself as a better choice than aspirin for body aches and pains.

In the case of prescription ibuprofen, the introduction of Motrin offered many features not then available in the existing products and of importance to prospective users of the drug: effective for pain relief and inflammation, less irritating to the stomach, nonaddictive, nonsedating, had relatively few other side effects and drug interactions, and was safe. Many of these features were not currently being offered by such products as butazolidin, high-dose aspirin corticosteroids, narcotic and nonnarcotic analgesics, and acetaminophen. Thus, both Motrin and Rufen utilized these features in their positioning strategies.

The OTC market represented a somewhat different arena. The unfulfilled needs were for a safe product that is effective for pain relief and inflammation, nonirritating to the stomach, has few other side effects and drug interactions, and does not cause Reye's syndrome. Aspirin, acetaminophen, and ibuprofen are approximately equally effective (ibuprofen *may* be slightly more effective in headaches); ibuprofen is less irritating to the stomach than aspirin but more so than acetaminophen. Both aspirin and ibuprofen provide anti-inflammatory effects yet cause Reye's syndrome. Thus, the newly introduced ibuprofen did not really fulfill the unfulfilled needs.

In the introduction, obviously promotion was the core strategic effort for Advil and Nuprin. Both companies blitzed consumers with coupons and spent at least $35 million each on introductory advertising. Later, product was a strong supporting strategy for Advil, as the focus of a $100 million promotion was its distinctive-looking tablet. AHP believed that consumers identified Advil so closely with the terra-cotta coating that it was part of the brand image. This promotional advantage actually was serendipitous—the coating was developed to protect against adulteration! In January 1986, Advil became the second best-selling pain reliever in the United States and AHP changed their strategy mix to emphasize distribution efforts in concert with its promotional efforts. They were looking to give Advil a sales force. They hoped strategically to increase endorsements by the medical profession through extensive sampling and promotion.

Johnson & Johnson, makers of Medipren and Tylenol, began a heavy ad campaign for Medipren to convince Americans to give up what they were using and give Medipren a try. It was promoted for use against body aches and pains, lest it pull headache customers away from Tylenol. Promotional effort was and is essential—McNeil offered coupons to customers and spent $50 million on a TV ad campaign. McNeil also flooded physicians with free samples for their patients, a tactic used successfully when introducing Tylenol twenty-five years earlier.

The two original ibuprofen licensers introduced ibuprofen-based pain relievers for menstrual cramps—Trendar by AHP's Whitehall Division and Haltran by Upjohn. Previously the OTC ibuprofen had not been promoted heavily for menstrual pain, a major market for Extra Strength Tylenol.

Upjohn spent an estimated $25 million on a magazine and TV campaign for "the tough cramps women get" and attempted to establish Haltran as a new product (not a line extension) with its pitch "A new generation pain reliever for menstrual cramps." The promotional messages were concentrated in journals read predominantly by women and during periods of high television viewership by the female sector. Upjohn claimed that Nuprin and Haltran do not compete against each other since Haltran is a menstrual cramp reliever and Nuprin is a regular pain reliever.

AHP's Trendar was positioned as "Today's choice for menstrual pain"—again, an attempt to establish ibuprofen as a new product by making the other options obsolete (but not necessarily less effective). Sterling Drugs' Midol-200 hoped to leapfrog the other two by name recognition. The company's aspirin-based Midol had been a leader in the cramp relief market. Recognizing that the pain relief market was a fairly mature market, these companies hoped that segmentation for menstrual pain relief would be one way to compete with Advil and Nuprin.

Packaging for OTC products is another form of promotion and should consider consumer likes, dislikes, preferences, convenience of use, and the ability of the package to command attention, deliver a promotional message, convey the proper company image, and stimulate purchase.

Three OTC ibuprofen packages are notable. Haltran, the menstrual pain reliever, is packaged in "ladylike" soft pink with neon, high-tech, red and blue print. This package conveys to the purchaser that it is for females but is a new-generation menstrual pain reliever. Advil, packaged in a blue and yellow grid pattern, also portrays a high-tech, new-generation image. Medipren's package shows several images of bodies in different positions, which demonstrates its attempt for the package to deliver the promotional message that it is for body aches and pains and for those who do not have time for the pain: "Let's get moving with Medipren!"

Glitches in Switches

The Rx-to-OTC switch was not as smooth as hoped. For example, when Actifed and Robitussin went OTC, they maintained the same brand names utilized when available only from the pharmacist. The strategies for Advil and Nuprin unfolded under fundamentally different conditions. First, their dosage changed when moving from prescription to nonprescription status, and, second, their prices fluctuated throughout their first year on the market, possibly confusing customers. On introduction, heavy couponing made the effective price per tablet approximately equal to aspirin and acetaminophen. In 1985, Advil (fifty tablets) cost $3.99 while Nuprin (fifty tablets) cost $4.39. Anacin and Tylenol sold for $2.99 per fifty tablets. Even though the dosage was different, i.e., one tablet for ibuprofen versus two tablets for aspirin and acetaminophen, the two ibuprofen brands seemed more expensive to the unfamiliar customers.

Another problem emerged from the licensing agreements with Boots/AHP and Upjohn/Bristol-Myers (B-M). Neither AHP nor B-M could use the established names, Rufen and Motrin, since Boots and Upjohn were still marketing their products under those names to physicians. Moving from prescription to OTC status often has a "made to order" market strategy—marketers are often ensured success by stressing the "ethical" history of the product. This strategy was foiled in the initial introduction of OTC ibuprofen. Anxious to present the drug as a new entity rather than a line extension, the two marketers devised new brand names. Consumers, however, could not graft their awareness of the prescription pain reliever onto the OTC form.

In addition, because of the Upjohn suit filed against AHP for using the name Motrin and Motrin's orange color in its initial advertisements, positioning messages moved from one claim to another with a net result of consumer confusion.

As if the companies were not having enough trouble, there was resistance in the field. As the products were reaching the shelf, certain local pharmacy associations took great pains to point out the dangers of ibuprofen. This adverse publicity was not completely altruistic. Many pharmacists saw $250 million in prescriptions threatening to evaporate, and they were angry that the drug had moved from Rx to OTC without being classed as an ethical pharmaceutical for a few years. This situation represented a dilemma for the two companies in attempting to satisfy all of their corporate publics with a company strategy. As shown, conflict may arise between two or more of these publics—in this case, the consumers, stockholders, and the public unique to the pharmaceutical industry, the decision maker/influencer/pharmacist.

Notes on Upjohn's Strategic Decisions

OTC ibuprofen could and did affect Rx Motrin. Motrin sales dropped by 20 percent during the first year of marketing OTC ibuprofen products.

Also, the 5 percent Upjohn would earn from sales of Nuprin as agreed with Bristol-Myers would not bring Upjohn enough to make up for what was happening to Motrin, which accounted for 40 percent of Upjohn's profits in 1983. A price war with Rufen was squeezing those profits, and Upjohn's stock dropped from $61 a share in early July 1983 to $45 in August 1984.

Upjohn's own OTC venture with Haltran was unsuccessful (down to $2 million in 1988), and it was not until 1989 that the name Motrin appeared on OTC shelves (as Motrin IB). Ads appeared in July. Consumer promotions included TV and print ads, sampling, and coupons. Professional journal ads to physicians and pharmacists were also planned. The TV ad from Motrin IB played on the strength of prescription Motrin's brand-name recognition, which studies showed was well over 85 percent. The ad, which intoned the Motrin IB name four times, stated in part:

You are about to see the most important words on pain relief in 100 years: Motrin IB.. No prescription needed. Now the doctor-recommended pain reliever in Motrin is available in nonprescription strength. . . . It's going to be the new generation of pain relievers.

Would this work? Why had Upjohn waited so long?

Upjohn made a major push into the OTC ibuprofen market partly because Motrin's prescription sales were off sharply, while its non-prescription competitors were selling briskly. "We will take the mark Motrin over the counter ourselves because we think the market is receptive to further analgesics of this type," said Theodore Cooper, then Upjohn's chairman and chief executive officer.

Partly because of generic substitutes, Motrin's 1988 prescription sales were off by about 20 percent from 1987. Meanwhile, the best-selling non-prescription brands of ibuprofen, Advil and Nuprin, were growing at a faster rate than any other segment of the $2 billion OTC analgesic market. Advil, sold by AHP, was the more popular of the two, with about 13 percent of the market. Nuprin, sold by B-M under a licensing agreement with Upjohn, had a 4.5 percent market share. Another ibuprofen brand, Medipren, sold by Johnson & Johnson, was a distant third.

In an article in *Medical Advertising News* (August 15, 1989), marketing consultant Hemant Shah called Upjohn's licensing of Nuprin the "goof of the century." He blamed it on a lack of commitment to the OTC market.

Observers have said that 1984 would have been the perfect time for Upjohn to launch a nonprescription ibuprofen and to associate its name with Motrin. Instead, the company launched a nonprescription product, named it Nuprin, and licensed Bristol-Myers to market it. Upjohn marketers abandoned the nonprescription ibuprofen market, thinking that they did not have the know-how to sell to consumers.

Then Upjohn CEO Theodore Cooper would see things differently:

Motrin is a good example of how Upjohn plans to develop the "full potential" of its more mature products—yet it also typifies the sometimes difficult task of getting such improvements through the regulatory process. A slow-release form, Motrin SR, is now under development at Upjohn, but its NDA filing—despite "early advice" meetings with FDA—seems bogged down in unresolved issues of pharmacokinetics that Cooper says have left both FDA staff and the company in a state of confusion.

Usually not mentioned in those discussions is the 1988 approval of Upjohn's Ansaid (flurbiprofen), a nonsteroidal anti-inflammatory drug (NSAID) of the same chemical family as Motrin.

At the FDA, Ansaid had to compete for attention with many other NSAIDs waiting approval and had only a 1C priority rating. In Europe, however, it has already been on the market for years, with an "excellent record," said Cooper. Competing with older medications in the United States, he noted, is thus a marketing advantage rather than a problem.

Unlike Motrin, Cooper said, Ansaid will suffer no early competition from an OTC form of the product. Although Upjohn also licensed Ansaid (flurbiprofen) from Boots, the originator of ibuprofen, the current product is protected against any OTC licensing to another company.*

*The contributions of Mohammed Rawwas and Patti Peeples to the development of this material are gratefully acknowledged.

Chapter 5

Responsiveness of the Pharmaceutical Industry to Its External Environment

Greg Perkins

As elaborated upon in Chapter 2, of all the stimuli to which the pharmaceutical industry is exposed in its external environment, the FDA is the most critical in determining its long-term profitability. Consequently, companies constantly reevaluate those processes which interface with the FDA and adapt whatever strategies necessary to sustain their return on investment.

In this regard, the pharmaceutical industry is no different from any other business sector. However, due to the importance and visibility of ethical drugs (a primary mainstay) within the public domain, discussion on how well they are doing frequently revolves around debates on pricing. These often assume the guise of pressure to curl or control prices, such as during the early months of the Clinton administration in 1993. More recently there has been a resurgence of such sentiments,[1,2] which appear to have bipartisan support.

Proposals to reduce the cost of pharmaceuticals have stimulated considerable debate about not only the real cost of drugs to the consumer but also the contribution that the pharmaceutical industry makes to society at large. Regarding the former, Figure 5.1 contains data compiled by PhRMA to illustrate that pharmaceuticals are a small part of daily expenditures.[3] Clearly, the amount spent for drugs is less for all items listed, with the exception of tobacco (this includes alcohol). When compared to those items which can be considered essential (i.e., food and housing services), spending for prescription drugs is less than 10 percent of either. Distracters, on the other hand, point to the fact that drug expenditures are now the fastest growing of health care costs, increasing at the rate of about 15 percent per year. [4-6]

Data intended to show the value of the U.S. pharmaceutical industry are captured in Figures 5.2 and 5.3. Both purportedly focus on innovation by demonstrating that the United States is the direct beneficiary of the revenues generated by the sale of drug products. Figure 5.2 displays the percentage of new drugs marketed in the United States as a function of time.[7] From a value

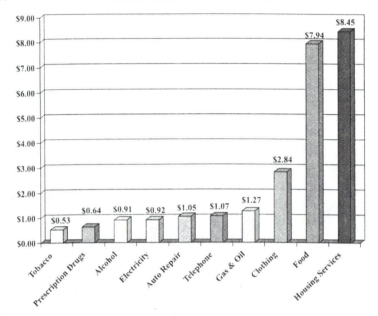

FIGURE 5.1. Consumption Expenditures Per Day, Per Capita

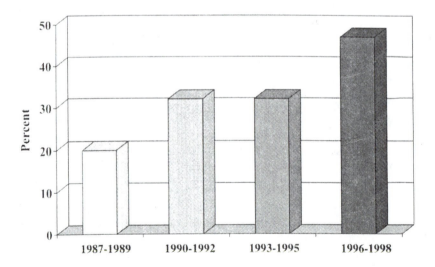

FIGURE 5.2. Percentage of New Drugs Marketed in the United States As a Function of Time

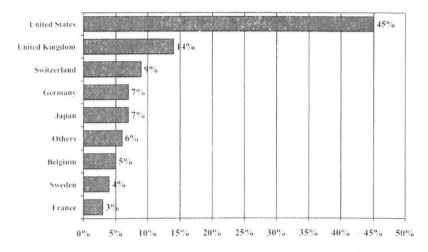

FIGURE 5.3. Development of 152 Global Drugs by Country of Origin, 1975-1994 (*Source:* Adapted from Paul E. Barratt, *20 Years of Pharmaceutical Research Results Throughout the World* [Rhone-Poulonc Rover Foundation, 1996].)

of approximately 20 percent in the first interval noted (1987-1989), the percentage stabilized at around 30 percent for 1990-1992 and 1993-1995, and rose to 50 percent in 1996-1998. This represents more than a doubling in the time frames shown.

Figure 5.3 is a chart showing the percentage of global drugs launched in individual countries.[8] Global drugs are defined as those being launched in the United States, Japan, France, Germany, United Kingdom, Switzerland, and Italy. It is apparent that the United States far exceeds any of the other countries with respect to the percentage of global drugs launched within the confines of its borders. In fact, the percentage is more than triple that of the United Kingdom, which falls into second place (45 percent versus 14 percent). Values for the remaining individual countries range from 3 percent for France to 9 percent for Switzerland. "Others" comprise 6 percent.

The pharmaceutical industry in the United States, indisputably, has played a key role in introducing new drugs into the marketplace. In so doing, the sector has been highly profitable, routinely outpacing many others.[9] Despite this record, however, most drugs developed do not produce revenues that match or exceed average R&D costs.[10] This is illustrated in Figure 5.4, where 1980-1984 pharmaceuticals are lumped in groups of ten and plotted against the after-tax present value (ATPV) in millions of 1990 dollars. The profitability of drugs is benchmarked against drug development costs in after-tax 1990 dollars.

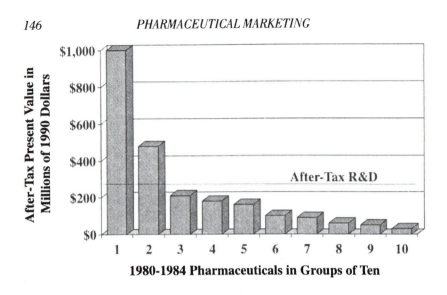

FIGURE 5.4. Profitability of 1980-1984 Pharmaceuticals Relative to After-Tax R&D Costs

Out of the groupings of ten, only three possess ATPVs that exceed the after-tax R&D costs. Of that number, one is approximately fivefold the threshold figure of slightly more than $200 million. The remaining two are roughly two and a half and one times the after-tax R&D costs. The balance, or vast majority, of the groupings (seven, representing seventy drugs) fail to regroup the expenditures necessary to bring the drugs to the marketplace. The shape of their regression from the threshold line appears to be geometric, as opposed to linear.[11]

FDA oversight extends through the life cycle of a new chemical entity, i.e., pre- and postmarketing. A. T. Kearney[12] developed a paradigm that graphically illustrates "drug life cycle cash flows" as a function of time and core capabilities. Cash flows are either negative or positive, depending upon whether revenues are being generated by sales of the drug, after its approval by the FDA, and subsequent marketing.

Figure 5.5 is a schematic representation of the model as it relates to the three core capabilities most critical to effective interfacing with the FDA. Operational excellence and organizational effectiveness, two additional core capabilities, are considered to be tangential to the current discussion and have been omitted accordingly. Obviously, cash flow is essentially negative until such time that approval is granted for marketing of the drug. Any improvement or enhancement resulting in a reduction of time to market would be beneficial, as would lessening the costs associated with individual

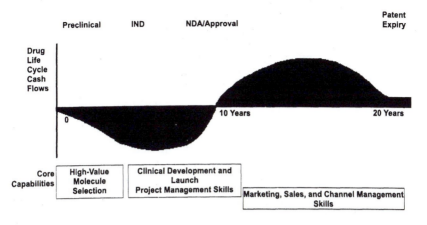

FIGURE 5.5. Cash Flows Across Core Capabilities

processes needed to reach that point. Conversely, cash flow after approval is positive, and hence it is advantageous to lengthen the time until patent expiry so that revenues can be increased over that time frame.[13]

High-value molecule selection is a critical element of drug discovery, given that the viability of a pharmaceutical company is often thought to be a direct reflection of its pipeline.[14] Aside from licensing drug candidates from the outside, the only means by which new chemical entities (NCEs) can enter the development stage is by screening a large number of potential candidates and choosing the most promising ones. Only 5 in 5,000 compounds screened in discovery/preclinical R&D and subsequent preclinical testing make it to human testing.

Clinical (or drug) development and launch project management skills are well-defined tasks associated with drug development that determine the approval cycle time. Any diminution of this interval would be highly advantageous from the standpoint of profitability. Although clinical development is a key player in this process, other functional areas, such as pharmaceutical development, preclinical R&D, and regulatory affairs, are critical as well.

Marketing, sales, and channel management skills represent a core capability that largely falls outside the realm of R&D. However, exceptions to this rule do exist, and these generally fall under the rubric of life cycle management. Extending the patent life by developing an alternate dosage form and extending exclusivity by acquiring additional clinical indications are illustrative of R&D involvement in this regard.

The manner in which the three core capabilities just described have been modified/enhanced by the pharmaceutical industry to better meet the needs and requirements of the FDA are described in the following pages. The chapter will conclude with a discussion of the fourth means by which the pharmaceutical industry has coped with its external environment, i.e., mergers.

HIGH-VALUE MOLECULE SELECTION

In order for Pharma and biotech companies to maintain double-digit growth rates through 2005, they need to multiply their productivity by a factor of five.[15] From a research perspective, the only means by which this can be accomplished is to maximize the number of viable NCEs selected in the discovery phase or before preclinical research begins. This entails being able to process an enormous amount of information in order to quickly eliminate irrelevant or inactive compounds.

Emphasis is placed on optimizing the number of potential NCEs in discovery, since this phase serves as the entry gate into the development process and has the fewest candidates that pass (1.25 to 2.5 percent). Also mentioned were the ability of combinational chemistry and throughput screening to provide such quantities, as well as genomics, which represents another potential source of therapeutics.

Figure 5.6 graphically illustrates the individual components of drug discovery. High throughput screening (HTS) entails testing massive numbers of compounds in simple binding assays. With the ability to use 1,536 well plates, companies are now able to run up to 100,000 screens a day, more

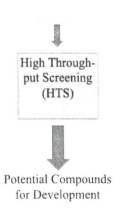

FIGURE 5.6. Interrelationship Between Individual Components of Drug Discovery

than a thousandfold increase in the past decade.[16] Potential NCEs are derived from two sources: combinational chemistry and genomics. The former provides the majority of candidates at present, and the latter is expected to play a dominant role as genomics and related fields are better delineated.

Combinational chemistry necessitates libraries that contain information on chemical compounds numbering from the hundreds of thousands to the millions.[17] Since sampling the entire range of chemical diversity has not proved appropriate for picking compounds with biological targets, compound data need to be integrated with information about such targets and their relevance to specific diseases. This has created more focused compound libraries and has been alluded to as the "Drug Discovery Factory,"[18] wherein the history and life cycle of each compound must be readily assessable and translated into leads as rapidly as possible. Lack of efficiency equates to immediate competitive disadvantage.[19]

Opposed to combinational chemistry, genomics is in its infancy as a source of major therapeutic breakthroughs. Notwithstanding such a qualification, however, the field possesses unfathomable potential, given that it will eventually lead to the delineation and understanding of disease processes. Figure 5.7 affords a representation of the pathway to marketable products, and the fledgling disciplines that need to provide vast amounts of information before genomics can be fully tapped.

The critical bottlenecks in translating genetic or genomic information into well-characterized therapeutic targets are twofold:[20] (1) understanding the underlying basis of disease pathways and (2) rapidly identifying the essential targets that are amenable to therapeutic intervention. At the beginning of the undertaking is the sequencing of the approximately 3 billion nucleotide base pairs comprising the human genome.[21] As of July 2000, such an undertaking was 97 to 99 percent. This has recently been completed.[22]

The first step in the understanding of disease pathways is genotyping, or the process of creating associations between single nucleotide polymorphs (SNPs) and disease.[23] On the estimated 30,000 human genes,[24] it is believed that there are approximately 300,000 such entities.[25] Either singly or, more likely, in combination, SNPs predispose a person to a given disease.[26] Establishing a linkage between SNPs and a disease response pattern enables progression to determination of a gene product variant.

Proteins are the end result of gene transcription and translation and, as a consequence, represent the gene product variant in question. It is estimated that more than 100,000 proteins are found in humans, only a fraction of which are expressed in any given cell type.[27] Proteomics seeks to provide functional information for all proteins and the manner by which this might be modified by the disease process. Suitable targets for intervention can then be identified, leading again to high throughput screening and eventual "winners" from the standpoint of drug candidates.

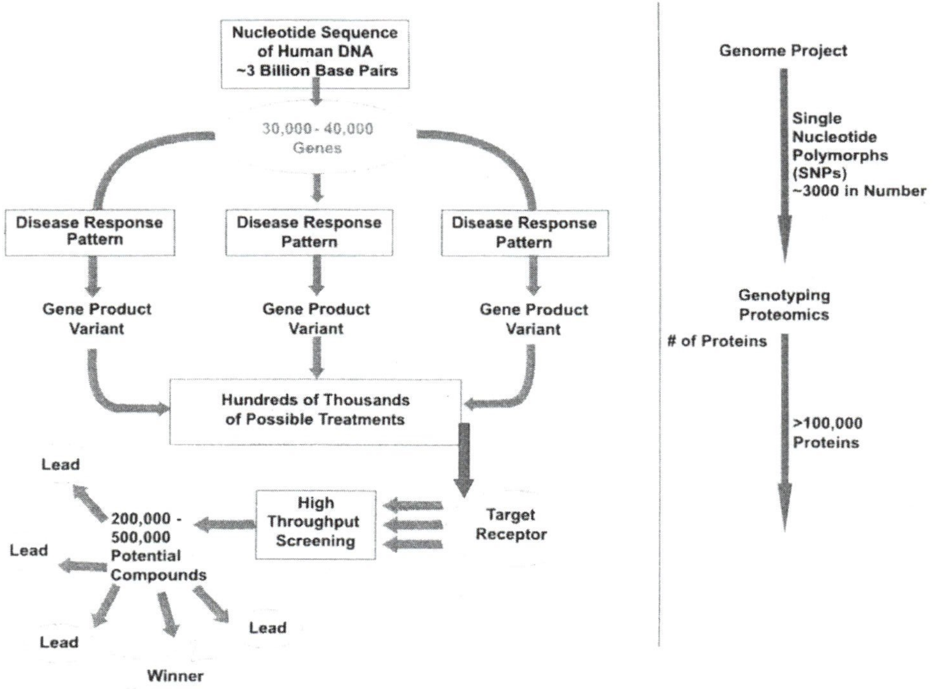

FIGURE 5.7. Genomic Pathway to a Marketable Product and Corresponding Disciplines (*Source:* Adapted and updated from Steve Gardner and Rich Hamer, "Informatics Magic—How to Turn Data into Knowledge," *Pharmaceutical Executive* 20(12): 64, 2000.)

CLINICAL (DRUG) DEVELOPMENT AND LAUNCH PROJECT MANAGEMENT SKILLS

For purposes of this section, drug development is defined as a set of inter-dependent tasks with the intended purpose of marketing a new chemical or biological entity (see Figure 5.8).[28] The specific tasks include preclinical testing, clinical phases I through III, registration (new drug application or product license), phase IV commitments particularly crucial for expedited drug development, and preapproval inspections.

Figure 5.9 depicts a model for the essential integrative/interactive components needed for successful accelerated drug development.[30] In this paradigm, regulatory affairs and project management are full partners in coordinating the drug development process.

The key element for execution of such a program is the avoidance or minimization of time gaps between sequential tasks that can be done.[28] This is best accomplished by pushing decision making down to the project team. Delay of product launch can result in enormous sums of lost revenues, as is illustrated in Figure 5.10.[31] For the average drug, the average lost prescription sales on a daily basis is $1.3 million. The corresponding figures for

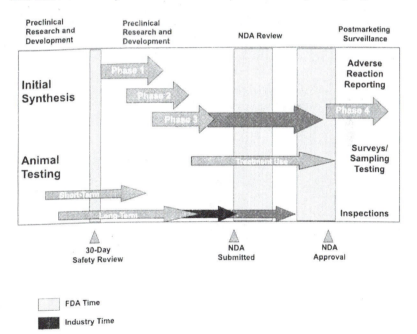

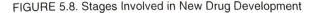

FIGURE 5.8. Stages Involved in New Drug Development

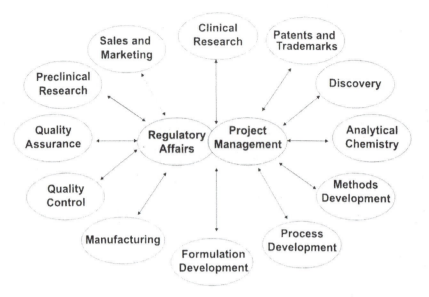

FIGURE 5.9. Schematic Representation of the Essential Integration/Interaction Components Needed for Successful Accelerated Drug Development

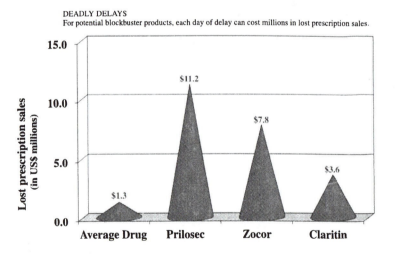

FIGURE 5.10. Lost Prescription Sales Incurred on a Daily Basis As a Result of Delay in Approval

blockbusters such as Prilosec, Zocor, and Claritin are $11.2 million, $7.8 million, and $3.6 million, respectively.

Certain companies have an inherent competitive advantage by being faster in development speed. For purposes of this discussion, development speed is defined as the time from IND filing to NDA submission. Five companies who excel in this regard are listed in Figure 5.11.[32] The industry-wide development time is 3.7 years. AstraZeneca is the industry leader, eclipsing the industry median by 2.0 years. Glaxo Wellcome is close behind with a speed advantage of 1.6 years. Merck, Pfizer, and Abbott comprise the balance and are 1.1 to 1.2 years faster than their competition.

Interestingly, the performances of the aforementioned five companies become even more striking when considering specific therapeutic areas (see Figure 5.12).[33] Viewed as a group, the five companies outperform the remainder of the industry by 8.3 and 8.4 years for the endocrine and anesthetic/analgesic areas, respectively. The central nervous system (CNS) area is 6.3 years better, followed by cardiovascular (5.7 years), antineoplastic (5.0 years), and finally anti-infective (2.5 years).

Although it is beyond the scope of the chapter to provide an exhaustive analysis of time savings measures adapted by all functions depicted in

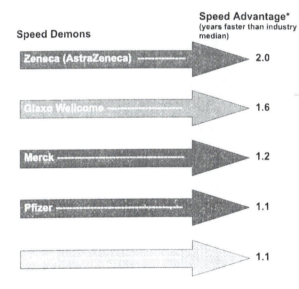

FIGURE 5.11. Top Five Companies in Terms of Development Speed (*Source:* CenterWatch Database of Approved NCEs 1981-1999, FDA. *Speed variability between company median development time and industry-wide development time.)

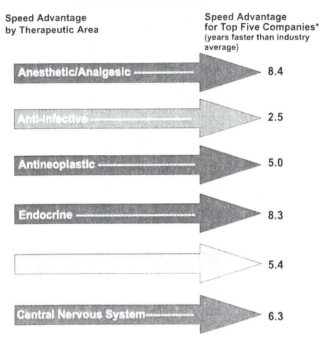

FIGURE 5.12. Performance of Top Five Companies (Figure 5.11) According to Therapeutic Area (*Source:* CenterWatch Database of Approved NCEs 1981-1999, FDA. *Speed variability between top five companies' average development time and industry-wide average development time.)

Figure 5.9, certain elements, such as the following, appear to be operative within the most successful companies:[34]

1. *Faster approval time after NDA submission:* median approval time for top-performing companies is 1.5 years compared to the industry average of 1.9 years.
2. *Global project planning:* development programs are integrated and harmonized from an international standpoint.
3. *Realistic protocols:* input is sought from physicians, consultants, and study staff before implementation.
4. *Active collaboration:* frequent feedback is solicited from regulatory agencies.
5. *Project and data management and communication technologies:* technology solutions are used to facilitate the development process.
6. *Project team cohesion:* project team enjoys a high degree of independence and empowerment.

Obviously, a theme pervasive throughout these entries is communication, whether it be with an outside entity, such as the FDA, or internal, among the various groups that need to interact to bring an NCE to the marketplace.

In addition to the previous list, the following are isolated examples of shortening development time by favorably impacting discrete tasks within the process.

Preclinical Screening

It has been estimated that approximately 40 percent of NCEs fail because of pharmacokinetic profiles, and 11 percent of failures are attributable to toxic effects in humans.[35] Another category lacking quantification, but representing the single most costly group from the standpoint of lost revenue and investment, includes NCEs possessing liver toxicity that fails to surface in human trials.[36] As a consequence, any preclinical tests that can be devised to detect such shortcomings early on are a definite advantage in the development scheme, as illustrated in Figure 5.13.[37]

Regarding pharmocokinetics, utilization of screens employing human cell lines and enzyme systems has resulted in enhanced predictability of successful candidates for development.[38-40] Process rate data generated in such screens are incorporated into suitable mathematical models. Another approach relies on bioinformatics or computer-based models. These rely on a multiplicity of parameters, including a compound's molecular weight, lipophilicity, number of hydrogen bond donors and acceptors, as well as properties that lead to toxicity or render a component inaccessible to cells. The latter characteristic is linked to high affinity to P-glycoprotein, a transmembrane transporter that pumps hydrophobic NCEs out of cells.[41]

Predicting liver toxicity that fails to surface in the NDA clinical program has proven to be somewhat more intractable. Even so, several areas hold the promise of a major breakthrough in the not so distant future. Liver cells are an intricate part of any approach, either as heterogeneous populations or homogeneous ones transfected with specific P450 enzymes.[42]

Clinical Trials

At the most basic level, any process that facilitates reduction in the amount of time needed to conduct individual clinical trials will shorten development of an NCE. One means by which this can be accomplished is by using an electronic-information-based system (see Figure 5.14).[43] Lag time between the generation of data at the site and their availability electronically is minimal. This is in sharp contrast to paper case report forms, which by their very nature accumulate gradually and necessitate laborious quality assurance prior to locking of a database. An example of such an approach was recently cited in the literature.[44] A company specializing in developing

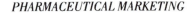

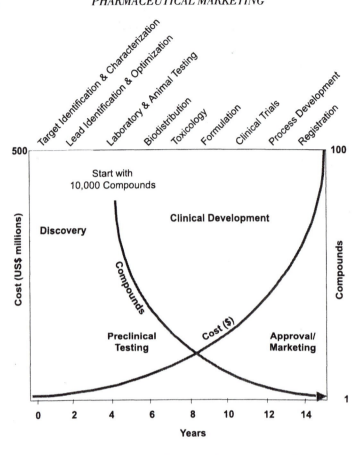

FIGURE 5.13. Relationship Between Cost and NCE Pool Size

electronic tools for clinical trials was used to shorten the amount of time needed to reach a decision about the viability of an NCE in lieu of conducting a traditional phase III study.

Considerable benefit can also be gained by focusing the development process on devising a draft package insert as early as possible. By doing so, experiments can be designed that can better address the desired profile of the potential drug. A whole part of such an approach is building a strong foundation of knowledge in the early I and IIa phases on which to construct the more expensive phase IIb and III programs. Aside from the measures already mentioned, the following are also important clinical considerations to assist in achieving these objectives:[45]

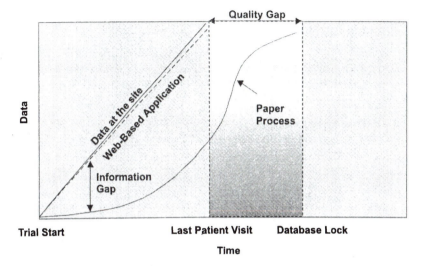

FIGURE 5.14. Comparison of Time Required to Generate Clinical Trial Data via Electronic and Paper Case Report Forms (CRFs)

1. Inclusion of surrogate endpoints in early trials
2. A phase IIa proof-of-concept program conducted to determine mechanism(s) of action, dose range, and optimum dose regimen prior to embarking upon phase IIb and phase III studies

Impact of the Internet

Implicit in a number of items discussed earlier is an increasingly pivotal role of information technology in implementation. With the advent of the Internet, this role can be expected to be amplified to a point at which it revolutionizes the manner in which R&D is conducted within the pharmaceutical industry.[46] Table 5.1 provides the results from a survey of R&D executives who were polled regarding the future impact of the Internet upon their jobs. Overall, the responses were generally positive and more than counterbalanced whatever reservations were voiced.

Beyond the results of any survey, however, is a pervasive view that the Internet will intensify the modifications already taking place in the pharmaceutical industry with respect to how it allocates resources to discover and develop drugs.[47] By virtue of the Internet's ability to simplify greatly the transfer of information between parties, it facilitates interactions between two companies. As a consequence, a number of tasks that traditionally have

TABLE 5.1. Assessment of Fifty R&D Executives' Opinions on the Internet's Current and Future Impact on Their Departments' Performance

	Pros		Cons
74%	Will use Netsource IT applications or application service providers versus 26% today	82%	Voiced concerns about the security of information on Internet-related systems
60%	Believe they will capture and transmit clinical trial data electronically compared to 14% today	58%	Say that patient privacy is an issue
56%	Envision recruiting clinical trial participants opposed to 10% today	44%	Agree that budget and staffing issues can be an obstacle and that Internet technologies sometimes create more problems than they solve
64%	Anticipate filing computer-assisted NDAs compared to 30% who currently do so		
80%	Think e-R&D will result in shorter time to market		
69%	Believe e-R&D will lower development costs		

Source: Pradip Banerjee and Fraser Skittow, "R&D Com—Research to Revenue," *Pharmaceutical Executive Supplement* December: 30, 2000.

been kept in-house can more easily be outsourced to specialists in a focused and well-defined area.

Whether to outsource and to what degree will be critical decisions facing all R&D organizations in a future where the Internet becomes more vital in order to function efficiently. One extreme is represented by the current model in which a company maintains all the skills required to discover and develop its own products. At the other are virtual companies maintaining only a few core skills. Partial virtualization falls somewhere in between.[48]

R&D LIFE CYCLE MANAGEMENT POSTAPPROVAL

R&D involvement in the life cycle management of an NCE usually begins in the development phase and is facilitated through interaction with the marketing component of the organization.[49] Basically, it involves anticipatory planning and direction of efforts toward development of novel forms of the drug and promotion for additional indications.

Novel dosage forms of the drug can encompass the pharmaceutically active ingredient (PAI) as well as the means of delivery itself. Regarding the former, chiral, or single-isomer, drugs are a primary means of extending the patent protection of an NCE. Table 5.2 illustrates this point quite well.[50] All therapeutic categories increased in global sales between 1998 and 1999 and are projected to continue upward in 2003. Chiral drugs now represent close to one-third of all drug sales worldwide.[51]

Delivery of the PAI to a specific biological target can be enhanced by several technologies that are designed either to increase a drug's stability or to facilitate its transport across physiological barriers, such as membranes. In

TABLE 5.2. Global Sales of Chiral Drugs

Drug Types	Global Sales (US$ Millions)		
	1998	1999	2003
Cardiovascular	21,906	24,805	26,012
Antibiotics/ antifungals	19,756	20,907	23,265
Hormones/ endocrinology	12,297	13,760	17,345
Cancer	8,006	9,420	13,360
Central nervous system	7,027	8,592	13,720
Hematology	6,730	8,680	11,445
Antiviral	6,131	7,540	13,446
Respiratory	4,305	5,087	8,795
Gastrointestinal	1,718	2,998	5,355
Ophthalmic	1,482	1,794	2,070
Dermatological	1,124	1,270	1,540
Analgesics	842	1,045	1,135
Vaccines	568	676	1,100
Other	7,947	8,527	7,425
TOTAL	**99,839**	**115,101**	**146,013**

Source: Adapted from Technology Catalysis International Corporation. From Anonymous, "Chiral Drugs," *Chemical and Engineering News* October 23: 56, 2000.

the past, drugs have been entrapped in polymeric microspheres and liposomes, which carry them through the body to where they are needed.[52] More recently, transporters, such as oligomers of arginine, have been developed that allow rapid entry of drugs into the cells.[53] Another modern innovation is nanotechnology, which has enabled more targeted delivery of PAIs by means of minute particles as carriers.[54]

The top fifteen companies that specialize in drug delivery technology generated more than $3 billion in sales during 1999 (see Figure 5.15).[55] In terms of new drugs approved for marketing, this translates to eleven out of seventy-seven approvals granted by the FDA.[56] Table 5.3 lists these eleven drugs as a function of indication, delivery system, and marketer. Noteworthy are that neither indication nor marketer is listed more than once as well as the diversity of delivery systems. Included in the latter are delayed-release tablets, extended-release tablets, transdermal patches, topical solutions, foams, depots, gels, and fast-dissolve tablets.

R&D involvement in the acquisition of new indications for the product labeling generally entails the generation of data in clinical trials. Therapeutic areas that are expected to realize striking growth in the future are as follows:[57]

- Nonsteroidal anti-inflammatory sales of $3.8 billion in 1998 are expected to reach $11.7 billion in 2008.
- Cholesterol-reducing therapeutic sales of $7.5 billion in 1999 are expected to surpass $13.0 billion by 2006.
- Hormone replacement therapy market is expected to grow from $2.7 billion in 1998 to $5.9 billion by 2008.
- Sales of drugs for inflammatory bowel disease are expected to reach $970 million in 2008.
- Sales of medicines used for ischemic stroke totaled $771 million in 1998. Combined sales of acute and secondary preventive therapies are expected to be $1.5 billion in 2008.
- Drug therapies for Parkinson's disease are expected to double in generated revenues by 2008.
- Sales of type 2 diabetes drugs, totaling about $4.6 billion in 1998, are expected to reach $7.5 billion in 2003.
- The urinary incontinence market, which was valued at about $250 million in 1998, is expected to grow to $1.4 billion in 2008.

Of these eight therapeutic categories, only the cholesterol-reducing therapeutics contained entries in the top-ten-selling U.S. drugs in 1999 (Lipitor and Zocor).[58]

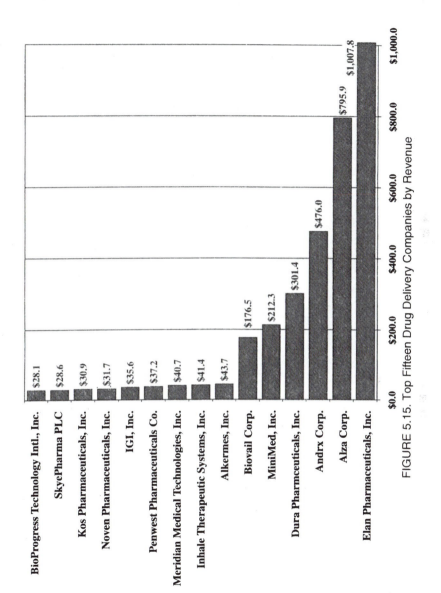

FIGURE 5.15. Top Fifteen Drug Delivery Companies by Revenue

BioProgress Technology Intl., Inc. $28.1

SkyePharma PLC $28.6

Kos Pharmaceuticals, Inc. $30.9

Noven Pharmaceuticals, Inc. $31.7

IGI, Inc. $35.6

Penwest Pharmaceuticals Co. $37.2

Meridian Medical Technologies, Inc. $40.7

Inhale Therapeutic Systems, Inc. $41.4

Alkermes, Inc. $43.7

Biovail Corp. $176.5

MiniMed, Inc. $212.3

Dura Pharmaceuticals, Inc. $301.4

Andrx Corp. $476.0

Alza Corp. $795.9

Elan Pharmaceuticals, Inc. $1,007.8

$0.0 $200.0 $400.0 $600.0 $800.0 $1,000.0

TABLE 5.3. Drug Delivery Products Approved in 1999

Brand Name	Indicated for . . .	Delivery System	Marketer
Aciphex	Ulcers	Delayed-release tablet	Eisai Co., Ltd., and Janssen Pharmaceutica, Inc.
Aggrenox	Stroke	Extended-release tablet	Boehringer Ingelheim Pharmaceuticals, Inc.
E2 III	Vasomotor symptoms related to menopause	Transdermal patch	Cygnus Corp.
Levulan Kerastick	Actinic keratoses	Topical solution	DUSA Pharmaceuticals, Inc., and Berlex Laboratories, Inc.
Lidoderm	Postherpetic neuralgia	Transdermal patch	Endo Pharmaceuticals, Inc.
Luxig	Corticosteroid-responsive dermatoses	Foam	Connetics Corp.
Metadate ER	Attention deficit hyperactivity disorder	Extended-release tablet	Medeva Pharmaceuticals, Inc.
Nutropin Depot	Pediatric growth hormone deficiency	Depot	Genentech, Inc.
Panretin	AIDS-related Kaposi's sarcoma	Gel	Ligand Pharmaceuticals, Inc.
Paxil CR	Depression	Extended-release tablet	SmithKline Beecham
Zofran ODT	Nausea and vomiting	Fast-dissolve tablet	Glaxo Wellcome, Inc.

Source: Taren Grom, "Annual Report: Drug Delivery Timed for Revival," *Med Ad News* June, 19(6): 1, 2000.

MERGERS

Mergers are primarily aimed at ownership of specific marketed drugs, strategic filling of drug pipelines, plugging of strategic holes in the R&D process, streamlining the organization by removing duplicated efforts across projects, and accelerating the development process through the use of newly acquired proprietary technologies.[59] In other words, consolidation is often deemed expedient in order to maintain a steady increase in profitability.

Of all the aforementioned factors involved in mergers (thirty in the past fifteen years),[60] an enhanced R&D department is the most critical consideration in joining forces.[61] An explanation that has been given for this resides in the escalating costs associated with the evolving fields of molecular genetics, cell biology, and the modern sciences.[62] Table 5.4 provides a listing of the 1999 R&D expenditures of the top eleven Pharma companies. It is interesting to note that companies involved in the most recent megamergers top the list.

Although consolidation can reduce costs and improve bottom-line performance on a short-term basis,[63] increasing questions focus on the long-term viability of such ventures, as is evidenced in Figure 5.16.[64] Without exception, merged companies realize a negative impact on the change in market share. This is in sharp contrast to those companies not electing to merge, which show increases ranging from 14 percent (Merck) to 100 percent (Eli Lilly).

TABLE 5.4. R&D at Top Eleven Pharma Companies

Company	Prescription Sales*	Total Revenues (in Billions)	R&D (1999)
Glaxo Wellcome/ SmithKline Beecham	$20.1	$26.3	$3.7
Pfizer/Warner-Lambert	18.7	29.1	4.0
AstraZeneca	12.6	18.5	2.5
Merck	12.5	32.7	2.1
Aventis	12.1	17.9	2.7 **
Novartis	11.5	21.6	2.4
Bristol-Myers Squibb	11.3	20.2	1.8
Johnson & Johnson	10.3	27.5	2.6
Roche	8.9	18.4	1.9
American Home Products	8.5	13.6	1.7
Pharmacia & UpJohn/Monsanto	8.3	16.4	2.8 ***

*   Twelve months ending 9/30/95; excludes mail order and sales in the Netherlands
**   1998
*** Includes $600 million in agricultural R&D

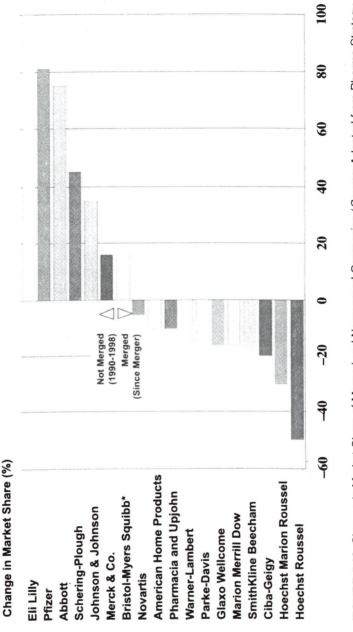

FIGURE 5.16. Change in Market Share of Merged and Nonmerged Companies (*Source:* Adapted from Pharma Strategy Consulting AG as reported in Wayne Koberstein, "The Mergers," *Pharmaceutical Executive,* 20(3): 50, 2000. *Reconsolidated.)

164

An explanation for the data contained in Figure 5.16 is that pharmaceuticals is an industry in which margins and returns in assets are largely independent of sales volume, and market share and size are independent of scale and output.[65] As a consequence, factors such as culture and management, rather than the size of the company or available cash, are paramount in determining the productivity of an R&D function. Table 5.5 compares such productivity for single, nonmerged, and merged (married) companies. The average revenue per high-value drug for the nonmerged companies is $1.31 billion, as opposed to $608 million for the merged.

Another perspective on the dilemma confronting the combined R&D functions from two merged companies is that of threshold level, i.e., the amount of revenue a new product must generate to have an impact on the companies' performance.[66] In the case of GlaxoSmithKline, the threshold level is estimated to be $800 million, or an amount representing 3.6 percent of total sales of $22.2 billion. Figure 5.17 shows that Glaxo Wellcome and SmithKline Beecham, as independent entities, launched two products with annual global sales potentially exceeding the threshold level between 1995 and 1999. To better cope with the task of meeting the quota of blockbusters in the future, GlaxoSmithKline has separated R&D into eight competing profit centers in an attempt to improve efficiency.[67] Concurrently, they are contemplating another acquisition.[68]

Finally, despite the trend toward big or mega-Pharma, one school of thought advances that such an approach will suffer the fate of the dinosaurs.[69] According to it, a confluence of factors will make it increasingly

TABLE 5.5. Average Revenues per High-Value Drug for Single and Married Companies

	Married	Single
Number of companies	10	10
Total number of high-value drugs from all companies	82	66
Total revenues generated by high-value drugs	$49.9 billion	$84.6 billion
Average revenue per high-value drug	$608.0 million	$1.31 billion

Source: Adapted from Pharma Strategy Consulting AG, as reported in B. James, "Tying the Knot," *Pharmaceutical Visions* Spring: 15, 2000.
Note: High-value drugs signify those with global sales of $500 million plus or new drugs forecast to reach $500 million within seven years of launch in a major market (1996-2002).

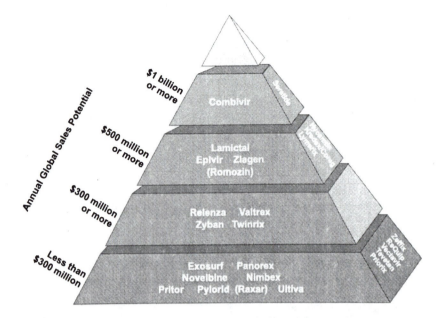

FIGURE 5.17. Products Launched by Glaxo Wellcome and SmithKline Beecham During 1995-1999 (*Source:* Adapted from John Ansell, "The Billion Dollar Pyramid," *Pharmaceutical Executive* August, 12(18): 70, 2000.)

difficult for large companies subscribing to the traditional, fully integrated business model to establish or maintain a dominant market position. These include changes in customer demands, new R&D technology, and new approaches to the delivery of care. As a consequence, they will have to "demerge" to be profitable. GlaxoSmithKline's R&D function has already established such a trend by its division into eight units.

CONCLUSION

The pharmaceutical industry engages in a broad spectrum of activities to maintain a steady stream of increased profitability. Given the confluence of a number of factors, it is adapting in various ways to continue to do so in the future.

Chapter 6

Product Research and Development Practices

Greg Perkins

Of all the external factors described in Chapter 5, the one influencing the pharmaceutical industry most directly is the FDA. As the Food, Drug, and Cosmetic Act has evolved over the years, the FDA has undergone an analogous process to arrive at its present stature as one of the most visible and well-known federal agencies. In regulating new drug development, probably its most important remit, the FDA has restructured and realigned itself multiple times so that it could better accommodate a changing set of expectations from not only Congress but also society at large. This is reflected in Figure 6.1, which depicts the composition of five offices of drug evaluation, which are primarily responsible for the review of new drugs in the United

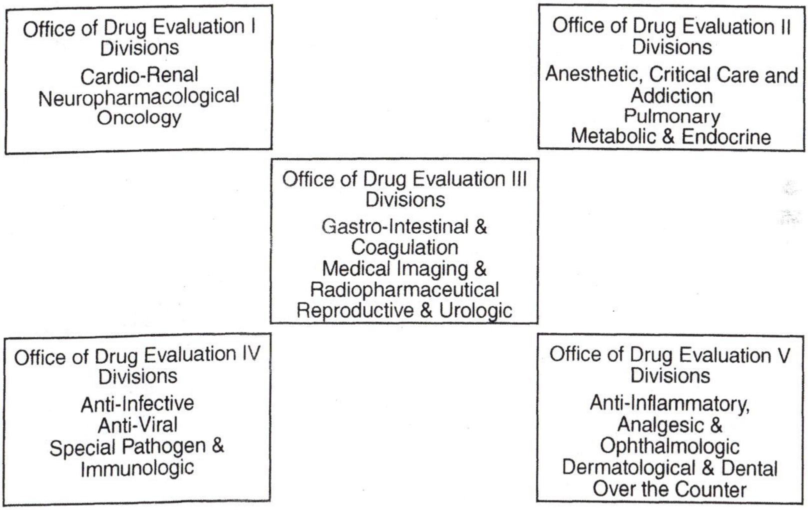

Office of Drug Evaluation I Divisions Cardio-Renal Neuropharmacological Oncology	Office of Drug Evaluation II Divisions Anesthetic, Critical Care and Addiction Pulmonary Metabolic & Endocrine
Office of Drug Evaluation III Divisions Gastro-Intestinal & Coagulation Medical Imaging & Radiopharmaceutical Reproductive & Urologic	
Office of Drug Evaluation IV Divisions Anti-Infective Anti-Viral Special Pathogen & Immunologic	Office of Drug Evaluation V Divisions Anti-Inflammatory, Analgesic & Ophthalmologic Dermatological & Dental Over the Counter

FIGURE 6.1. Review Divisions Comprising the Office of Drug Evaluation (*Source:* Adapted from *2000 FDA Directory* July-December (2): 40, 2000.)

States. These comprise a portion of the Office of Review Management within the FDA's Center for Drug Evaluation and Review (CDER).

Figures 6.2 through 6.5 encapsulate the various stages of nonexpedited drug development.* For purposes of this discussion, the development process is defined as a set of interdependent tasks with the intended purpose of marketing an NCE. The specific tasks include discovery, preclinical testing, clinical phases I through III, and registration of the NDA. The discovery phase (see Figure 6.2) serves as the entry gate into the development process

Years	2-10
Test Population	Chemical Synthesis Cell-Screening Assays Genomics
Purpose	Search for Any Experimental Drug
% of All New Drugs That Pass	1.25-2.50 (based on 250 out of 5,000-10,000 drug candidates)

FIGURE 6.2. Tasks Associated with the Discovery Phase, Its Duration, and the Percent of All New Drugs That Pass (*Source:* Adapted from *PhRMA Industry Profile,* 2000, Chapter 3, Figure 3, p. 2.)

Years	1	2
Test Population	Laboratory and Animal Studies	
Purpose	Assess Safety and Biological Activity	
% of All New Drugs That Pass	2 (based on 5 out of 250 drug candidates)	

FIGURE 6.3. Preclinical Testing (*Source:* Adapted from *PhRMA Industry Profile,* 2000, Chapter 3, Figure 3, p. 2.)

---

*Expedited drug development will be discussed in later sections.

	Phase I	Phase II		Phase III		
Years	3	4	5	6	7	8
Test Population	20 to 80 Healthy Volunteers	100 to 300 Patient Volunteers		1,000 to 3,000 Patient Volunteers		
Purpose *File IND*	Determine Safety and Dosage	Evaluate Effectiveness, Look for Side Effects		Verify Effectiveness, Monitor Adverse Reactions from Long-Term Use		
% of All New Drugs That Pass	70% of INDs	33% of INDs		27% of INDs		

FIGURE 6.4. Clinical Testing of New Chemical Entities (*Source:* Adapted from *PhRMA Industry Profile,* 2000, Chapter 3, Figure 3, p. 2.)

	Years	9	10	
Purpose *File NDA*		Review Usually Takes About 1-2 Years		Postmarketing Safety Monitoring
				Large-Scale Manufacturing
				Distribution
				Education
% of All New Drugs That Pass		20% of INDs		

FIGURE 6.5. Registration and Approval Phase of New Drug Development (*Source:* Adapted from *PhRMA Industry Profile,* 2000, Chapter 3, Figure 3, p. 2.)

and has the fewest candidates that pass (1.25 to 2.5 percent). As a consequence, emphasis is placed on optimizing the number exposed to testing.

From the standpoint of chemical synthesis, combinatorial techniques have dramatically increased the number of new chemical entities that could be produced.[1] The present-day output of 500 new compounds in a day contrasts sharply with the 50 to 100 new compounds per year that a medicinal chemist was able to synthesize a decade ago. Such volume requires that companies specializing in combinational chemistry possess libraries with the capacity to store information about compounds ranging from the hundreds of thousands to the millions.[2]

Given the number of compounds that need to be evaluated, it is imperative that the means be developed by which they can be tested. Fortunately, high throughput screening has progressed to a point at which pharmaceutical companies are able to perform up to 100,000 screens on a daily basis. Such a number represents more than a thousandfold increase in the past decade[3] and has necessitated the development of software to maintain the disposition of the vast number of compounds synthesized.[4]

Genomics, or genome-based drug discovery and development, is a more recent advance and has the potential to supercede the more traditional procedure just described.[5] This has been made possible by the delineation of the human genome and competition within the industry to define variant base pairs that predispose some people to disease and protect others.[6] It is estimated that such pairs occur with a frequency of 0.001 percent and hold the potential of leading to the discovery of variant genes.[7] Delineation of the manner in which such genes are expressed could lead to new treatment modalities.

Elements of the preclinical testing phase of drug discovery are contained in Figure 6.3. Lasting approximately two years, this phase involves animal testing and has a success rate comparable to the discovery phase (2 percent versus 1.25 to 2 percent). Approximately 40 percent of new chemical entities are rejected because of poor pharmacokinetics (i.e., absorption, distribution, metabolism, or excretion). Topical effects in animals account for the elimination of an additional 11 percent.[8] The balance of the candidates do not proceed to clinical testing because of a failure to measure up to a preconceived profile of biological activity.

Figure 6.4 adds the stages of human testing that commence after an IND Application is filed for that purpose. Phase I consists of limited testing in healthy volunteers (twenty to eighty in number). Usually a maximum tolerated dose is determined, as well as the pharmacokinetic profile. Seventy percent of drug candidates survive this phase. Phase II involves testing in 100 to 300 patients and monitoring of side effects. From an effectiveness standpoint, dose response relationships are determined. Almost half of the drugs entering phase II advance into phase III.

Phase III represents the chief expenditure of the drug development process, requiring the same amount of time to complete as phases I and II combined (three years). Enrollment involves 1,000 to 3,000 patient volunteers to establish the efficacy of the recommended dose and to define an adverse reaction profile. Only 6 percent of the drugs entering phase III are rejected as a result of this expanded testing.

The registration and approval phase of new drug development is depicted in Figure 6.5. After compilation of the safety and efficacy data, an NDA is submitted to the FDA for review. One out of five, or 20 percent of NCEs for which INDs are filed, eventually gain approval. On the other hand, 7 percent of drugs completing phase III fail to do so. Before approval can be granted, a firm must first undergo a preapproval inspection, in which the FDA checks adherence to good manufacturing practices and validation of manufacturing practices. After the drug is approved, there are usually phase IV commitments.

Figures 6.6 and 6.7, respectively, afford a glimpse of how the drug development process has changed over time as it relates to number of patients needed for an NDA and the length of the development process itself. The number of patients needed to file an NDA actually decreased approximately 16 percent in the interval between 1981 and 1984, compared to the five years preceding it (1,321 patients compared to 1,576). However, in the following five years, the number more than doubled, to 3,233 patients. After remaining fairly constant between 1989 and 1992 (3,567 patients), the number then increased by over 650 patients, to 4,237.

The burgeoning number of patients required to file an NDA has had a very distinctive impact on development time, namely, that it has remained constant in the 1980s and from 1990 through 1998, despite a reduction of nine months in the approval phase. The amount of time required to conduct the preclinical phase was identical for the two intervals. Thus, the decrement in approval time is offset by an increase in the clinical phase from 5.7

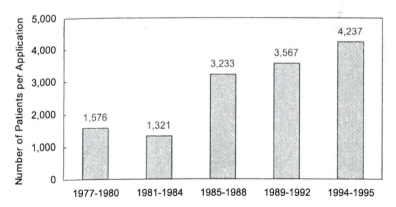

FIGURE 6.6. Number of Patients Needed for a New Drug Application (*Source: Adapted from Salvatore J. Giorgianne, "Perspectives on Health Care and Biomedical Research," The Pfizer Journal* 3(2): 23, 1999.)

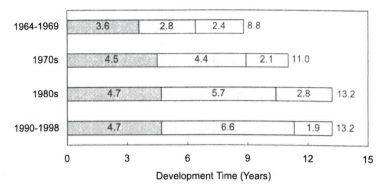

FIGURE 6.7. Development Time As a Function of Time (*Source:* Adapted from Salvatore J. Giorgianne, "Perspectives on Health Care and Biomedical Research," *The Pfizer Journal* 3(2): 22, 1999.)

to 6.6 years. Similarly, the length of the clinical phase had the greatest influence on development time between 1964 to 1969 and the 1970s. Although the review time again showed a decrement in the later interval, actual development increased by 25 percent. Unlike in the 1980s and 1990s, the preclinical phase also showed an increase, which was smaller than that of the clinical phase.

The previous description of the development process applies to post-1962, or after passage of the Kefauver-Harris Drug Amendments to the Food, Drug, and Cosmetic Act. This represented a significant milestone, since it meant that companies had to establish efficacy, as well as safety, for new drugs. As mentioned previously, the FDA has also undergone a significant evolutionary process in adapting to changing expectations. A number of such expectations have been applied to the development of NCEs, and the ease with which new drugs pass through the process to become available for patients. The following attempts to describe how the FDA has responded to those instances.

ORPHAN DRUG ACT

Orphan diseases and disorders (1) affect fewer than 200,000 persons in the United States or (2) affect more than 200,000 persons in the United States and for which there is no reasonable expectation that the cost of developing and making available drugs for such diseases or conditions will be recovered from sales in the United States.[9] Approximately 20,000,000 U.S. citizens are inflicted by the over 5,000 rare diseases so categorized.[10]

Prior to passage of the Orphan Drug Act in 1983, it was commercially nonviable for the pharmaceutical industry to develop drugs to treat orphan diseases. As a consequence, a significant number of individuals were deprived of effective medications for their illnesses. Fortunately, their plight was recognized, and a lobbying effort to focus attention on the problem was initiated in the 1970s by an organization founded by Abbey Meyers. Her organization, named the National Organization for Rare Disorders (NORD), was instrumental in pressuring Congress to pass legislation conducive to the development of orphan drugs.[11] In 1982, Congressman Waxman's Subcommittee on Health and Environment held hearings that resulted in passage of the act the following year.

The law was enacted only temporarily in 1983 and reenacted periodically thereafter until it expired in 1994. It was permanently reinstated three years later.[12] Industry incentives resulting from the legislation are as follows:

1. The sponsor receives seven years exclusivity if its NDA remains unique for the product, and if no significant improvements are instituted by a competitor.
2. If requested, the sponsor can have help with protocol assistance from the FDA during development.
3. An orphan product manufacturer is entitled to tax credits up to 50 percent of qualified clinical research expenses incurred in developing the product. This tax credit was permanently extended by Congress and signed by President Clinton in August 1997.[13]
4. Researchers may apply for grant funds to support pivotal clinical trials. Amounts may total up to $200,000 for a phase II or III study.[14]

To accommodate the act, the FDA formed the Office of Generic Drugs. In order to pursue this option, a company must first seek FDA agreement that a drug qualifies for orphan designation. As mentioned earlier, one key criterion for qualification is that the disease in question has prevalence no greater than 200,000 individuals in the United States. If this requirement is fulfilled, the company must defend the drug's uniqueness in relation to the disease. Otherwise, the company may find itself competing with a similar drug that has also earned an orphan indication. In this eventuality, unless the two drugs in question can be shown to be distinct, an NDA will be granted to only one.[15]

The impact of the Orphan Drug Act on the number of new orphan drugs approved is provided in Figure 6.8. In the decade prior to passage (1972-1982), a total of ten orphan drugs were approved. This compares with 193 approved between 1983 and 1998. The cumulative number of orphan drugs

Number of Approved Orphan Drugs

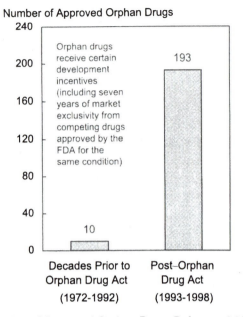

FIGURE 6.8. Number of Approved Orphan Drugs Before and After Passage of the Orphan Drug Act (*Source:* Adapted from *PhRMA Industry Profile,* 2000, Chapter 3, p. 11.)

approved after enactment of the act is contained in Figure 6.9. Looking at the shape of the line—i.e., the number of cumulative approvals divided by time expressed as individual years—the rate of change is not linear, or constant, over the interval. Rather, it steadily increases, with the greatest increments coming in the later years. A compilation of the twelve orphan drugs approved by FDA in 1999 is as follows:[16]

1. Alitretinoin (Panretin): a topical treatment of cutaneous lesions in patients with AIDS-related Kaposi's sarcoma
· 2. Bexarotene (Targretin): for treating manifestations of cutaneous T-cell lymphomas in patients who are refractory to at least one prior systemic therapy
3. Epirubicin HLC (Ellence): a component of adjuvant therapy in patients with evidence of axillary node tumor involvement following resection of primary breast cancer
4. Exemestane (Aromasin): for treating advanced breast cancer in postmenopausal women whose disease has progressed following tamoxifen therapy

5. Lidocaine patch (Lidoderm): for relief of allodynia (painful hyper-sensitivity) and chronic pain in posthepatic neuralgia
6. Temozolomide (Temodar): for the treatment of recurrent malignant glocoma
7. Busulfan (Busulfex): a preparative therapy in the treatment of ma-lignancies with bone marrow transplantation
8. Caffeine citrate (Cafcit): for apnea of prematurity
9. Cytarabine (DepoCyt): for neoplastic meningitis
10. Nitric oxide (INOmax): for the treatment of persistent pulmonary hypertension in newborns
11. Poractant alfa (Curosurf): for the treatment of respiratory distress syndrome in premature infants
12. Somatropin (Nutropin Depot): for the long-term treatment of growth failure

EXPEDITED DRUG APPROVAL

Expedited, or "fast track," drug approval dates back to the early 1970s when Dr. Richard Trout and senior staff in the Bureau of Drugs coined the term. It was applied to any NCE offering significant improvement over ex-isting available therapies for serious or life-threatening diseases. After 1973 to 1974, these drugs were identified as IA and received priority over other applications.[17]

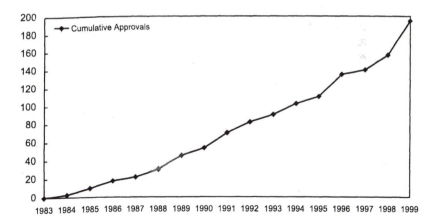

FIGURE 6.9. Cumulative Number of Orphan Drugs Approved After the Enactment of the Orphan Drug Act (*Source:* Adapted from *PhRMA Industry Profile,* 2000, Chapter 3, p. 11.)

With the advent of the AIDS epidemic, the need to further refine the process became apparent. As a consequence, the FDA introduced two mechanisms for providing new therapies for patients in 1987: expanding patient access during clinical trials (treatment IND) and accelerating the testing and review process (Subpart E drugs).[18] Figure 6.10 is a schematic representation of the manner in which both can impact the drug development process.[19]

Such a scheme places heavy emphasis on frequent and early discussions within the FDA in the early stages of drug development. This enables agency buy-in and participation in the design of key studies. Equally important is the generation of sufficient studies in phase II that would allow the conventional phase III testing to be deleted prior to FDA evaluation and approval. Patients are afforded access to the drug via a treatment IND until availability by means of commercial distribution. Firms have the option of charging for the drug under a treatment IND. If the data generated in phase II are insufficient to warrant approval, the drug enters phase III and normal development. Drugs developed according to this process are referred to as either Subpart E or Subpart H drugs.

Subpart E Drugs

AZT (azidovudine), the first drug authorized for the treatment of AIDS, was the prototype for the formulation of Subpart E. Approval largely was based on the only placebo-controlled trial conducted in relation to AIDS,[20] which necessitated not only a subsequent diminution of dose after approval

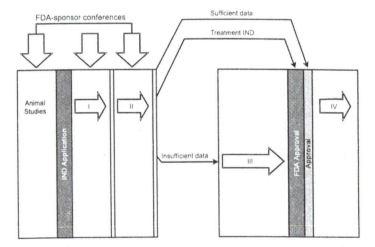

FIGURE 6.10. Drug Development Process Involving Products for Life-Threatening Illnesses

but also Wellcome's commitment to, and execution of, an extensive phase IV program.[21] The latter is illustrative of the need to defer until phase IV the generation of data normally required for approval.

Twenty-eight Subpart E approvals occurred between October 1988, or immediately after promulgation of the regulation, and December 1994.[22] Three of these were biologicals, and twenty-five were NCEs. A vast majority (two-thirds) were for the treatment of cancer, AIDS, or other HIV-related conditions. Figure 6.11 contains comparative data on the time lapse between submission of the IND to the FDA and approval for Subpart E NCEs versus non–Subpart E NCEs.[23] The average interval for the former was 3.3 years shorter than for the latter. Most of the disparity was attributable to the clinical phase (2.7 years shorter for the Subpart E approvals), although the FDA review phase was briefer, as well, by 6.3 months.

To further encourage the faster review of breakthrough drugs, the FDA adapted the classification contained in Table 6.1 on January 1, 1992.[24] By differentiating between routine (standard) and expedited (priority or AIDS), the FDA was better able to concentrate their resources on facilitating the availability of new drugs to patients infected with HIV and other diseases, such as Alzheimer's. The new system replaced the old classifications of

- "A" drugs, with significant therapeutic gain over existing therapies;
- "B" drugs, with modest therapeutic gain; and
- "C" drugs, with little or no therapeutic advance.

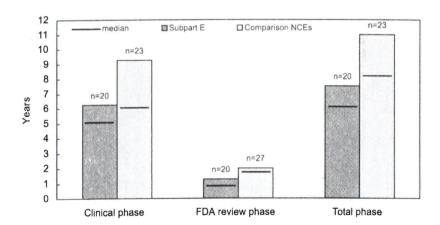

FIGURE 6.11. Mean and Median Clinical, FDA Review, and Total Phase Lengths for Subpart E and Comparison NCE Approvals (*Note:* Excludes new formulations and supplemental approvals.)

TABLE 6.1. Classification System

Types	Therapeutic Value
1. New molecular entity 2. New salt 3. New formulation 4. New combination 5. Already marketed drug product duplication 6. New claim for already marketed drug product	S = Standard P = Priority AA = AIDS V = Orphan drugs

Subpart H Drugs

Enacted on January 11, 1993, as a reaction to the worsening AIDS crisis, Subpart H of the Code of Federal Regulations enables the FDA to grant "conditional" approval on the basis of a drug's effect on a surrogate endpoint.[25] The most important provision under Subpart H was the linkage of approval with the company's concurrence that it would later demonstrate a correlation between the surrogate and a more traditional endpoint, such as slower disease progression, longer survival, or fewer opportunistic infections. Additional differences between drugs approved under Subpart H and either conventional drug development or Subpart E pertain to the following:

1. Restrictions of the drug's distribution and the conditions under which it can be administered
2. Preapproval of promotional materials while the NDA or PLA (product license application for biologicals) is under review
3. Six conditions or circumstances that could result in the FDA withdrawing its approval

The latter apply to failure of the drug to live up to its anticipated safety and efficacy profile, failure on the part of the company to live up to restrictions on usage and distribution, and false and misleading promotional materials.

Between January 1993 and December 1995, twelve approvals were granted under Subpart H. These included seven NCEs, two new biopharmaceuticals, and three supplemental applications for already approved drugs. AIDS or HIV-related indications accounted for eight approvals, whereas the balance covered therapies for multiple sclerosis, cystic fibrosis, pancreatic cancer, and cardioprotection from doxorubicin toxicity in breast cancer patients.[26,27] The average clinical development and FDA review times for the nine new drugs were five years and 10.3 months, respectively.[28] The corresponding figures for Subpart E drugs (from Figure 6.11) are about 6.3 years for clinical development and 1.3 years for FDA review time.

Parallel Track Policy

Implemented on April 18, 1992, the Parallel Track Policy was intended to extend the availability of promising investigational therapies for AIDS and HIV-related diseases beyond the provisions of the preexisting treatment IND regulations.[29] Basically, this policy allows access to an investigational drug without change as early as the end of phase I if patient enrollment in FDA-approved phase II controlled clinical trials has been initiated.[30] Given that distribution of drugs in this manner involves community-based physicians, any data generated by such means are restricted to safety and limited in terms of being able to support the application. Three AIDS drugs have been distributed by means of parallel track (only one after official publication of the policy statement).

Expanded Access and Accelerated Approval for Cancer Drugs

In March 1996, the FDA, in conjunction with the Clinton administration, announced a program to increase the availability of cancer drugs.[31] The initiative was necessitated by underutilization of Subpart H for this class of drugs, resulting from lack of general agreement on surrogate markers. This obstacle has been refined, while maintaining many of the aspects of accelerated approval previously described. Two months after the announcement, Taxatere was approved for the treatment of refractory breast cancer based upon data showing that it effectively reduces tumor size. Survival time and quality of life were to be evaluated in postapproval studies.

PRESCRIPTION DRUG USER FEE ACT OF 1992 (PDUFA)

Resulting from the pharmaceutical and biotechnology industries lobbying for more rapid approval of their applications, the enactment of PDUFA in 1992 inaugurated a new era of FDA-company interactions.[32] PDUFA originally was a five-year program that enabled the FDA to collect fees for the review of certain NDAs, PLAs, and supplemental applications. User fees were renewed for an additional five years in the 1997 FDA Modernization Act (see the following section). The fees enabled the hiring of additional personnel to review applications.

Table 6.2 lists the amount of revenues collected for the first four years of the program.[33] From an initial amount of $36 million, the total increased by approximately $20 million over each of the next two years. After that, the

TABLE 6.2. Revenues Generated by User Fees As a Function of Fiscal Year

Fiscal Year	Revenues Generated
1993	$36,000,000
1994	$56,284,200
1995	$77,415,000
1996	$79,981,200

rate of increase slackened by approximately three-fourths, to reach an amount of $79,981,200 by 1996.

In 1992, the FDA agreed to performance goals for the following five categories of submissions pertaining to NDAs:

1. Original new drug applications
2. Resubmissions of original NDAs
3. Efficacy supplements to already approved marketing applications
4. Manufacturing supplements to already approved new marketing applications[34]

Figures 6.12 and 6.13 depict a number of performance parameters related to the FDA's review of NDAs.

Figure 6.12 plots the percentage of drugs approved over two years and under one year during PDUFA. At the time of enactment, or 1993, slightly less than 50 percent of new drugs required more than two years to approve. This contrasted with the approximately 20 percent that were approved in less than one year. By 1998, the percentage of drugs approved in over two years had decreased steadily to less than 5 percent. On the other hand, drugs approved in under one year had increased to a plateau of roughly 50 percent by 1996, where it has remained since that time.

The FDA's ability to meet its performance goals under PDUFA as they relate to reviews of NDAs is captured in Figure 6.13. The last year such goals were not in place was fiscal year 1993, during which 65 percent of the eighty-four reviews were completed within the twelve-month review window. Every year thereafter, the FDA was able to surpass the performance objective that it had set for itself. Although this was very much in evidence between fiscal years 1994 and 1997 for drugs subjected to a twelve-month review, improved performance goals were a key element of the reauthorization of user fees in 1997.[35] As a consequence, standard drugs began a phase-in to ten-month reviews in fiscal year 1999 (30 percent goal),

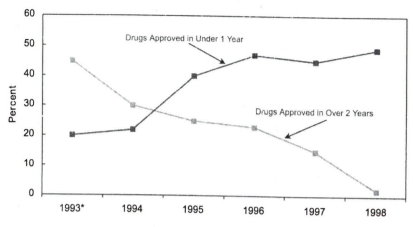

FIGURE 6.12. Percentage of Drugs Approved Over Two Years and Under One Year During PDUFA (*Source:* Adapted from Tufts Center for the Study of Drug Development, "Faster Approval of New Drugs Does Not Compromise U.S. Public Safety," *Tufts Center for the Study of Drug Development Impact Report* 1:3, 1999. *Prescription Drug User Fee Act enacted.)

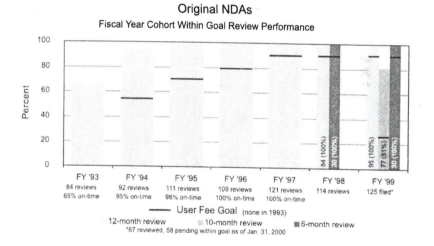

FIGURE 6.13. Percentage of Reviews Completed on Time According to User Fee Goals (*Source:* Adapted from CDER 1999 Report to the Nation: Improving Public Health Through Human Drugs, p. 17.)

whereas priority drugs had a performance goal of 90 percent reviewed and acted upon within six months, dating back to fiscal year 1998. The FDA was able to exceed these objectives as well.

To meet its objectives, the FDA has exercised increased consistency in applying its authority to refuse to file an application. This obligated sponsors to enhance the quality of NDAs in general in order to diminish the risk of having an application returned. Figure 6.14 graphically illustrates the percentage of NDAs subjected to refuse-to-file actions since PDUFA was enacted.[36] From a peak of 26 percent in fiscal year 1993, the percentage has dropped steadily to approximately 4 percent in recent years.

FDA MODERNIZATION ACT OF 1997 (FDAMA)

FDAMA amended the Food, Drug, and Cosmetic Act and the biological products provisions in Section 351 of the Public Health Service Act.[37] It essentially enacted many FDA initiatives implemented under the Reinventing Government Program.[38] The following are the most important provisions of the act related specifically to enhancing the drug development process.

Prescription Drug User Fees

As was alluded to previously, FDAMA reauthorized the original PDUFA of 1992 for an additional five years.

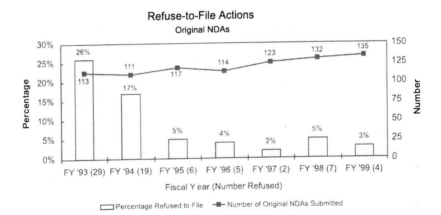

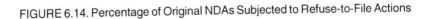

FIGURE 6.14. Percentage of Original NDAs Subjected to Refuse-to-File Actions

Speeding Drug Development

FDAMA's fast-track drug development established a more formal system for accelerating drug development and approval for critical therapies than has been described preivously.[39] This was accomplished via several means. First, the definition of "severe disease" was modified to encompass diseases that have substantial impact on day-to-day functioning and are associated with "persistent or recurrent" morbidity. In addition, animal data can be used as a basis for fast-track designation, and approval can be granted on the basis of surrogate endpoints that are not well established.[40]

What could be viewed as an ancillary provision of FDAMA stipulated that the National Institutes of Health work with the FDA to establish a database of information on clinical trials for therapies to treat serious and life-threatening diseases. The listing will include eligibility criteria for studies, location of investigational sites, and points of contact for enrollment.[41]

Revised Standard of Evidence

Reliance on the traditional two well-controlled demonstrations of safety and efficacy for approval was modified by FDAMA so that the FDA could conceivably approve NDAs based on data from an adequate and well-controlled investigation plus confirmatory evidence. This affords greater flexibility in dealing with therapies studied in one large multicenter trial or in large studies with different clinical endpoints.[42]

Establishment of Standard Regulations Worldwide for Regulated Products—ICH Initiative

ICH is the abbreviated name for the International Conference on Harmonization of Technical Requirements for Registration of Pharmaceuticals for Human Use.[43] Established in 1990, ICH has brought together the regulatory authorities of the European Union, Japan, and the United States, as well as experts from the pharmaceutical industry in these three regions. Their objective is to produce a single set of technical requirements for the registration of new drug products so that the development process can be streamlined on a global basis.[44] Three important projects under ICH are Medical Dictionary for Regulatory Activities (MedDRA), Common Technical Document (CTD), and Guidances.

MedDRA is an international medical terminology that is intended to facilitate the electronic transmission of regulatory information and data on a worldwide basis.[45] Its primary utility will be twofold: (1) to process information on medical products during clinical and scientific reviews, as well as marketing, and (2) to enhance the ability to transmit electronically adverse event reports and coding of clinical trial data.

The CTD is an international effort to harmonize the format of dossiers to allow for more efficient registration in the three ICH regions. When finalized, the CTD will greatly reduce the duplication of effort that is currently common practice in global registration. Figure 6.15 is a diagrammatic representation of the ICH Common Technical Document.[46] Module I contains information specific to each of the three regions. Examples include application forms as the proposed labels for use in individual regions. Individual regulatory agencies have the latitude of defining the content and format of the module.

Modules II through V constitute the CTD and are common to all three regions. Analogous to the organization of an NDA, the degree or organization increases as one proceeds from the base of the triangle to its apex. For the clinical and nonclinical areas, the most basic component is the report, whereas for quality it is the information stipulated by a specific guideline. All these data are eventually distilled into a comprehensive recapitulation that justifies the dosage regimen, indication(s), shelf life, containers, and validation of the manufacturing process for the drug being proposed for marketing.

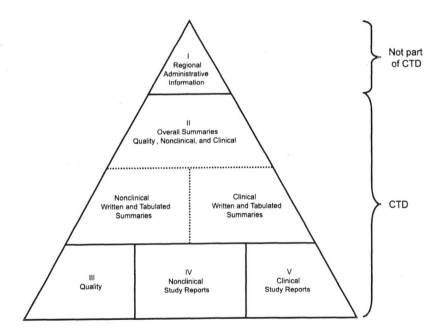

FIGURE 6.15. Diagrammatic Representation of the ICH Common Technical Document

Guidance documents are intended to provide consistency in the requirements for new drug approval among the three regions (see Figure 6.16).[47] They essentially contain the regulatory agencies' thinking on the processing, content, evaluation, and approval of applications. The documents also outline policies not only to facilitate consistency in regulatory approaches but also to establish inspection and enforcement procedures. They are neither regulations nor laws and, as a consequence, are not enforceable.

CONCLUSION

As described previously, the FDA has undergone an intensive evolutionary process over the years in order to be responsive to the public's need for major therapeutic advances. It is anticipated that such a process will continue in the future.

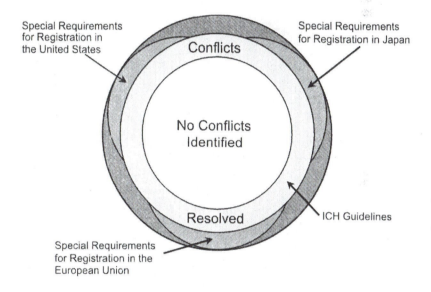

FIGURE 6.16. Resolution of Conflicts by ICH Guidance

SECTION III:
PRICE

Chapter 7

Pharmaceutical Pricing Principles

Mick Kolassa

The primary principle that should guide every pricing decision is that the price should reflect the value of the product to the customer. The other elements of the marketing mix—product, promotion, and distribution—each add or create value. The physical product itself should have clinical and economic value. Through distribution the value of the product is enhanced by providing "place utility." Having the product available where and when it is needed adds tremendous value. With effective promotion, the value of the product is enhanced by explaining to the customers the best use of the product. Pricing should not only reflect the value created by the other elements of the marketing mix; it should be used by the firm to capture some of the value that has been created. Profitable pricing decisions allow the firm to generate the funds necessary to continue to perform the research necessary to remain viable.

Pricing decisions are reached in a number of ways, using a varied range of considerations, types of information, and internal processes. Each pricing decision is unique, depending on the company, the medication, and external factors that affect both. In this chapter, the factors that should be considered when making pricing decisions are discussed. There is no one "best" or "right" manner in which to set prices, but certain considerations and processes do provide the company the best chance of making informed, and profitable, pricing decisions.

ESSENTIAL FACTORS IN THE PRICING DECISION

There are no quick and easy approaches to pricing, no "magic" models that deliver the precise price or formulas that, when solved, render the optimal number. Although some consultants may offer such miracle cures for pricing problems, they simply do not exist. Attempts to reduce the pricing process to a simple model or formula are not only misleading but reflect an absolute lack of knowledge about the pricing of medicines, or the pricing of anything else.

It is unlikely that any two pharmaceutical companies set prices using the same thought processes—or even consider the same issues when establishing a price. Moreover, it is unlikely that a single company would price any two different products in the same way, given differences in markets, timing, market entry dynamics, and other environmental factors. This lack of singularity, which critics may question, is actually quite appropriate—no two companies have exactly the same needs, philosophies, or resources, and no two separate products will be marketed using precisely the same strategy, even if sold by the same company. These basic differences demand different pricing criteria and different prices.

The pricing of pharmaceutical products, as with the pricing of any product or service, should be market based. Contrary to the widely held notion that pricing is simply a matter of adding up costs and establishing a markup, pricing experts agree that costs may help to establish a price floor but the market provides most of the information for the pricing decision. As competition within pharmaceutical markets, especially price-related competition, heats up, the need for market-based pricing will continue to grow.

The following are some general rules, or considerations, that should be included in every pharmaceutical pricing decision:

1. The prices, product features, and past actions of the competition
2. Specific patient characteristics
3. The economic and social value of the therapy itself
4. The decision-making criteria of prescribers and those who influence that decision
5. Characteristics of the disease treated by the medication
6. Company needs, in terms of market position, revenue, and other issues
7. Company abilities, including available budgets and willingness to support the product
8. The current and anticipated environment for insurance reimbursement
9. The public policy environment

These factors must be addressed, either formally through adherence to a company policy or informally by a product manager or other individual charged with developing a pricing recommendation. The failure to address these factors has contributed to many pricing missteps in pharmaceutical markets.

To further complicate the process, it is likely that the elements of this simple model will vary greatly among different companies and company affiliates, as local variations in health care delivery, reimbursement, and regulations compound the problems. Still, these issues must be investigated and addressed.

COMPETITION

Typically, the first pieces of information gathered when arriving at a price recommendation are the prices of competing drugs. If a new product is to be launched into a therapeutic area that is already served by one or more agents, the prices of those agents should provide initial guidance in price selection. Which prices to use for this analysis (e.g., ex-factory prices, discount prices, prices per dose, per day of therapy, per package, per course of therapy) will depend upon the perspective of the analysis and the product under study. Generally, list (or ex-factory) prices for a comparable unit of therapy, whether that be a single day's therapy for a chronic disorder or a complete course of therapy for an acute treatment, are an appropriate place to begin. Discounts and other considerations are tactical in nature, and the first steps in any analysis of initial pricing should be focused on strategy.

In addition to the current prices of competitive agents, the price histories of products in this class should be examined, to assess any recent changes in the price positions of the various products. Anticipated competitive product launches must also be considered. The range of prices for branded products in this market, from highest to lowest, should also be examined. If the price levels seem to be related to relative market success of the agents (e.g., those with the highest market shares seem to have prices that are either higher or lower than their less successful competitors), this could indicate the presence or absence of significant price sensitivity. High-priced market leaders imply little or no price sensitivity, whereas lower-priced leaders may imply the opposite.

The prices of other products sold by the major competitors and recent entrants in this market should also be investigated, to determine whether their pricing in this market reflects a company pricing policy or a deliberate pricing strategy for this specific market. If the prices reflect a departure from a firm's typical approach to pricing, that may be a signal that price sensitivity is at work in this market, or at least that the company believes that is the case.

Other competitive factors that must be assessed at this stage are the level of promotion by other agents, their rates of growth, and the extent of discounting in price-sensitive markets, such as managed care and hospitals. Here again, the level of discounting must be compared with the success of the products in those discounted markets. High levels of promotional spending in a market make it difficult for a new agent to break through. If the decision makers can be swayed with a low-price appeal, markets with significant promotional spending may be good targets for a low-price strategy—if you can determine how low the price must be to gain prescribers' attention. This approach usually requires high levels of spending as well.

Low levels of promotional spending imply a satisfied or mature market, which may be less responsive to low-price positioning. Conversely, they may imply a mature market with little true competition and patients with unmet needs. In such markets, a new agent that offers improvements over those currently available can often command a premium with no negative effect on prescribing levels. In some cases, products launched at discounts are perceived by physicians to be priced at premiums because of the improvements in quality—the prescribers assume that the better product must cost more. In such cases, prescriber decision making plays a major role in the pricing decision.

Relative market share, compared with price levels, is also a telling statistic. In markets in which the leading products are also those with the lowest prices, it may mean that the markets are extremely price sensitive. Figure 7.1 portrays this relationship graphically. The market leader is also the product with the highest price, and the lowest-priced agent holds the lowest share of market. In this case, it can be concluded that the market is not price sensitive.

In Figure 7.2, the opposite holds true: the market leader is also the product that has the lowest price. Note that this does not automatically imply that the market is price sensitive, only that the competitors appear to be price sensitive. However, indications suggest that the market is aware of, and responds to, price differences.

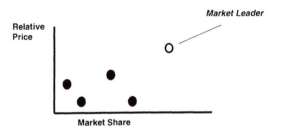

FIGURE 7.1. Graph of Non-Price-Sensitive Market

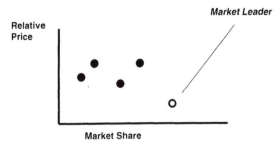

FIGURE 7.2. Graph of a Potentially Price-Sensitive Market

The importance of competitive analysis in pricing cannot be overstated. It has been suggested by many researchers that the pricing and presence of competitors together with the uniqueness or therapeutic value of the new product are the major determinants of launch prices. Reekie, in his book *Pricing New Pharmaceutical Products,* found that the price levels of current competitors and the anticipation of future competitors were the driving factors in setting prices for pharmaceuticals.[1] New entrants that offered significant benefits over current competitors were consistently priced above the prevailing prices in their therapeutic class. Those products offering little or no therapeutic advantage tended to be priced at or below prevailing levels.

An interesting finding of Reekie's study, however, was that even for unique products offering improvements, those which had close or superior competitors entering the market within two years of their launch tended to be priced lower than those which anticipated little or no competition from new products in the near future. The general rule can be seen graphically in Figure 7.3.

The rule portrayed in Figure 7.3 is a simple application of the three basic pricing approaches:

1. *Skimming:* The product, anticipating little direct competition, is priced above prevailing levels to maximize profits. Prilosec, the first proton pump inhibitor, was priced in this manner, substantially above the price levels of the H2 antagonists, although consistent with the value that it delivered.
2. *Parity:* The product is priced equivalent to the prevailing price levels in the market. This is the most common approach used by firms launching products into already established markets.
3. *Penetration:* The product is priced below the prevailing market level. Many products have been launched with this approach. Because the market is generally unresponsive to price differences, it may be concluded that the majority of firms using this approach have chosen to make price a "nonissue" in the marketing of their products.

These approaches, as can be seen, also depend on other factors, such as the needs and abilities of the company, the sensitivity of the specific market segment to price levels, and the therapeutic value of the product itself. Thus, the factors presented here are not discrete entities to be considered separately, but a complex system of elements that must be evaluated together.

Reekie and others have noted that even though it appears that most pharmaceutical markets are not price sensitive, most companies act, and price, as though this were the case. The lack of responsiveness to the deep discounts in many markets in the United States implies that

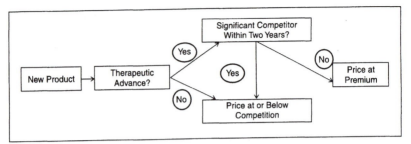

FIGURE 7.3. Typical, but Flawed, New Product Pricing (*Source:* Adapted from discussions within and throughout the text of W. Duncan Reekie, *Pricing New Pharmaceutical Products* [London: CroomHelm, 1977].)

1. these markets do not respond to price, and
2. the companies marketing many of the products act as though they believe the markets are responsive to price.

Belief in price sensitivity, as opposed to an objective measurement of price sensitivity, appears to have led many pharmaceutical companies to underprice their products. A "me too" product priced at a 30 percent discount and achieving a market share of 2 to 5 percent, which can be expected of most such products, regardless of price, implies that the 30 percent discount represents an opportunity cost to the company of nearly 50 percent. This means that a price 50 percent above that charged may have delivered the same level of unit sales as the lower price, but with significantly greater dollar sales and profits. That is a very high cost to pay for such timidity.

The following are key questions to answer concerning competitors:

1. What are the current competitive alternatives?
2. Are new competitors anticipated?
3. Do the competitors have a history of responding to the pricing actions of others?
4. What steps might competitors who feel threatened by this new product take?

PATIENT CHARACTERISTICS

Although in many markets the patient bears no direct financial burden, this is not the case in all markets. In markets without universal coverage for pharmaceuticals, the patients who will be the final users of your new agent must be considered in the pricing decision. If the bulk of the patient population is elderly, a great proportion of whom in the United States have no third-party coverage for medications and must pay for them out of pocket, their ability to afford the product, in addition to other medications, must always be considered. Although a product may seem relatively inexpensive at $1.50 per day, if a patient on a fixed income must take three or four such prescriptions on a daily basis, the total cost can be prohibitive.

Such considerations are not simply altruism—although there is room for compassion in every strategy. The fact is, patients who are unable to afford a medication will often not take their medications. Compliance, both with the daily dosing and the length of therapy, is a growing concern and a source of significant unrealized revenue.[2,3] It is not uncommon for 50 percent of patients prescribed a medication for a chronic disorder that is relatively asymptomatic to "drop out" in the first year.[4,5] How much of this is due to failure to understand the importance of compliance versus inability to afford the medication is not yet known, but if a significant proportion of this can be eliminated through a lower price, the product may earn more with a lower price than a higher one.[6]

Some patient groups are highly organized and able to exert political and economic pressure on a company. The areas of mental health, Parkinson's disease, HIV, and cancer all have active support groups who are playing a growing role in therapy selection. The degree of patient involvement in therapy decisions appears to be growing across most major therapeutic categories, and the market power of these groups must play an ever-growing role in pricing decisions.

Yet even in markets in which patients are shielded from the financial consequences of medication use, patients can, and do, play a role in the adoption of many agents, and their demand for some products can provide price flexibility. In the United States, the most price-sensitive buyer may be the giant health maintenance organization (HMO) Kaiser Permanente, a staff model HMO with many restrictive policies and the ability to limit drug use. Schering-Plough refused to grant Kaiser the major price concessions they demanded, and Kaiser then refused to list the Schering antihistamine Claritin on their formulary—denying Schering access to Kaiser patients. In doing so, they also denied Kaiser patients access to Claritin, and the protests from patients were overwhelming. In the end, Schering was able to get Claritin on the Kaiser formulary without granting major discounts. In many such cases, when patients are involved with treatment of their disorders (diseases such as diabetes, asthma, allergy, and many others), patient pull-through may enable the company to command higher prices than pricing authorities may be initially willing to grant. It is wise to examine this when the launch of appropriate medications is anticipated and perhaps wait for patients to demand reimbursement for the product.

The following are key patient characteristic questions:

1. What is the potential for patients to view the drug positively (i.e., it will offer relief of symptoms, disease reversal, or a cure)?
2. What is the extent to which patient protests over the price are likely?
3. Is the patient population likely to have trouble affording this new product, and it is possible to make affordability a key feature of this product?

VALUE OF THERAPY

Early in the clinical development process, it is wise to begin economic as well as clinical studies. Among the first pieces of "outcomes" work should be a financial profile of the disease for which the agent is being investigated. Doing this allows the fitting of the agent into this financial profile, to determine its potential effect on the cost of treatment.

Ideally, any new agent will help to reduce the cost of treatment, especially if other pharmacologic therapies are already available. In theory, the value of a new agent is equal to the cost reduction it provides. Should the use of your new agent reduce the cost of treatment of the disorder by $1,000 per year, before considering the price for the product, its "economic value" is $1,000.

If this new agent has significant clinical or quality-of-life advantages over current therapy, which would provide better overall patient care and outcomes for the same cost, pricing the product to "capture" its entire economic value of $1,000 would be appropriate. Unfortunately, it is not always this straightforward, and certainly not this simple, and many in the marketplace appear to resist the use of such information in product adoption decisions. A study by Kolassa and Smith, for example, found that hospital pharmacy directors in the United States were incapable of fully understanding and processing the results of pharmacoeconomic studies and, although they believed these studies would become important in the future, found them to be of little value today.[7]

It is unlikely that any new agent could be documented to reduce costs by a precise figure. Instead, savings ranges are the more likely result, due to regulatory, patient, and provider differences. These ranges do, however, provide a range for pricing as well and can certainly help to establish a price "ceiling," or maximum reasonable price. Costs and margin requirements, based on unit cost or "standard cost" figures, would provide the price floor.

Given the focus on, and need for, health care reform and cost containment, an agent that can deliver documented cost savings should (in ideal circumstances) be well received. One must look to other issues as well, however, to ensure the acceptance of this argument. The reimbursement and public policy environments will both affect this.

The following key questions relate to the value of the therapy:

1. What does this disorder cost the health care system and society?
2. What is the potential to reduce this cost with the new product?
3. What information will be needed to document and demonstrate any savings?
4. What is the potential of this product to increase costs but improve outcomes?

THE DECISION-MAKING PROCESS

The specific decision maker for the use of the agent plays a large role in the effectiveness of any pricing approach. Products that will be used primarily on an in-patient basis will be subjected to significant price scrutiny, as the institutional market is, perhaps, the most price-sensitive single pharmaceutical market. Because of the influence of multiple decision makers, including pharmacy directors and hospital administrators, the cost of any new agent will be considered carefully before it is adopted. Several studies have shown that clinical pharmacists, through various outreach and educational efforts, can bring about a significant change in physician prescribing behavior.[8,9,10,11] Lazarus and Smith (1988) reported that 52 percent of pharmacist interventions in response to reviews of prescriptions written in an Alabama medical center resulted in changes in medications.[12] That pharmacists can, and do, intervene in and influence the prescribing decision, then, is well-established. Their potential role in the use of a new product must be seriously considered.

In the outpatient setting, the practitioner can often choose therapies without regard to cost. Not that an outpatient drug is not subject to price sensitivity—the growth of managed care in the United States, local fundholders in the United Kingdom, local budgets in Germany, and other initiatives elsewhere have the potential to increase the level of price sensitivity over time.

Primary care physicians are often more "risk averse" than are their specialized colleagues, and they are unlikely to adopt a new medication as rapidly as would a neurologist or cardiologist.[13] New agents whose use will be limited to specialists are unlikely to come under any price scrutiny by the prescriber, since specialists tend to be less concerned with (or aware of) the costs of the treatments they order. It stands to reason that they would be less likely to receive feedback on drug costs from patients than would primary care physicians, who see the patients more regularly and are more likely to operate under systems that force them to bear (or share) the costs of their decisions.

Unfortunately, another consideration in this area is the potential for competition by and with prescribing physicians. In several cases, the use of a new agent is a direct "threat" to a procedure relied upon by one or more physician specialties. Routine use of some thrombolytic agents has been resisted by vascular surgeons, who may perceive the drugs as threats to their own livelihoods. Studies comparing thrombolytic use with vascular surgery are interesting in that those performed by vascular surgeons tend to conclude that surgery is not only safer and more effective but also less costly than the use of thrombolytics alone. Studies performed by radiologists and other nonsurgeons, however, show the opposite. While the situation is, as yet, not resolved, several more studies will be done to clarify the issue. This lack of resolution has allowed many decision makers to assume that the prices of thrombolytics are too high, without benefit of adequate documentation.

The key questions regarding decision-making processes in the marketplace are as follows:

1. What role does price play in the decision to prescribe, dispense, consume, or purchase drugs in this category?
2. How likely are prescribers to receive negative feedback on the cost of the drug?

DISEASE CHARACTERISTICS

The characteristics of the disease itself can provide some of the most valuable guidance in establishing a pricing strategy. Experience shows that disorders of an acute nature, such as minor infectious diseases and pain due to injury, tend not to be accompanied by price sensitivity. Patients receiving a prescription for an antibiotic or analgesic usually receive no refills and often do not follow up with the physician. Even in situations in which the patient pays the full cost of the prescription, this appears to hold true. For chronic disorders, however, patients pay the price every month and often complain to the prescribing physician about the cost of medications. In the United States, retail pharmacists, for competitive reasons, usually apply lower markups to chronically used medications than to those for acute therapy.[14]

Research indicates that this could have an additional dimension—that of the symptoms of the disease.[15] Physicians appear to overestimate the cost of medications that treat chronic, asymptomatic diseases, such as hypertension, and underestimate the cost of medications that treat more symptomatic disorders, such as arthritis and acute infections. It has been postulated that this is due to the type of patient feedback received by the physician. A patient paying $1.00 each day to treat a disease he or she does not feel, such as hypertension, should be expected to complain of the cost more than a patient whose NSAID is relieving the pain of arthritis and allowing him or her to lead a more normal life.

Thus, it is likely that the prescriber will overestimate the cost of a product if it treats a relatively asymptomatic chronic disorder and generates a large amount of negative feedback. This overestimation may result in fewer prescriptions. Figure 7.4 graphically portrays the general findings of a study of physicians' price estimates.

These are the key questions concerning disease characteristics:

1. Will the symptoms or severity of the disorder affect price sensitivity?
2. What is the position of the disease on the payer's, provider's, or public's "radar screen"?

THE REIMBURSEMENT ENVIRONMENT

In highly regulated health care systems, such as many European systems, reimbursement and pricing are nearly synonymous—the price is what the agency is willing to pay. Care must be exercised in dealing with these agencies, and it is worthwhile to remember that success depends on being a

	SYMPTOMATIC	ASYMPTOMATIC
ACUTE	Tendency to underestimate actual cost. Average estimate 35 percent below actual. Examples: antibiotics, analgesics.	N/A
CHRONIC	Generally the most accurate estimates. Examples: NSAIDSs, anti-ulcerants	Tendency to overestimate, often by 100 percent or more. Examples: Antihypertensives, hormone replacement.

FIGURE 7.4. Physician's Price Estimates and the Nature of the Disorder (*Source:* E. M. Kolassa, "Physician's Perceptions of Drug Prices and Their Effect on the Prescribing Decision," *Journal of Research in Pharmaceutical Economics,* 6:1, 1995.)

"price maker," and not a "price taker," in such markets. Understanding the needs and motives of the reimbursement authorities, and their history with specific firms, often determines the difference between receiving a good price or a not-so-good one.

The reimbursement environment must always be considered. Agents used in the inpatient setting are often reimbursed as part of the total hospital charge. Costly agents, or those perceived as so, could be restricted in their use, either by the hospital or the insurers. Many agents are placed on prior authorization lists in hospitals, and their use is restricted to certain physicians. Although these situations are not yet routine, economic studies that support the price and reimbursement assistance programs may relieve some pressures and allow a price higher than would otherwise be accepted by the market.

Insurance reimbursement status has been shown to affect drug product selection in the inpatient setting. Some researchers have found that patients with comprehensive coverage receive more, and more expensive, medications than those with less adequate insurance coverage.[16]

Finally, a major consideration in the reimbursement environment is the effect of managed care formularies. Securing placement on these formularies has often required discounting from list prices. Should a significant portion of the potential market be subject to such formulary management, and this portion is growing rapidly, setting a price that is acceptable in the "open" market may render the product overpriced in managed settings. Appropriate discounts to some segments may be useful in these cases, but the legislative and judicial moves favoring "uniform" pricing for pharmaceuticals may make this more difficult in the near future. It may be wise to establish the appropriate price for managed care and use this price for all market segments.

The key questions about the reimbursement environment are these:

1. How is this product reimbursed?
2. Who stands to make or lose money with the new product?
3. Are any elements of reimbursement in this area out of the ordinary?

COMPANY NEEDS

Although the cost of goods and company-established minimum selling margins play a role in the establishment of a price floor, other company-specific issues must also be addressed. New research investment or activities that are expected to require significant amounts of funding might well necessitate the charging of a higher price for agents about to be launched, providing the higher price would not negatively affect the sales of the product.

Conversely, a new agent may be seen as simply providing the company with experience in a therapeutic category prior to the introduction, some years later, of an agent that is believed to be superior. In this case, a low-price strategy on an agent without significant advantages could allow the company to develop this experience and important relationships with prescribers and key thought leaders in this market.

Finally, an innovative pricing strategy that may offer savings or guarantees or some other feature could result in positive press coverage for the company, and this may be seen as valuable for investor or customer relations.

The following key questions concern company needs:

1. How vital is this new product to the future of the company, or to a current franchise?
2. Will the pricing of this product complicate, or be complicated by, the pricing of other company products?

COMPANY ABILITIES

The ability and willingness of the company to support the pricing strategy must always be considered. A high price in a sensitive market requires significant resources, by way of economic studies and, often, senior management time, to alleviate much of the price resistance. Similarly, a low-price strategy in an outpatient market is likely to cost more in promotional expenses than would parity pricing, if the strategy is to be successful. This is because physicians, as has been previously mentioned, tend not to respond to low-price appeals. A successful low-price approach requires significant promotional expenditures to saturate the market with the message that the product is less costly and to induce physicians to consider cost.

Prescribing physicians do not actively seek out price information, and often they do not respond to low prices even when they are aware of them.[17] A penetration strategy requires greater promotional coverage and more creative selling messages in order to instill a sense of economic responsibility (or guilt) in prescribers than would be required of the approach of simply charging whatever the competition charges.

Whether you choose a price that is significantly above or below the prevailing prices in the market, top management must be willing to spend the time and the money necessary to support the pricing strategy.

These are the key questions concerning company abilities:

1. What would be the cost to the company of a pricing mistake for this product?
2. Is senior management prepared to address controversy if the price is seen by the public as too high?
3. Will senior management supply the necessary financial support to make an innovative approach to pricing successful?

PUBLIC POLICY CONSIDERATIONS

Last, but certainly not least, is the public policy environment. For the foreseeable future, the response and actions of government officials and patient advocates must be considered when setting a price. Criticism by one of these individuals, no matter how unfounded, can result in severe limits on the potential success of a new drug. Once a "working price" has been developed for a new agent, if it is a potential target for the attention of a highly placed critic, constituent, or other individual, investigate ways to avoid the problem or be prepared to address the issue directly with the critic.

The key public policy question is this:

1. What is the likelihood that the price of this product will attract the attention of the press or legislators?

These factors and issues will affect every new pricing decision made. Figure 7.5 provides a summary of these issues in schematic form, with the final price at the center of the chart. Note that the public policy environment surrounds the other considerations. This must be a major consideration in every pharmaceutical pricing decision.[18]

PUBLIC POLICY		
Competition	Disease Characteristics	Value of Therapy
Prescriber Decision Making	PRICE	Patient Characteristics
Company Needs	Reimbursement Environment	Company Abilities

FIGURE 7.5. Pricing Considerations for New Pharmaceuticals

SUMMARY

Pharmaceutical pricing is a complex area with no simple answers to the important questions. Although each pricing decision is unique, many issues are common to every decision. Failure to address each of the elements discussed in this chapter can lead to poor pricing decisions.

Chapter 8

The Pharmaceutical Pricing Environment

Mick Kolassa

The pricing of any product is problematic. Competing objectives drive the price in different directions simultaneously. Senior managers and corporate headquarters often want the highest prices possible to maximize profits, while local managers and sales personnel argue for lower prices to ease the task of selling. These issues are the same regardless of the product under consideration, but the problems grow when it is a pharmaceutical agent that must be priced. For pharmaceuticals, the typical buying patterns are dislocated, as the user of the product (the patient) is not the one who selects it, and the individual making the selection does not, usually, bear any financial burden for the choice. Pharmaceutical pricing on a global basis is even more complicated, as managers must deal with different regulatory systems, each seeking to minimize drug expenditures.

One must keep in mind that *price is the only element of the marketing mix that produces revenue;* the others produce costs. The task of price setting requires balancing these many demands, attempting to please several different constituencies, but it must also be consistent with the objectives and the message of the marketing program. To accomplish this, managers must question old methods and learn new ones. Too often, prices are set based on simply copying the prices of a competitor, or by following the findings of a marketing research study. As the pricing decision becomes more and more important, those charged with recommending prices must quickly identify the most important questions and issues and purposefully reach decisions that are aimed at achieving a solid objective—the best definition of an "optimum" price.

Three distinct forces are exerting a powerful effect on the pharmaceutical pricing environment:

1. Large, organized buyers wield power over pharmaceutical marketers, demanding lower prices, proven value, or both.
2. Markets have become more competitive, as new agents enter the markets at a faster rate, causing many firms to turn to pricing as a means of maintaining or garnering sales.

3. Governments at all levels have zeroed in on pharmaceutical prices as a political issue, introducing, and even passing, new legislation aimed at controlling the prices of medicines.

These forces have created an environment in which pricing mistakes are costlier than ever before. In the near past, a firm that realized it had under-priced its new product could make corrections in a rapid time frame, bringing the price up to levels equal to its competitors. Today such price increases bring protests from legislators, threats of formulary exclusion from managed care organizations, and new contracting activities from competitors who are eager to take advantage of any misstep. Every pharmaceutical pricing decision confronts the marketer with a "trilemma."

More than 70 percent of outpatient prescriptions are now covered by some form of third-party payment, concentrating buying power among a smaller number of customers. In the late 1980s, most firms established account management groups, to market (or, rather, sell) to managed care and other buyers perceived to be large and influential. These account managers then set out to define and describe managed care and its growing influence. Because selling to managed care was their job, they made sure the company took this emerging market very seriously—and overstated the importance of managed care in product selection.

Convinced that managed care organizations care only about price, it became virtually impossible in some firms to resist discounting to this segment, and account managers continually provided horror stories of closed formularies and "NDC lockouts"* that required huge discounts to ensure product use. Most firms in the United States have responded to these threats by offering discounts in exchange for favorable treatment and generally have not realized the gains they had expected.

Although it is true that managed care now accounts for more than 50 percent of the outpatient prescription market in the United States, data from IMS indicate that few of the managed care plans have actually restricted the use of branded pharmaceuticals. In fact, there are indications that the growth of managed care is responsible for a significant proportion of the growth of sales for branded pharmaceutical products over the past few years, and that the discounts provided these payers have had little, if any, effect on product use.

---

*An "NDC lockout" is a mechanism by which pharmaceutical benefits managers (PBMs) and other benefits processors try explicitly to prevent a prescription for a nonformulary drug from being filled by preventing the processing of the claim. Because the NDC (national drug code) number is used for most claims processing, locking out the NDC number would, in theory, prevent the claim from being processed. Many providers, however, have found ways to bypass these lockouts and have the claims processed and paid.

Some managed care organizations, specifically the staff models, do have the ability to affect sales because they take possession of the products and dispense the prescriptions that are written by employee physicians. However, this type of managed care organization (MCO) is declining in importance, losing "covered lives" to network, IPA, and PPO model systems, which contract with physicians rather than employ them. It has been estimated that the average physician in the United States participates in more than three such plans, which dilutes the influence on any one MCO. More important, those working with the majority of these plans, including the pharmaceutical benefits managers (PBMs), do not have the capability of significantly affecting product use. It is estimated that only 17 percent of outpatient prescriptions are covered by plans that can have any meaningful affect on the sales of specific branded products. The rest either simply allow the reimbursement for prescriptions, with no restrictions at all, or offer incentives to dispense generics when out-of-patent drugs are prescribed. This means that the bulk of the business for branded products is effectively free of MCO constraints.

The recent implementation of three-tier copayment schemes by many MCOs as a means of controlling prescription use does have the potential to affect product use. But there is no set configuration for these programs, with each organization establishing different parameters for its system. Some researchers have raised the issue of potential harm to patients from these programs, which shift the ultimate responsibility solely to the patient. A necessary and appropriate prescription that had formerly been "managed" through prior authorization but is now shifted to a higher tier with a substantial copay may go unfilled, and the patient's condition will deteriorate because of lack of treatment. The jury is out on these programs, for the verdicts on their effect on patients, their effect on product use, and their effect on the pharmacy budget. Still, many firms have set goals of favorable placement of their products on lower tiers and have chosen to "buy their way" to those tiers with lower prices.

Most firms have been eager to contract with MCOs based on the threat of their ability to control use. Pharmaceutical marketers have bemoaned the shrinkage of the unrestricted "cash market," where patients pay for their own prescriptions, believing that this market offers greater opportunities for pricing flexibility and a higher rate of profit. This segment declined from over 50 percent of the market just two years ago to less than 25 percent in 2000. Yet this segment appears to be much more price sensitive than the "managed care market," which uses generics at a lower level than does the cash segment and offers costlier agents higher shares than does the cash market. But how can this be?

Two facts must be understood: First, when the patient must pay for the prescription, he or she must be sensitive to the cost, as the ability to pay will determine the likelihood of the purchase. The bulk of the cash segment is senior citizens on fixed incomes, who tend to use more prescription drugs than do younger patients. They request products with generic alternatives and lower-cost agents. A patient covered by a prescription plan, just as patients in most European nations, cares nothing about the cost of the medications. Physicians routinely ask patients whether they have prescription coverage, knowing that a "prescription card" means that the patient will have the prescription filled, regardless of the cost.

But what about "managed care," will they not intervene? The head of pharmacy for a major plan that covers nearly 10 million people stated that the most common question asked in his operation is, "How do we deny payment for this claim?" This question is asked because the prescription for the "restricted" drug has already been dispensed. Retail pharmacists know that they can override most restrictions, fill the prescription, and receive reimbursement. The plans tend to focus on reducing use of big-ticket items, such as Prilosec and Prozac, in their attempts to achieve savings. They simply cannot control hundreds of thousands of physicians, 50,000 pharmacies, and millions of patients, not to mention the thousands of prescription products that achieve sales lower than the blockbusters. Over half of MCOs find that their efforts at cost control amount to nothing more than asking physicians to consider costs while prescribing.

More important, competition among managed care plans has become intense, and the appearance of restrictiveness on the part of a plan, manifested by refusing to pay for prescriptions ordered by their doctors, results in dissatisfied members, who will look for a less restrictive plan. Member satisfaction has become a key performance measure among managed care plans, and losing members while trying to restrict pharmaceuticals, which account for approximately 10 percent of MCO spending, makes little sense.

Discounts to MCOs have been declining, mainly because of the costly requirement that equal discounts be given to the federal government, which accounts for approximately 15 percent of sales, and the price discrimination suit against manufacturers. Many, but not all, companies have reigned in their discounts to managed care in response to these external stimuli. Those who have reduced discounting, however, have discovered that lower discounts often bring higher net sales, with little impact on unit use.

NEW PRODUCT PRICING

Many pharmaceutical firms have adopted the tactic of setting prices for new products at or below the prices of competitive agents, apparently in the belief that lower prices lead to increased unit sales. Although this practice has become generally accepted, no definitive evidence supports that lower prices have proved to be financially prudent for firms. Products such as

Lipitor and Celebrex, whose lower-than-expected prices have garnered much attention (especially among pharmaceutical marketers), are perceived by the majority of their loyal prescribers as being the most costly agents in their respective classes.[1] Prescribers are often unaware of the "price advantages" of popular agents and simply assume they are more costly if they perform better than similar products.

Although some firms appear to believe that setting prices somewhat lower than competitive products may provide some benefit, no evidence suggests that such pricing helps improve the performance of these products in the marketplace, makes prescribers or patients more satisfied with them, or affects the degree of scrutiny with which critics address the products. This final point is discussed in the next section.

PHARMACEUTICAL PRICING AND PUBLIC POLICY

Many public forces, including liberal legislators, national news media, and retail pharmacies, have attacked industry pricing practices, using the courts or legislation to remedy real and imagined problems. Some legislators at the federal level, such as Representatives Waxman and Stark and Senators Kennedy and Wyden, have long records as critics and opponents of the pharmaceutical industry. Others, such as Representative Allen, have recently emerged as vocal critics. On the Republican side of this aisle, criticism of the industry's pricing practices emerged from Representatives Coburn and Gansky.

Recently, forty-five members of Congress formed the Prescription Drug Task Force, cochaired by Arkansas Representative Marion Berry. This group of mostly Democratic legislators has focused on prescription medicines, and their costs, as one of the major issues on their agenda. On their Web site (http://www.house.gov/berry/prescriptiondrugs/index.htm), they state their purpose as follows:

> The Prescription Drug Task Force is working to bring focus to issues involving the cost and availability of prescription drugs. The Task Force pursues policies that will improve the quality of life for seniors and other consumers who are forced to choose between food, medicine, and paying their bills.

The members of this group take advantage of every opportunity to criticize the pricing practices of the pharmaceutical industry. They also conduct and publicize many "studies" that are also critical of the industry, misstating many key aspects of the marketplace as a means to bring about more criticism. Among the most blatant of the "studies" was a series of reports released early in 1999 that claimed to discover that seniors are overcharged several hundred percent for their prescriptions relative to the best customers of pharmaceutical firms. These reports were published to coincide with, and provide support for, Representative Allen's bill, which would make Federal Supply Schedule prices available to all seniors.

These and other critics can be counted on to continue to put pressure on the pharmaceutical industry and its pricing practices. The political section of this report details much of the legislation, and its history, aimed at pharmaceutical pricing.

The pricing of pharmaceuticals will continue to be closely scrutinized by regulators, the media, and public "advocates." It is incumbent on the industry, and all its members, to make pricing decisions in full awareness of this scrutiny. Pricing decisions must be supported with arguments that emphasize the value delivered by new products, rather than the cost of research. This means that the firms must have a better understanding of the value they deliver, and the financial effects of their products on the health care system. Such information will not silence all criticism but will provide firms with a more defensible position.

PRICING ON PURPOSE

Many of the problems encountered in the domain of pharmaceutical pricing have occurred because those involved in the decision were not proficient in the field of pharmaceutical pricing, and because erroneous, but often logical, assumptions were made concerning the role and effects of price in the market. Pricing mistakes emerge from failure to consider all the potential consequences of pricing actions—failing to "price on purpose."

Pricing on purpose means that each price considered has been evaluated for its effect on the health care system and members of that system and balanced with a realistic assessment of the willingness and ability of those members to take action. As the cost of pricing mistakes increases, the need to price on purpose grows as well.

Chapter 9

Pharmaceutical Pricing in Practice

Mick Kolassa

> ... pricing is the moment of truth—all of marketing comes to focus in the pricing decision.
>
> Raymond Corey[1]

Pricing, as with many aspects of business, can simultaneously be overwhelmingly complex and surprisingly simple. As discussed in the two previous chapters, there are many different facets of the environment to think about, many elements to consider, when arriving at an appropriate pricing decision. The chronicle of pharmaceutical pricing is filled with examples of firms taking simplistic approaches to pricing when more deliberate consideration was needed, and of cases when firms agonized over pricing decisions that were really quite simple. There are also many examples of good, even great, pricing decisions in the pharmaceutical market, and some of these will be examined here, along with some decisions that, in hindsight, were not so great. Why is this important? Failure to develop and execute an appropriate pricing strategy usually results in the failure of the firm to capture an appropriate share of the value of the product, which translates into lower profits.

Most experts in the field of pricing agree that very few people in the pharmaceutical industry (or any industry, for that matter) pay close enough attention to their prices. To be certain, account managers, contract managers, and others spend a great deal of time bringing prices down, but very few people are charged with ensuring that the prices charged are appropriate—and profitable.

The failure to manage pricing within the industry is a symptom of a much larger problem, one that is also shared with other industries: the rampant lack of knowledge about the market and the competition. It is astonishing how little product managers, marketing researchers, and their superiors know about the markets in which they compete. Failure to understand customers and competitors is certain to lead to poor pricing decisions. This failure in understanding is compounded by the failure of many to learn and apply basic pricing principles in pharmaceutical markets.

NEW PRODUCT PRICING TRENDS

The typical approach to pharmaceutical marketing itself has fed this problem because those involved in the marketing of pharmaceuticals tend to focus on their products and to view every aspect of the market through the filter of their own impression of their products. This is the reason many promotional campaigns focus on a drug's mechanism of action rather than its end benefit. But what the market values, and what should be priced, is not the mechanism of action or unique chemical structure, but the outcome of the therapy, the end result, and how that differs from competitive products. When a product delivers better outcomes, it deserves to be priced at a premium relative to competitors. Should the outcomes not differ from competitive products, a parity price is in order. Worse relative outcomes should be reflected by a price that is lower than prevailing levels.

Setting the price according to the relative value of the product is pricing at its most basic, and most logical. This basic price-quality relationship has, traditionally, not been used to guide pharmaceutical pricing decisions. In 1977, Duncan Reekie, an economic researcher in health care markets, noted that pharmaceutical companies appeared to believe their markets were much more sensitive to price differences than they, in fact, were. Recent pricing decisions by many firms imply that Dr. Reekie's observation continues to hold true more than twenty years later. Figure 7.3 in Chapter 7 displays graphically the pattern most firms have exhibited in their pricing—to the detriment of profits (see p. 192).

Many, if not most, new pharmaceutical products entering into competitive markets are priced at or below the prices of their leading competitors. One explanation for this is Reekie's observation that the companies believe their markets to be sensitive, and responsive, to price differences. It must be assumed that companies which choose to set a price equal to or lower than their competitors are seeking either to make the price a "nonissue" in the marketplace (in the case of pricing parity) or to use a low price as a competitive advantage, thereby securing higher unit sales levels. The cost to the firm of these decisions can be measured in the opportunity cost of failing to price a product at a level commensurate with its value.

Leading products that have recently been launched at prices below, equal to, and above their primary competitors are listed here.

Products priced below competitive levels

- Lipitor
- Prevacid

- Baycol
- Allegra

Products entering the market at competitive parity

- Diovan
- Avapro

Products priced at premiums compared to their major competitors

- Vioxx
- Flonase

A more thorough examination of the pricing of recently launched products is presented in Table 9.1. The first of the new products is Lescol, by Novartis. Much has been written and said about Lescol, which may be the only successfully discounted product to hit the U.S. market thus far. As we will see, it cannot be argued that discount prices have been especially helpful to any of the other products under investigation that appeared to attempt this tactic. The Lescol discount of nearly 50 percent and its relative share of

TABLE 9.1. Recent New Product Launch Prices

Product (Launch) Comparator	New Rx Share	Price at Launch (AWP)	Price at Launch (Ex-Factory)	Difference @ AWP	Difference @ Ex-Factory
Lescol (4/94)	15.6%	$1.02	$0.85	– 49%	– 46%
Mevacor	29.7%	$1.98	$1.59		
Univasc (6/95)	0.4%	$0.50	$0.40	– 50%	– 50%
Vasotec	27.0%	$1.00	$0.80		
Prevacid (6/95)	3.4%	$3.25	$2.64	– 10%	– 13%
Prilosec	22.0%	$3.63	$3.03		
Zyrtec (1/96)	N/A	$1.71	$1.37	– 11%	– 15%
Claritin	53.0%	$1.93	$1.61		
Effexor (2/94)	4.9%	$2.00	$1.60	– 4%	– 8%
Prozac	27.8%	$2.09	$1.74		
Serzone (1/95)	3.2%	$1.66	$1.38	– 23%	– 23%
Prozac	27.8%	$2.16	$1.80		
Flonase (1/95)	15.6%	$38.88	$32.40	20%	20%
Vancenase AQ	28.8%	$32.40	$27.00		
Rhinocort (6/94)	8.1%	$27.00	$22.50	– 13%	– 13%
Vancenase AQ	28.8%	$31.01	$25.84		

the market (15 percent after its first year on the market versus 30 percent for its major competitor, rendering a competitive index of 0.5 [.15/.3]) will be used for comparative purposes. Achieving a share equal to half its biggest competitor's is a major accomplishment for the fourth product into a market, and Sandoz's (producer and manufacturer of Lescol) combination of low price and intensive, high-spending promotion was essential in achieving this.

Univasc, the Schwarz Pharma angiotension-converting enzyme (ACE) inhibitor, was also launched at a 50 percent discount. This product, being the ninth ACE inhibitor brand to enter the market, would not be expected to capture a significant share, but even with its massive discount, Univasc has failed to achieve even a half point of share. The ACE inhibitor market is a "loud" one, with a considerable amount of promotional noise. I believe that the lackluster performance of Univasc is testament to the observation that a product still requires a compelling clinical reason for being prescribed, and a low price will not overcome this shortcoming. A successful low-price strategy requires a significant amount of promotional spending—and a fair amount of luck. Univasc, apparently, has neither. Univasc's competitive index of 0.01 (one-fiftieth that of Lescol) is testament to the need to do more than simply have a low price.

TAP Pharmaceutical Product's proton pump inhibitor Prevacid is the next product to review. Launched at a 10 percent discount to Prilosec, Astra Merck's pioneer product that is on its way to becoming the biggest pharmaceutical brand in history, many believed that a significant discount for Prevacid would be disastrous to the Astra Merck product. TAP, however, seems to have understood the costly mistake of deep discount pricing and chose to price only slightly below Prilosec, allowing the representatives to claim that it is a little less costly, but not attempting to devalue the therapeutic class (and leave a lot of money on the table while doing so). Prevacid's competitive index of 0.15 is respectable, but not fantastic.

Another product with potential is Pfizer's Zyrtec, which competes with Schering's Claritin in the nonsedating antihistamine market. Pfizer, too, chose a small discount (11 percent) versus the competition, essentially removing price as an obstacle to sales (a choice that will be addressed later). Although the share data used for this analysis were collected too early to be of use in assessing Zyrtec's performance, many expect Zyrtec to capture a substantial share of the market, as much as half that of Claritin's. This success, again, comes from promotional might, not deep discounting.

Next we will consider two products that entered a very large, competitive market: antidepressants. Wyeth-Ayerst's Effexor and Bristol-Myers Squibb (BMS)'s Serzone entered the market about a year apart, but miles apart in terms of pricing strategy. Effexor was launched at essentially the same price as Prozac, the biggest competitor, with a discount of less than 10 percent.

Serzone, which was launched later, came to market priced 23 percent below Prozac. Although Effexor has earned a higher share of prescriptions than has Serzone, its year-long head start makes for an unfair comparison between the two. One would expect, however, that if the market were price sensitive, Serzone should be enjoying a much higher share than it is. Serzone's competitive index of .115 compares with Effexor's index of .17. Effexor's sales are 50 percent higher than Serzone's, and its price is 20 percent higher, a combination that argues against the efficacy of price in moving products.

Another market with similar competitive entries is the inhalable steroids. Schering's Vancenase leads that market with a share of nearly 29 percent. Astra launched Rhinocort into this market in mid-1994, at a 13 percent discount, achieving a respectable 8 percent share, for a competitive index of .275. Glaxo then launched Flonase into this market at a substantial premium of 20 percent over Vancenase and has captured a 15.6 percent share in its first year, a competitive index of .54. The unarguable success of this product, with unit sales nearly twice those of Rhinocort's at a price about 40 percent higher, again argues against the routine use of price as a selling point.

Because we are not privy to the reasoning behind the pricing of the products that have been discussed here, it is difficult to evaluate the success of their approaches. From this sample, however, we see more high-price successes than low-price successes, and no high-price "failures." The role of price in the success of a pharmaceutical product may be more related to the firm's confidence in the product and its ability to market it than in a physician's decision to prescribe it. Some firms, as stated earlier, apparently believe that a price slightly below the competition's will provide them with some advantage, or at least help them to avoid a potential pricing problem.

The decision to price a new product 5 to 15 percent below the competition, and thus avoid pricing problems altogether, might be considered a lazy approach to pricing. Essentially, it is an admission that the competitor has already set a good price, and the firm has chosen to avoid problems by parking below it. It could also be construed as an admission that the new product is not quite as good as, or at least no better than, what is already on the market. If that is the truth, then it may not be a bad choice. If the team selling the product believes they have any clinical advantages, however, the price chosen for the product argues against any such suggestion.

The benefits of such a choice may be in peace of mind, but it must be admitted that, for most of these products, a 10 percent discount represents an opportunity cost of 10 percent of sales.

Deep discounting, in the 20 percent-plus range, can be construed as either a bold move or an act of desperation. One could conclude that Novartis exhibited boldness, with a deep price differential and a big budget to sell the advantage of its low price. Others who have used deep discounts may not deserve the appellation of boldness, as these prices appear to have been set in hopes that the lower prices alone would sell the products—and this did not work.

Some, if not most, products that were launched into the market at premiums compared to their primary competitors have done quite well. In fact, one is hard-pressed to identify any recently launched products that could be considered to be handicapped by a high price. Perhaps the best recent example of such a product is Merck's cyclooxygenase-2 (COX-2) inhibitor Vioxx, which entered the market six months after Searle's (now Pharmacia's) Celebrex and was priced at a premium. Within a year Vioxx had garnered sales nearly equal to those of Celebrex, and at this writing it had surpassed it in total prescriptions. The premium, apparently, has had no negative effect on the sales of Vioxx, and the slight price advantage of Celebrex does not appear to sway the market in its direction.

Those who understand pricing make informed, and profitable, decisions; those who fear pricing make mistakes!

THE NEED TO PRICE ON PURPOSE

The failure to take pricing seriously results in lower profit margins—it is that simple. Many firms appear to have surrendered their own pricing authority to their competitors or their customers—neither of whom are at all concerned about the financial success of these firms. They may, in fact, benefit from their demise. Companies must make serious commitments to invest in pricing skills, and to use prices to capture the value of their products, not to lower their value. Profitable pricing requires constant attention and continual learning, and it requires an understanding within the firm that the role of price is to secure the financial well-being of the firm, not as a means to move more unit volume.

SECTION IV:
PLACE

Chapter 10

Principles of Place, Channel Systems, and Channel Specialists

Bruce Siecker

INTRODUCTION

You can discover, test, and market the most amazing "wonder drug" of the world, but if it is not in the right place when the patient needs it, it will not do anyone any good.

A core objective of marketing is to make sure that the right amount of the right product reaches the final customer when it is needed or wanted. Sounds simple, but it is not.

The choices and activities necessary to make sure that the right amount of products are available when and where they are needed constitute the place part of the four Ps of marketing. In economic terms, place has to do with the utility[1] or usefulness that a customer derives from having possession or use of the

- *right product,*
- at the *right time,*
- in the *right form* (color, size, shape, flavor, composition, grade, class, fashion, texture, etc.), and
- in the *right amount.*

The ways to accomplish these aims are infinitely combinable and constitute the challenge of managing place in the marketing equation.

CHALLENGES OF MANAGING PLACE

Managing place involves three major challenges. The first major challenge in managing place is that the assortment, form, and quantity of each product needed by a specific customer at a specific place in a given point in time has little, if any, relationship to the amount that can be produced, stored, and shipped economically and efficiently.

Production engineers, for instance, know that manufacturing lines are most efficient when allowed to run for long periods of time—to produce a single strength and type of antibiotic capsule, for instance, for a month at a time, then package it as a single bottle of 500,000 capsules—because changing them over to produce another product is very costly and time-consuming. Although such a choice is obviously untenable, the example serves to demonstrate an equally unrealistic alternative: that is, for the same manufacturer to produce, pack, and ship a single antibiotic capsule directly to an individual pharmacy each time a single patient needs to take a dose. Practical reality lies somewhere between these extremes. Combining the in-gredients to satisfy the marketplace in an effective and affordable manner is the task of marketing.

A second major challenge of managing place is that decisions regarding place tend to have longer-term implications, take longer, and are harder to accomplish and change once they are implemented. For these reasons, place decisions are made less often than those concerning the other three Ps.

A decision to outsource product production, when a company already has a fully functioning, paid-for production facility, is a very complex pro-cess. The effort, risk, and cost for a pharmacy to change its primary pharma-ceutical supplier (a place decision) are much greater than when changing which brand of penicillin it stocks (product decision) or how it will an-nounce a new service to area physicians (a promotion decision). The impor-tance and implications of place choices and decisions are major challenges for managing the marketing function and need to be made carefully.

The third major challenge of managing place lies in the tendency of some marketers to overlook its crucial importance in marketing management. In spite of example after example in which place played a key role in the suc-cess of products, companies, armies, and even national economies, there ap-pears to be a natural tendency to favor the other three Ps over place.

The longtime success of Frito-Lay, the largest marketer of snack foods, is attributed more to its phenomenal record of keeping its products freshly and fully stocked (100 percent of the time) in every store, restaurant, and vend-ing machine possible, than to its products per se. Quite simply, Frito-Lay outdistributes its competitors.

Many companies (e.g., L.L.Bean, Dell Computer, Merck-Medco) owe much of their success to the skill, dependability, and efficiency of overnight delivery services—UPS, FedEx, Roadway RPS, USPS, etc.—that allowed access to much larger geographic areas and target markets at an affordable cost. Much of the World Wide Web (WWW) is nothing more than a giant catalog with keystroke order entry convenience. These are all facets of place.

Military historians agree that many battles fought by U.S. armed forces (e.g., World War II's Battle of the Bulge, Gulf War's 100-hour Desert Storm) were decided more because of superior U.S. logistics—the ability to move people, weapons, and supplies to where they were needed on the battlefield—than exceptional strategy, tactics, training, personnel, or equipment.

Business historians now attribute a major share of the unparalleled business growth of the U.S. economy in the past forty-five years to the foresight of former President Dwight Eisenhower, who insisted that Congress pass the Interstate Highway Act in the mid-1950s. The interstate highway system was a substantial and highly unusual investment in transportation infrastructure that produced the single most efficient transportation network in the world. In essence, the federal interstate highway system was, and still is, a competitive advantage for the United States, in that goods and services get to the right place faster and less expensively than in any other country in the world.

Much of what constitutes place issues involves discrepancies—of form, quantity, time, place, possession—which are best thought of as mismatches that marketers can alter to meet specific customer needs. For example, assume that a customer needs a knee brace in Oxford, Mississippi; the local pharmacy only has a wrist brace; the closest knee brace is in Jackson, more than two hours away by automobile. The knee brace gathering dust in Jackson is a medium; the Oxford customer needs an extra large. One of the components of the Jackson knee brace is nylon; it turns out the customer is allergic to nylon. All of these mismatches (though admittedly overstated here to make a point) exist every day in the marketplace. It is the marketer's job first to recognize then to rectify such discrepancies (and minimize them in the future), so that the customer is satisfied *and* the marketer stays in business.

Place Discrepancies

These mismatches are *place discrepancies* that few people ever notice or think much about. Why? Because thousands of decisions and actions by tens of thousands of people are involved in producing, buying, shipping, and displaying goods and services needed in local markets. Marketing involves managing discrepancies of key customer utilities, including the following:

- *Accumulation*—amassing enough product in a local market to meet demand for as long as it takes to get more, plus provide a cushion, i.e., extra quantity if demand is above average (as may be the case during extreme weather, in an unusually bad flu season, or with unexpected popularity of an item). Besides the cost of the products themselves, accumulated products cost money to hold, i.e., holding costs, which is one reason why cushion or safety stocks cannot be unlimited.

- *Assortment (sorting)*—the degree to which accumulation involves or requires a variety of products to meet the demand for choices and varying needs. Different products have widely different assortment needs; e.g., shoes, jewelry, and pharmaceuticals are high-assortment products, whereas coffee shops, photocopy centers, and self-serve gasoline stations have relatively few different items.
- *Allocation*—economics and space placing limits on how much and how many different kinds of products a marketer can accumulate and assort. At any one given time, more than 500,000 health products (drugs, health and beauty aids, etc.) are available. Few, if any, pharmacies ever have more than 20,000 different items on hand at any given time; most have about 5,000 to 8,000. The choices of which items to stock to meet local needs involve allocation.
- *Breaking bulk*—correcting discrepancies in terms of size, amount, or quantity. As products move from manufacturer to final customer, each handler may break bulk. A manufacturer may ship forty-eight cases of twenty-four bottles of antihistamines to one wholesale drug distributor because that is what the distributor needs to meet customer (pharmacy) demand. The pharmacy, to fill a prescription, will order a bottle of 100 capsules of the antihistamine. The distributor sells one bottle at a time to its customer. Assuming a prescription for twenty capsules, the pharmacist counts out and repackages the medicine to dispense it to a specific patient. The process (in both situations) is that of breaking bulk, and it is one of the most important processes in the market mix of many products, including pharmaceuticals.
- *Repackaging*—packaging products differently (type, strength, durability, safety, protectiveness, size, etc.) to meet individual customer needs (and legal and regulatory requirements). Repackaging involves changing a package size or type to increase a product's usefulness. Few people, for example, could deal with (or even use) a whole beef hindquarter, so butchers "repackage" them into meal-size packages of Styrofoam trays and clear plastic wrap. A unique aspect of pharmaceuticals is that they are dispensed in patient-specific quantities or amounts. Pharmacists repackage pharmaceuticals into child-proof, custom-sized quantities and containers with patient-specific labels (and auxiliary labeling and information as necessary).
- *Reformulating*—changing the form of a product to meet the need of the customer. Gasoline refiners engage in reformulation when they refine oil into fuel. Tire manufacturers (rubber and synthetics into tires), bakeries (flour, sugar, and eggs into cakes and pastries), and pharmacies (powders and liquids into creams and ointments) do as well.
- *Disbursement*—movement (distribution) of selected products to defined accumulation points (e.g., warehouses, retail stores, outlet

stores). Disbursement involves moving goods and services closer to the customer.

The marketplace must address and decide fundamental questions involving place functions, including which functions need to occur, which market entity will do which function, how each will be done, and when each function will occur—e.g., at what point in the entire process will products be formulated into their final form? Such questions may seem inconsequential—or foreign to pharmacy and the drug industry—but they are not.

An excellent example of why these place decisions are so important may be found in the history of pharmaceuticals in the United States. In the first half of the twentieth century, pharmacists "compounded" virtually all prescriptions at the time they were dispensed to individual patients. This meant that they formulated various materials into the final form that the patient would use using techniques of compounding. "Inventory" at that time was very limited and consisted primarily of botanical roots, bark, and powders and various refined chemicals, e.g., sulfur, zinc oxide, etc. There were few, if any, ready-to-use dosage forms with the exception of simple topical powders and plant materials that were steeped in hot water for various ailments.

By the 1940s, pharmaceutical manufacturers began to produce "finished dosage forms," i.e., specific drugs produced in a form meant to be used directly by patients, in large-scale production lines using tablet-making and capsule-filling machines. The finished dosage forms—tablets, capsules, syrups, elixirs, creams, ointments, drops, sprays, etc.—were in turn sold to pharmacies. Subsequently, pharmacists dispensed them intact to patients (as tablets, capsules, syrups, premixed/prepackaged creams and ointments, etc.).

Although many more patients could be accommodated faster and at lower overall cost, which meant higher pharmacy sales and pharmacists' incomes, this change produced major upheaval in the industry. What might seem to have been an inconsequential change today actually took many years to occur and resulted in a great deal of doomsaying, debate, and consternation along the way. Even today, a vocal, activist minority in pharmacy supports and encourages a compounding countertrend. Pharmacist compounding, it is said, better provides for special patient needs. It is also a means of creating a specialty or niche practice of pharmacy and getting reimbursement by drug plans when commercially available products are not covered.

Most changes in place are neither minor nor easy!

CHANNEL SYSTEMS

Channel systems (a.k.a. *distribution systems, distribution channels,* and *supply chains*) are pathways from product producers (manufacturers, fabricators) to end users. They develop in response to the characteristics and needs of particular products and services, customer needs, and the capabilities and business goals of channel members (various types of businesses that play various roles in a channel system). A channel system is a set of independent, but interacting, and to some extent interdependent, business entities that exist to make products and services conveniently available to consumers and businesses.[2]

Although channel systems appear rigid and static, they are actually evolving and changing all the time. The rate and degree of change in how place is addressed in each industry is usually less than is evident for the other three Ps, but it exists nonetheless.

Efficiency (cost) and effectiveness (customer well served and marketer recovers its costs), along with legal and regulatory requirements and advances in technology, are the guiding forces that define and shape channel systems. Channel systems most often evolve to minimize the number of transactions necessary to serve customers because doing so makes them more efficient, but only if consumers and businesses continue to have convenient access to products and services.

Channel specialists exist to play particular roles within a channel system. Examples include manufacturers, repackagers, brokers, agents, wholesalers, retailers, direct sellers, importer-exporters, and storage and transportation specialists. Each is a specialist in a group of related functions that the channel has determined over time, by trial and error, to be necessary and efficient. The number and types of channel specialists in a channel system vary greatly in different product categories.

Characteristics of Channel Systems

Direct versus Indirect Channels

Channel systems are described as direct when one or no intermediaries are between the producer (the manufacturer) and the end seller (the retailer) to the customer, and indirect if intermediaries are in between (e.g., brokers, agents, wholesalers).

Channel Systems May Share and Shift Functions

Channel functions can be shifted and shared between and among various channel specialists, and even customers and suppliers. What they cannot be is eliminated.

Functions may be undertaken by more than one market specialist; e.g., pharmaceuticals are packaged by manufacturers and repackaged by repackagers and pharmacists. A manufacturer may ship its products to a contract warehouse, which in turn ships smaller quantities to a wholesaler. The wholesaler then delivers still smaller orders to its customers. Four different entities, plus one or more shipping services, undertook the same function, i.e., moving products from one place to another.

Channel Systems Evolve

Channel systems evolve continually in response to the following:

- *Changing needs:* e.g., target market includes fewer children and is composed mainly of older individuals necessitating smaller package sizes and product redesign for easier use.
- *New ways of doing business:* e.g., competitors are staying open around the clock and able to get special items overnight.
- *New services:* e.g., catalog items may now be ordered over the Internet twenty-four hours a day, 365 days a year.
- *New entrants (competitors and specialists) into the system:* e.g., vitamin-nutritional specialty shops now compete with pharmacies.

Traditional channel systems are made up of independent market specialists that act in a somewhat interdependent and somewhat adversarial manner. As independent business entities, each market specialist follows its own operating objectives and policies. Independence and separate "masters" (self-interest) tend to keep market specialists from controlling or bullying one another and to improve each entity's efficiency.

Emerging channel systems exist today that consist of vertical market specialists (manufacturer, wholesaler, and retailer) acting in a cooperative, interdependent manner to develop and foster joint objectives. The idea is to increase the "partnership's" combined efficiency by reducing counterproductive and redundant behaviors and costs. Whether such systems have competitive staying power has yet to be determined.

CRUCIAL PLACE FACTORS

Marketing must help decide a number of important questions that largely determine how well the target market will be reached (penetrated) and served (market share), and whether a company's objectives are met. These include (but are not limited to) the following:

- What is the best way to reach and service various target markets (distribution channel and physical distribution methods)?
- What services will be needed initially and on an ongoing basis?
- What distribution methods exist and what are the trade-offs of speed, effectiveness, control, and cost?
- Should a direct, indirect, or hybrid channel of distribution be used?

- What is the best way to communicate with channel entities (market channel specialists)?
- What steps should be taken to ensure that intended results are the actual results (i.e., how to control the process)?

Market Coverage

An important aspect of attaining and increasing sales is how best to reach intended customers. This is the question of market coverage. One measure of market coverage is the number or percent of customers in a group who are contacted or sold products. Another might be the geographic coverage of a given territory. Another might be percent of market share, i.e., the percent of total sales for this type of product.

Using the percentage of customers contacted to the total number is not a particularly good measure of market coverage because customers are not all equally important. Everybody needs to eat, but not everybody needs or wants a particular food all the time. Knowing this, it makes sense that simply saying that the message reached 1,000 people or 75 percent of all consumers is less useful (and therefore less powerful) than saying that a pain reliever message and product reached 75 percent of people who had a headache and were looking for an analgesic at the time. The former is a gross measure of unqualified consumers, whereas the second is a targeted measure of qualified and ready customers. Embodied in the statement is the idea of targeting specific market segments and readiness to buy.

Customer Service

The types and level of product and customer services needed to be successful differ greatly from customer to customer *and* in different markets. They also differ by type of product and by competing channel specialists. More affluent, higher educated, and more experienced customers tend to require more and higher levels of product and customer services, but even these tendencies vary over time.

Product information, warranties, repair services, replacements, return privileges, help desks and technical service may each be part of a service package. Each has a cost (that needs to be taken into account), and the ability to deliver each depends on other place decisions. For example, on-site product repair of a product sold by mail order is more difficult than if it is available in every pharmacy in the country.

Distribution Methods and Costs

Distribution involves weight, amount, distance, and time, which have to be considered simultaneously with customer needs and cost. Shipping 144 bottles of cough syrup all at once from Puerto Rico to Virginia is less expensive on a per-piece basis than shipping each bottle individually every time a single customer needs it. The trade-offs are not that simple, however; costs are associated with buying and storing 144 at a time when a customer only wants one today, so marketers must balance the trade-offs or develop mechanisms to offset them.

On first glance, it may seem attractive to ship everything from one huge warehouse in the market center of the country by overnight express (rather than have so many retail stores). But, does it make sense to pay $16 to "overnight" a single $1 battery or a box of facial tissues, and will someone in cardiac arrest today really benefit if it takes twenty-four hours to "overnight" the materials and equipment to start a lidocaine drip?

Obviously, these examples are extremes. They do, however, serve to illustrate two things: (1) different products and situations demand different solutions, and (2) the combinations and the permutations to address place discrepancies are almost limitless. Marketers spend a great deal of time on decisions involving how to distribute products, and they are hesitant to make sudden or precipitous changes because, once made, such decisions permeate the entire place arena and are expensive and difficult to change.

Choice of Market Channel

Another important choice is whether to sell directly to the end user or to use one or more intermediaries. Or, does it make sense to do both (a hybrid model) or one or the other depending on the target market or geography? The drug industry provides several good examples.

A drug manufacturer that wants to sell its products to pharmacies has a choice of marketing to 28,800 independent pharmacies; 19,000 chain drug stores; 7,500 hospital pharmacies; 220 mail-order operations; 7,800 food stores; 5,200 mass merchandisers; and 4,000 long-term care pharmacies and facilities, or 74 wholesale drug distributors that will in turn service the pharmacies. The first choice is the direct choice. It means developing and maintaining business relationships with 64,520 pharmacies; it means accepting orders from, shipping to, and collecting from 64,520 pharmacies. The second choice is the indirect choice. It involves an intermediary between the manufacturer and each pharmacy and implies less control, but it is dramatically less work at a much lower cost.

Channel Control

In this context, control is defined as the degree to which a marketer can take steps to bring desired and actual results closer together. It may involve such things as how quickly a manufacturer can get its products onto the shelves of every pharmacy once the product is approved for sale by the U.S. Food and Drug Administration. Having good relationships with few, large accounts makes such control easier than trying to get 64,520 pharmacies to move quickly. Getting product to 245 wholesale drug distribution centers, which will in turn ship overnight to 64,520 pharmacies, has proven to be much faster, less expensive, and more effective.

Market Information and Feedback

Market information is increasingly important to marketers and includes competitor activities; the attributes, attitudes, and actions of customers; why a product is successful or having difficulty; what intermediaries and retailers are doing to support and encourage sales; and so on. Good business relationships, supply agreements, and various contracts and cooperative efforts encourage and support market feedback. Still, all of these activities have costs and all take time. What the marketer must decide is how much of each type of information is needed and at what cost.

CHANNEL SPECIALISTS

Channel specialists develop in response to specific market needs. The U.S. marketplace is very large in terms of people and dollars; it is also quite diverse and growing more so every day. Because the marketplace is, to a large degree, free to respond to need, the numbers and types of U.S. market specialists are unusually large and varied. It is also becoming increasingly difficult to locate pure types, i.e., those which fall neatly into a single category. Despite periodic predictions that markets and products are converging, or will converge, just the opposite is true—markets are becoming ever more diversified; product and brand proliferation appear to have no end.

- *Market proliferation:* Mail order and the Internet did not (and will not) replace retailing; both have added to the number of market channels. TV home shopping is in reality another way (channel) to get products to customers.
- *Product proliferation:* Minivans did not replace or converge with station wagons; they created a whole new product category. NSAIDs did not replace aspirin or acetaminophen; they simply became another new type of pain reliever.
- *Brand proliferation:* Once soft drink distributors serviced small self-serve racks with two or three different products in several different sizes. They delivered products in small panel trucks. Today, the same distributors stock fifty or more different products, flavors, sizes, and packages from double trailer-sized behemoths. A dramatic example of brand proliferation is the estimate that more than 5,000 different cough and cold remedies are on the market today.

Because of constant change in the marketing landscape, taking a valid snapshot is difficult. On the other hand, continual creation, evolution, and hybridization add to the dynamism of U.S. marketing and fuel further innovations in drug marketing.

Retailers and Service Companies

The most prevalent and probably best-known market specialists are retailer and service companies. Examples include JCPenney, Kmart, Texaco, Staples, Goodyear, Safeway, 7-Eleven, Avis, H&R Block tax service, pharmacies, beauty salons, dry cleaners, and film developers. Retailers sell products and services primarily to individual consumers (but also to other businesses). The United States has more than a million retailers, and their size, character, and makeup are difficult to grasp, let alone describe completely. They range in size from several football fields to tiny kiosks and stands.

Most retailers are fixed-address specialists, meaning that they conduct business from a known, fixed location or address. Traditional fixed-address retailers (a.k.a. "bricks and mortar" retailers) can be

- free-standing, meaning that they are housed in self-contained or complete structures (Wendy's, Borders Books, Pizza Hut, Red Lobster) (even though they may be located in the parking area of a shopping center);
- occupying a separate but integrated space within a larger shopping center structure (Sears, the Gap, Nordstrom);
- operated from within a kiosk or stand (film and developing, jewelry, cell phone dealers); or
- existing as a store within a store, meaning they are subleased (and sometimes licensed separately) from a larger operator (a subleased bank branch within a grocery store, an eyeglass shop within a department store).

Several newer forms of retailing are appropriately referred to as floating-address retailers, in that they offer no permanent, fixed address for conducting business.[3] Examples include individual commercial operators at trade and products shows (technology, home remodeling, auto shows, garden, antiques) and those which are best described as transient weekend sellers. These retailers are most often located at local hotels, parking lots, or business intersections and offer seasonal and/or unique goods (artwork, furs, computer parts, plants, and holiday products, e.g., Fourth of July fireworks and Christmas trees) often at supposedly low prices.

Franchises, Co-Ops, and Buying Clubs

The category of franchises includes several different types of specialty end sellers. Some differentiate themselves by selling a single or exclusive line of products (Amway, Hallmark stores, Dairy Queen) or a unique product assortment or service model (Medi-Cap Pharmacies, Medicine Shoppe).

Co-ops, short for cooperatives, are less prevalent than they once were, but they still play a role in assembling, offering, and selling goods and services. The best description of a co-op is a user-owned marketer, formed by its members to offer products at a lower cost or to obtain those which are difficult to get. The co-op itself is more a convenience, or group buying mechanism, than a separate marketing specialist that exists for its own benefit. Examples include agricultural products co-ops, fresh fruit and vegetable co-ops, and buying clubs.

A buying club is similar to a co-op, differing mostly in degree of organizational and operational formality and sometimes size (most are smaller than co-ops). Buying clubs are typically formed by individual consumers, who see value in sharing information, making joint purchases, and/or consolidating their purchasing power.

Another form of buying service was originally developed to serve other businesses but quickly expanded to include individual consumers too. These marketing specialists behave, to some extent, similar to retailers and, in other respects, resemble co-ops and buying clubs. They tend to be very large, handle thousands of items, move inventory very quickly, not always have the same items week to week, and sell products in large amounts or quantities (family sizes, cases, bulk sizes) at very low prices. "Customers" typically pay an annual "membership" fee for the privilege of being able to shop there (Costco/Price Club, BJ's, and Sam's Club).

Internet-Based Selling—E-Tailers

The newest market specialists are Internet-based marketers, sometimes referred to as e-tailers or dot-com retailers. They may operate only on the Internet or as both retailers and e-tailers. Internet-based selling offers several advantages that are reshaping retailing in general. E-tailing can be an effective way to reach very large customer geographic regions—the entire United States, North America, or even the world—at an affordable cost. It is well suited for highly specialized items that have few customers per capita and/or when the product required to be successful is so large that the cost to assemble and maintain it in a small local market is prohibitive (vis-à-vis the sales that would be generated in that market).

E-tailing pioneers, to a large degree, have learned some economically painful lessons about the exigencies of place in the marketing equation. The Internet can indeed be an economical and effective information and promotion pathway to legions of consumers. It can also be one of the most efficient ways to take orders from individual consumers (as opposed to business customers). However, the Internet offers no advantages whatsoever in terms of accumulating and maintaining inventory, order fulfillment, or transportation to the customer.

Direct Marketers

Direct marketers are those which sell directly to individual customers (including individual consumers and businesses). In short, they include marketing specialists that sell to end users and are not retailers. As a category, direct marketers have grown in terms of the percentage of total sales faster than retailers.

Mail-Order Operators

Mail-order companies sell to individual customers from remote locations by using public or private carriers to deliver products. Typically, customers can only read, see, or hear product descriptions by telephone, fax, or catalog. Though a sizable number of mail-order operators rely on print advertising in various periodicals, most use printed catalogs in lieu of retail locations to attract and consummate sales. Most now augment printed catalogs with online Internet catalogs.

Everything can be bought by mail order! Vitamins, herbals, nutraceuticals, homeopathics, nonprescription drugs, and prescription drugs can be purchased by mail order. Most, if not all, major drug plans offer (encourage or even require) mail-order prescription services. Their advantage is economy of scale in purchasing, prescription processing, shipping, and billing. Their disadvantage is slower, less personal service.

Door-to-Door Operators

Although in long-term decline and hardly a factor anymore, still a few market specialists offer products and services door-to-door. Examples include home cleaning supplies, frozen ice cream novelties, and lawn care services, i.e., the neighbor who offers to mow the lawn. Several door-to-door operators still offer a number of nonprescription drugs, including a variety of "cough remedies."

In-Home Marketers

A variant of door-to-door selling is in-home marketing. Most such marketers offer high-quality and often high-margin specialty products and operate under the aegis of getting others to host a "party" to create a market in the home. Plastic storage containers, cosmetics, vitamins, decorative baskets, greeting cards and stationery, and plush toys are examples of products sold by in-home marketers. Several vitamin and natural product lines are sold in-home as well.

TV Sellers

A phenomenon of the growth of TV cable services, TV sellers represent another direct-selling marketer that offers a wide variety of products. They operate on cable channels as regularly scheduled programs or appear irregularly as what have become known as infomercials, "programs" lasting thirty to sixty minutes that are best described as program-advertisement hybrids. An increasing variety of medical-surgical, personal care products are being marketed by TV sellers.

Telemarketers

With so many Americans working during the day and door-to-door selling losing favor, telemarketers have learned that calling people at home is not only a more economical but also surprisingly successful way to sell many different products and services. The list of products and services offered by telemarketers is almost endless and includes more health and health-care related products and services than most people realize.

Direct Factory Outlets

Ostensibly, direct factory outlets are special marketers that are owned and operated by manufacturers (which makes them de facto direct sellers). This distinction is less true today, in that more and more are not owned by, or linked in any way to, a manufacturing plant, except that they stock items which carry the manufacturer's brand name. In short, many direct factory outlets have become retail operators instead of direct sellers. Supposedly, they offer first-quality overstock, factory "seconds" (have minor flaws), and/or manufacturer closeouts at very low prices. In some cases, seconds are fraudulently offered as first-quality items, and prices are indistinguishable from retail marketers.

Brokers

Brokers are market specialists that exist to deal with large quantity and/or price discrepancies or uncertainty in the marketplace. Brokers do not usually take title to products, meaning that they serve only to facilitate sales between two other parties that do not realize the other exists; e.g., one has something to sell, and the other wants to buy that same something. Their role is much like that of a marriage broker in that they serve to create market transactions where none previously existed. Brokerlike activities exist in the drug industry to dispose of large overstocks and short-dated products (those about to expire), and as a hedge against future price increases.

Wholesalers

Wholesalers and distributors (a more exclusive term for wholesalers, used to distinguish wholesalers that provide a myriad of services above and beyond what most wholesalers provide) are sometimes known as middlemen. They exist to sort out discrepancies of product, quantity, place, and possession and function in much the same way as a hub airport facilitates the transfer of people and products and reduces the number of flights (i.e., transactions) necessary to carry the traffic. Wholesalers search the marketplace and buy a wide assortment of products from a few to thousands of manufacturers and suppliers. They then sell those products to retailers and others, who will in turn sell them to end users (individuals and businesses) in customer-specific assortments and amounts. Although not apparent to the casual observer, wholesalers are one of the most important market specialists in making individual channels successful. Wholesale drug distributors are particularly important to the success of the drug industry.

Importer-Exporters

Importers and exporters are market specialists that move products into and out of a country by crossing national borders. To a large degree, importer-exporters are regulation and transportation facilitators, in that they know the complex and often arcane and conflicting rules and requirements to export or import products and how to ship products so that they actually arrive and are intact. U.S. marketers are able to export finished-dose drug products to other countries but may only import drugs and drug products that have been approved by the U.S. Food and Drug Administration. As a result, exports represent more than 75 percent of all international pharmaceutical shipments. By a large margin, drug imports are raw materials instead of finished products.

Storage and Transportation Specialists

The last group of market specialists includes storage and transportation specialists. Storage specialists exist to mediate quantity discrepancies, such as when a manufacturer produces a large quantity of antibiotic capsules in anticipation of flu season and needs extra storage for this seasonal buildup of orders. Storage specialists help by providing economical, short-term storage (that meets regulatory requirements, of course), rather than the manufacturer having to build or lease storage space.

Transportation specialists include long-distance (over-the-road trucks, trains, air freight, and other commercial carriers) and local delivery specialists. They range from overnight express services to local delivery services and may be common carriers (accepts anyone's shipments) to contract carriers (shipments limited to contracted arrangements for or to specific customers). In other cases, manufacturers, wholesalers, and retailers have their own transportation department, which owns (or leases) and operates transport vehicles for its own use.

CHANNEL RELATIONSHIPS AND CONFLICT

There are many compelling reasons for members (various market specialists) of a marketing channel to cooperate in serving customer needs. The opposite is true also—because of conflicting goals and objectives, there are many obvious reasons for conflict between and among channel members. By its very nature, some conflict is inherent in a competitive marketplace. Conflict is natural and well tolerated by marketers until it begins to outweigh cooperative needs. When this happens, channel efficiency decreases and customers are not served as well.

Most horizontal channel conflict, that is, conflict between the same or similar market specialists providing roughly the same utilities, manifests itself as competition. This is true when two different food stores (same-type competitors) compete for the same customer, or when a chain drugstore, convenience store, and a vitamin store (mixed-type or intertype competitors) compete to sell aspirin to customers. Unless such conflict becomes extreme, harmful, or unsafe, it is welcomed as healthy rivalry because it tends to make everyone better at what they do and customers get a better deal. Competition most often results in customers choosing which marketer, method, and policy they prefer and directing their business there. Each competitor is free to respond to, or ignore, a competitor's move—the essence of free markets.

When horizontal competition turns hostile or destructive, however, it can harm channel effectiveness and efficiency. Price and service wars, in which local competitors continually reduce prices in response to price reductions by competitors, rarely result in any new real business but typically harm all channel participants. As a result, customers' long-term needs are not met as well. However, much of what longtime competitors view as "uncompetitive" behavior is, more often than not, new ways of doing business that challenge and upset the status quo.

By far the more interesting type of conflict is vertical channel conflict—conflict between two or more functional levels of market specialists. It is interesting because it often affects the entire industry and is essentially a power conflict. Balance of power relates to the notion of a channel captain and explains many vertical channel conflicts. Several examples taken from the drug industry serve to illustrate vertical conflict:

- Manufacturer A wants pharmacies to stock its newest product but refuses to give return credit for partially filled containers. With new products, pharmacists are concerned about whether they will sell and are sometimes reluctant to open a sealed container to fill a small-quantity prescription.
- Pharmacies want to order inventory well past the evening cutoff time, then get angry when their wholesaler order is late the next morning because the wholesaler started processing two hours later as a result of tardy pharmacy customer orders.
- Manufacturers want community pharmacists to dispense their products (over competing choices) but charge other types of competitors much lower prices or give large fees to other types of pharmacies for getting prescribers to switch to their brands.
- It is December 12 and a community pharmacy is out of a product needed for a continuing-therapy refill; local pharmacies and wholesale drug distributors are out of stock too. The pharmacy calls the manufacturer only to find out that its office and order department are closed for a three-week year-end holiday.

CHANNEL ACCESS

An important aspect of managing place is access to a channel. With so many different products on the market, channel intermediaries, retailers, and direct sellers have to decide which products to stock. Manufacturers also try to induce down-channel partners to promote their products (rather than competing products) and not to stock competitive products. Wholesaler and retailer house brands compete for space and attention, which restricts channel (shelf space, catalog listing) access.

In some industries, very large marketers are able to "lock out" competing products through exclusive, long-term customer agreements or sheer size. Market access and balance of power are two-way streets, however, and everyone is free to respond to attempts to restrict or deny channel access or to shift the balance of power. Recent innovations involving new channels of distribution and new ways of distributing products are acting as countervailing forces that foil most attempts to restrict channel access or consolidate power.

PHYSICAL DISTRIBUTION

Physical distribution involves the movement of goods within individual firms and throughout the channel system. Products in a warehouse have little or no use to those who need or want them. Their usefulness (dollar value) increases substantially, however, when they are moved to where the customer can have possession of them. A substantial part of the marketing dollar is spent on distribution, nearly half in many industries (much less in the drug industry).

Physical distribution involves receiving, storing, handling, order filling, packing, and shipping products to other channel specialists or customers. In addition, a number of essential ancillary processes and requirements are involved in distribution, including buying and properly storing raw materials and inventory, physical and product security, receiving and processing orders (including invoices, credit memos), picking and packing orders, staging shipments, and producing shipping documents.

Physical distribution may involve *vertical integration.* A channel is vertically integrated if two or more successive levels of market specialists are combined into one operation. A retailer may integrate "up the channel" by acquiring or starting a wholesale operation and eventually adding a manufacturing capability. Manufacturers who own and operate factory (retail) stores and/or outlets have integrated "down the channel" as direct sellers.

Vertical integration is not a new phenomenon; it seems to resurface about once every twenty years. What is new are the control and communication technologies and new ways of thinking that foster vertical systems. The drug industry has experimented recently (since 1994) with vertical integration. It is too soon to decide whether it will be a sustainable marketing model.

The Challenges of Marketing Compression Stockings

Pharmacists have been advised to involve themselves in other health care products besides prescription and nonprescription drugs. A major growth opportunity is compression stockings, designed to alleviate or lesson poor circulation and prevent blood clots in the lower body. They are used by the elderly, people with poor circulation or congestive heart failure, those at risk for thromboses, and pregnant women.

A single pair of compression stockings sells for $50 to $95. The challenge is how to accommodate the permutations that exist without investing every dollar and every square foot of a pharmacy in compression stockings. The possibilities include:

Factor	Possibilities	Number
Brands	Four major lines	4
Styles	Waist, thigh-high, knee, sock, leotard	5

Compression levels	8-15, 15-20, 20-30, 30-40	5
Compression	Uniform, graduated	2
Sizes	Small, medium, large, extra large	2
Lengths	Regular, extra length, petite	2
Toes	Open, closed	2
Top brands	Regular, lingerie type	2
Colors	Black, taupe, beige, navy, black, white	6

To stock *just one of each possibility* in one pharmacy would mean finding space for 19,200 different boxes of compression stockings, representing from $960,000 to $1,824,000 in sales. Needless to say, this would be a physical and fiscal impossibility for even the largest pharmacy.

Based on place principles, what are some ways to meet both customer and pharmacy needs?

Chapter 11

Place Factors in the U.S. Drug Market: The Environment

Bruce Siecker

DRUG AND RELATED HEALTH CARE PRODUCTS

The legitimate drug market[1] in the United States is composed of three major components:

1. Prescription drugs
2. Nonprescription drugs
3. Alternative drugs

Prescription drugs are also called "legend" drugs because they are labeled with the federal legend composed of words that say, in effect, this drug cannot be dispensed without a prescription or by Rx only. They are also generally referred to as pharmaceuticals, though not everyone restricts the term to mean legend drugs (those which require a prescription). Drugs are determined to require a prescription from an authorized medical practitioner because they are deemed dangerous to use without medical supervision and/or may become habit forming without proper supervision. Some new drugs are designated as requiring a prescription as a precaution in that substantive safety questions were unanswered during preapproval clinical research.

Prescription drugs are regulated by the U.S. Food and Drug Administration (FDA) and state agencies that enforce the Prescription Drug Marketing Act. All prescription drugs must be approved by the FDA before they may be sold in interstate commerce and are either dispensed or administered by approved health care practitioners.

Nonprescription drugs are also regulated and must be approved by the FDA. The difference is they have been determined (by the FDA) to be safe enough for users to self-medicate. The primary differentiation is contained in the name—nonprescription drugs do not require a prescription to be sold to the public. This difference forms the basis for an earlier name for nonprescription drugs—over-the-counter (OTC) drugs—in that they were originally available from pharmacists "over the prescription counter." Nonprescription drugs are sold virtually everywhere.

Alternative drugs is not really an accurate name for the third major component of the U.S. drug market. Alternative drugs include herbals, homeopathics, "nutraceuticals," and what some call functional foods. The term is a misnomer in that it fails to accurately describe what is included or, more important, how such products are viewed and used today by most consumers. Although the smallest component of the drug market in dollars and dosage units, alternative drugs are the fastest-growing segment with consumers.

An allied component of drugs are devices and what are loosely known as medical-surgical supplies. Medical devices and supplies are also approved and regulated by the FDA and are increasingly thought of as a normal extension of pharmaceutical care.

USE OF PRESCRIPTION MEDICATIONS

The U.S. population continues to grow as a result of resurgent birth rates, longer life expectancy, and immigration (and illegal border crossings). The U.S. population in 1990 was approximately 250 million. In Census 2000 281.4 million people were counted as residents in the United States, a 13.2 percent increase in ten years. A population growth of 32.7 million people between 1990 and 2000 is the largest census-to-census increase ever recorded in American history—and it is not projected by the U.S. Census Bureau to repeat by 2010. Table 11.1 shows a projected growth in population to 300 million by 2010. A projected increase of about 18.5 million more people, though substantially less than the record-breaking 1990 to 2000 period, still means substantially more prescriptions.[2]

The average age of the U.S. population is increasing and is projected to continue increasing for the foreseeable future. Equally important in understanding drug usage is a bulge in U.S. population known as the "baby boomers." Baby boomers represent the substantial increase in births that occurred after the end of World War II. The leading edge of the baby boom generation turned fifty in 1996, and the numbers right behind them are even larger. The importance of an aging population (with a major age bulge entering middle age) is this—drug use increases with age! An older population means more prescriptions per capita and much greater spending (see Table 11.2.)

The use of pharmaceuticals has grown steadily over the past fifty years; however, the rate of increase has accelerated in the past five years and is expected to increase even faster in the next five. In fact, the U.S. pharmaceutical industry and pharmacy will have to produce, pack, ship, and dispense an additional 1 billion prescriptions by 2005!

Prescription volume has increased dramatically since 1990. According to information published by IMS Health, total pharmaceutical sales continued

TABLE 11.1. U.S. Population, 1950-2050 (in thousands)

Year	U.S. Population	U.S. Projections
1950	152,271	
1960	180,671	
1970	205,052	
1980	227,726	
1990	249,949	
2000	281,422	
2010		299,862
2020		324,927
2030		351,070
2040		377,350
2050		402,687

Source: U.S. Bureau of the Census. Census 2000 and Components for Change for Total Resident Population, 1999-2100.

TABLE 11.2. Health Care and Drug/Medical Supplies Spending (in Millions) by Age Group, 1997

Age (Years)	Total Health Care Dollars	Drug and Medical Supply Dollars
Under 25	$ 425	$ 65
25-34	1,236	169
35-44	1,605	210
45-54	1,945	303
55-64	2,187	407
65-74	2,900	594
75 and more	2,799	691

Source: U.S. Bureau of Labor Statistics.

to rise briskly again during calendar year 1999, increasing 19.3 percent to $125 billion (retail value). The number of prescriptions dispensed (at retail) increased 9.0 percent to 2,821,770,000. The total translates into somewhat more than ten prescriptions per capita (see Table 11.3).

A significant part of pharmaceutical sales growth is the result of price increases for an average prescription, which in turn is related to the mix of drug products prescribed, the substantially higher prices of newly intro-

TABLE 11.3. U.S. Prescription Volume, 1999

Trade Channel	Total Rxs (in Millions)	% Total Market	% Change versus 1998
Chains and mass merchandisers	1,492.0	52.9	+9.8
Independent pharmacies	737.7	25.5	+4.4
Food stores	357.5	12.9	+16.9
Mail-order pharmacies	133.6	4.7	+9.0
Long-term care pharmacies	114.9	4.1	+7.1
Total	**2,835.7**	**100.1***	**+9.44** (average)

Source: IMS Health.
*Due to rounding

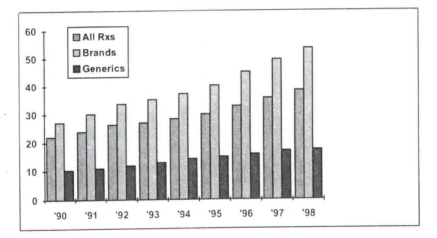

FIGURE 11.1. Average Prescription Retail Price, 1990-1998 (*Source:* IMS Health.)

duced drugs, whether a brand or generic product is used, and the quantity prescribed and dispensed. As can be seen in Figure 11.1, the average prescription price has continued to increase steadily in the past decade. Further, the average prescription price gap between brand and generic prescriptions continues to widen.

In 1990, the average prescription price was $22.06. The equivalent brand-name prescription average price was $27.16, and the average generic prescription was $10.29. Eight years later in 1998, the average prescription was $38.43. The average brand-name prescription charge in 1998 was $53.51, with many new drugs costing well over $100 for one course of therapy. The average generic prescription in 1998 was $17.33.

Although consumers continue to place great value on medicines, the continuing rise in pharmaceutical prices and the fact that prices are lower in other countries for the same drugs have gotten the attention of major consumer groups, employers, politicians, and the government.

DRUG PRODUCT IMPERATIVES

Place variables are affected by drug product imperatives, which means that marketing solutions for others types of products do not necessarily apply to drug products. Primary factors to consider include the following.

Wide, Highly Customized Assortment

Despite the fact that a limited number of pharmaceutical categories make up the majority of all prescribing, serving a patient population requires having a wide assortment of products. Individual drugs (active ingredients) can be solid oral dosage forms (capsules, tablets), oral liquids (liquids, elixirs, tinctures, drops), and injectibles. They may be topical forms (creams, ointments, gels), products for ears, noses, or eyes. Pediatrics represent another assortment.

The typical pharmacy stocks more than 1,000 different pharmaceutical products, which creates a significant fixed overhead. As pharmaceuticals continue to get even more expensive, drug wholesalers and pharmacies are doing all they can to minimize inventory levels (while not compromising service). Because of having to anticipate the seasonal and varying pharmaceutical needs of several thousand people, pharmacies necessarily stock a wide assortment of drugs. Unless patients would be willing to wait longer than they do today for their medicines—and they generally do so only when required to by their insurance plan or offered a substantial economic incentive, e.g., no copay if they use a mail-order service—there are limits to how low a pharmacy can reduce its inventory and still serve the public good.

Continuous Availability; Quick, Reliable Access

The U.S. market is accustomed to being able to get a prescription filled without making an appointment. Consumers expect to be able to find pharmacists available for long hours during the day and evening (ten to sixteen hours a day in many communities) and for six or seven days a week. More than a few twenty-four-hour pharmacies are open every day of the year. Marketers wishing to compete in the U.S. market must address these time and place imperatives.

Unique Handling and Storage Requirements

Pharmaceuticals are adversely affected by extreme temperatures, especially heat. Though small and light, pharmaceuticals are easily damaged if handled or stored casually or packed or shipped carelessly. Marketers must recognize these imperatives when making place-related decisions.

Very Highly Regulated Products

Pharmaceuticals per se are highly regulated products; how and under what conditions they are made available to the public are as highly regulated. The wide variety and complexity of regulations that affect place are often underestimated or even overlooked by new market entrants. Because of the high cost and relative inflexibility of place decisions, marketers need to understand all regulatory hurdles before making marketing decisions.

PHYSICAL AND FISCAL PRODUCT CHARACTERISTICS

In considering place factors, marketers should take into consideration several unique physical and fiscal characteristics of pharmaceuticals.

Small Cube, High Dollar Value

Pharmaceuticals are small products with relatively high dollar values. They require little space to store and ship. At the same time, their size and value make them vulnerable to theft and diversion into illicit channels. Their high value and small size also allow them to be shipped economically by specialty carriers, meaning they can reach the desired destination or site quickly.

Quantity Customization

By definition, a prescription is one of the highest customizations of quantity in the universe of other products. Any given prescription can range in size from one dose (or less) to whatever the prescriber, patient, and pharmacy can tolerate. It is virtually impossible for a manufacturer to produce package sizes that meet every patient situation, so physicians (as prescribers) and pharmacists (as dispensers) play an important role in customizing the physical quantity for patients.[3]

Safety and Security Concerns

Despite numerous safeguards, pharmaceuticals are not risk free. They are referred to as dangerous for a reason. Using pharmaceuticals is a calculated risk wherein the benefits are felt to outweigh the risks. Prescription drugs are those which are considered too dangerous to allow unrestricted availability and use. Who may prescribe, possess, dispense, and administer pharmaceuticals is therefore highly controlled and regulated.

Unsalables, Investment Losses, and Liability

Pharmaceuticals are "dated" products, meaning that they carry an expiration date. Outdated drugs cannot be dispensed. Unlike most other products, pharmaceuticals have traditionally been distributed with return privileges. Manufacturer returned-goods policies vary by company. Some only take back (and give credit for) unopened packages; others accept opened containers (called "partials"). Return processing and costs must be factored in by marketers in making distribution decisions.

LEGAL AND REGULATORY REQUIREMENTS

Unlike industrial and consumer products, not every drug can be marketed in the United States and not everyone can market drugs or designate them as they wish as prescription or nonprescription. Drugs and drug marketers are subject to numerous restrictions and requirements.

The control and regulation of the manufacture and marketing of prescription and nonprescription drugs is handled primarily by the federal government. Primary authority rests with the FDA, which is part of the Department of Health and Human Services. Major federal legislation passed in 1906, 1938, 1951, 1962, and 1989 addressed health and safety issues to protect Americans from impure, ineffective, mislabeled, misused, and even counterfeit drugs. Interestingly, most federal legislation is traceable to public sentiment that resulted from serious threats to public safety and questions about the effectiveness of certain drugs and combinations of drugs.

The FDA was created by the passage of the 1906 Pure Food and Drugs Act, which established federal authority and jurisdiction to regulate and control most aspects of drug marketing. The agency was also given powerful administrative sanctions to control the legitimate drug industry, including extensive authority to confiscate and destroy misbranded and adulterated drugs. The FDA can levy severe monetary and criminal penalties, giving it powerful control over every aspect of which drugs are approved for marketing in the United States and how they can be marketed.

The reach of the FDA was extended with a major amendment in 1938 (Food, Drug, and Cosmetic Act) as a result of the public outcry when forty people died from taking proprietary drugs that contained a poisonous industrial solvent. Though difficult to appreciate today, it was not until 1938 that drug marketers had to prove that the drug they wanted to be approved was safe when used according to the indicated uses and instructions.

The Durham-Humphrey Amendment to the Food, Drug, and Cosmetic Act, in 1951, established definitive criteria for what constituted a prescription versus a nonprescription drug. Prior to that time, the FDA used internally developed guidelines that were not well understood by the industry, or anyone else. The Food, Drug, and Cosmetic Act was amended substantively again in 1962 when the Kefauver-Harris Drug Amendments were passed. These amendments gave authority to the FDA to regulate all promotion and advertising of prescription drugs (to professionals and to the public). They also contained new requirements that drug marketers would henceforth have to prove that their drugs were not only safe but effective too.

Federal requirements define what constitutes a drug, and whether it is available with or without a prescription. They also proscribe procedures and practices for importing, storing, handling, and manufacturing drug products in a body of regulations and FDA requirements and guidelines that are known as good manufacturing practices (GMPs).[4]

The FDA defines how a natural or synthesized drug is to be identified (qualitative) and assayed (quantitative), and how it must be stored. Even the characteristics of the containers that drugs may be packaged in are defined in detail by federal requirements and regulations. The FDA controls what information must and may be printed on a drug package itself, what is required in the package insert, and what drug manufactures can and must say in advertising.

The requirements of the 1987 Prescription Drug Marketing Act (PDMA) are federal, but day-to-day requirements are vested with state agencies (which may be a state board of pharmacy or a separate office). The PDMA resulted from serious industry abuses involving importing and reimporting pharmaceuticals, diverting drugs from one market segment to another, diverting and selling drug samples, repackaging, and outright drug counterfeiting.

The PDMA prohibited anyone but the manufacturer from importing or reimporting its own drugs and established elaborate new requirements, controls, and record keeping for storing, handling, and shipping drug products. As a result of the PDMA, sellers have to provide substantive, written assurances (to buyers) that drugs have been stored and handled properly. They also must, if requested, provide details to a buyer about each entity that handled the drug since it left the possession of the original manufacturer until the time of the present sale—a written history that has come to be known informally as the "drug pedigree."

The PDMA established a series of new restrictions and controls, plus record-keeping and auditing requirements, for drug samples. It prohibited pharmacies and pharmacists from receiving and having possession of drug samples, and drug wholesalers from receiving open (partially filled) containers of prescription drug products.

Another major factor in how drugs are marketed in the United States is the Comprehensive Drug Abuse Prevention and Control Act of 1970, otherwise known as the Controlled Substances Act, or CSA. This legislation authorized the creation of the Drug Enforcement Administration (DEA), which was divided into two major enforcement branches. DEA agents work for the criminal section and focus their attention on illicit drug activity. It is the drug diversion branch of the DEA, staffed by drug diversion investigators, that affects how controlled substances can be marketed in the United States. Despite differences in what they do, both branches of the DEA function more as law enforcement agencies than regulatory bodies.

Controlled substances represent a separate level of federal (and state) control of certain FDA-approved drugs. These drugs are deemed (by the CSA and subsequently by the DEA) to require additional restrictions because of their potential for abuse, misuse, and diversion into illicit markets for nonmedical uses.

Controlled substances are divided into "schedules" according to their abuse potential and how much added control is thought to be necessary to prevent drug diversion. Schedules II to V may be marketed in the United States. Producers, distributors, repackagers, pharmacies, and other handlers must be registered separately with the DEA and meet additional process, storage, handling, ordering, record-keeping, and reporting requirements to avoid administrative, civil, and criminal penalties. DEA regulations and requirements are detailed; some are easily overlooked. Each violation of the CSA, whether willful or accidental, can cost up to $25,000.[5]

Marketers also need to be aware that controlled substances are regulated by individual states. The majority of the states adopted a model DEA act that aligns them with federal requirements; i.e., fulfilling a federal requirement also satisfies the state. *However,* almost every state has a few differences, most of which are more restrictive than the federal requirements and easy to overlook. A marketer is responsible for adhering to the more restrictive requirement.

Besides the FDA and DEA, which have substantial effects on drug marketing, drug marketers are affected by a number of other federal requirements. The Consumer Products Safety Commission (CPSA) regulates how drugs must be identified when in transit and whether they are hazardous substances. The federal Environmental Protection Agency (EPA) has jurisdiction if and when a drug product becomes a waste product, while the federal Department of Transportation (DOT) has myriad rules and regulations when drug products are shipped or stored in transit.

As part of the federal hazardous materials communications standard, drug marketers are required to provide what are known as material safety data sheets and poison control center information for every drug they market.

State and Local Laws and Regulations

Individual states and local jurisdictions have numerous requirements and regulations affecting how drugs may be marketed within their jurisdictions. Historically, state and local requirements have aligned well with federal requirements, and marketers have had to contend with few exceptions or additional requirements for states and local jurisdictions.

Although not documented, this may be changing. States are increasingly passing different and more restrictive regulations that affect how drugs may be marketed.

State Boards of Pharmacy

Although the manufacture and marketing of prescription and nonprescription drugs are regulated primarily at the federal level, marketers should not get the idea that nothing else affects their degrees of freedom. States have primary jurisdiction in regulating pharmacists and the practice of pharmacy—and *what regulates and controls pharmacy and pharmacists affects everyone up the supply channel,* even if indirectly.

Regulatory authority at the state level is vested with a state board of pharmacy on the basis of protecting the health and welfare of state residents. A state board of pharmacy is usually constituted as a separate state department or, less often, as a defined jurisdiction or subsection within a larger professional registration and licensure agency.

As with all professions, the practice of pharmacy is considered a privilege, not a right. To exercise the privilege, pharmacists must meet minimum educational qualifications and adhere to defined standards of practice and laws and regulations affecting the practice of pharmacy. Pharmacists must be properly registered, complete required continuing education requirements, and behave in a manner consistent with the public good. Further, they may not engage in, or associate with, people or activities involving the illicit use of drugs and compounds, especially controlled substances.

State boards of pharmacy typically define the conditions and requirements pharmacists must meet to dispense pharmaceuticals to the public or to distribute them to other registered health care professionals or entities. Board rules and policies define how drugs are to be stored and safeguarded in the pharmacy, what constitutes a prescription, what information must appear on the prescription label, what information and counsel pharmacists may or must give to patients, and what records are required and for how long. State board rules also address a pharmacy's operating characteristics, required equipment and professional references, housekeeping, physical security requirements, and, more than ever, the allowed uses of pharmacy technicians.

A fundamental of drug marketing is the longtime duality of the distribution channels—with the upper end (manufacturing and distribution) regulated by the federal government, while the patient interface (pharmacies) is regulated by individual states. Understanding the limitations and opportunities of place in the marketing mix requires an appreciation of the entire channel and the unique characteristics, practices, and requirements of each industry segment.

Chapter 12

Place Applications in the U.S. Drug Market

Bruce Siecker

The elements and practices of *place factors* in the U.S. drug market continue to evolve into an ever more complex panoply of choices and possibilities to serve 281 million U.S. consumers and facilitate the efforts of more than a million health care providers.[1] Understanding how place principles are applied in the market requires a deeper understanding of those elements and practices.

The primary elements or components of the U.S. drug market include suppliers, wholesale distributors, chain warehouses, and pharmacies. Secondary channel components include reverse distributors, clinics and laboratories, and pharmaceutical sampling.

DRUG SUPPLIERS—PRODUCERS, LABELERS, AND REPACKAGERS

Producers

Drug *producers* or *manufacturers* are the predominant type of drug *supplier* and the largest source of most finished-dosage-form pharmaceuticals in the U.S. market.[2] They are licensed by the FDA to manufacturer and market, i.e., promote and distribute, approved new drugs to appropriate down-channel entities. Drug manufacturers acquire new drugs through discovery, purchase, or licensing. Drug manufacturers fund and maintain by far the largest new drug discovery effort in existence. Such research is responsible for a very high proportion of all new drugs that eventually reach the market, i.e., achieve FDA marketing approval.

The rights[3] to market new drugs are also acquired through purchase and licensing. Drug manufacturers may purchase the right to drugs from other manufacturers (both foreign and domestic), independent development laboratories, colleges and universities, and individual discoverers. They also (but to a much lesser extent) may pay licensing fees for the right to market drugs that another company or organization (the licenser) owns. Licensing fees typically represent permission to market a drug for a limited period of time or to defined portions of the marketplace. Ownership rights, however, do *not* transfer with the license.

Drug manufacturers are responsible for complying with considerable federal, state, and local regulations concerning the production, handling, exporting, importing, storage, promotion, and selling of approved pharmaceuticals. Failure to comply can result in a loss of marketing approval, seizure of noncomplying drugs, fines, and even criminal charges.

Labelers

Another type of supplier (and the second largest source of finished-dosage-form pharmaceuticals) is a *labeler.* Drug labelers are licensed by the FDA in the same manner as manufacturers and often appear to be the same as drug manufacturers, at least to the outside world. A labeler is different from a manufacturer in that a labeler does *not* manufacture or produce the drugs it markets. Finished-dosage forms are *purchased* from other manufacturers, then "labeled" as being by, or from, the labeler. With the exception that a labeler purchases drugs from other sources, it must do everything that actual manufacturers do to market drugs and must comply with all government regulations (with the obvious exception of adhering to GMPs).

Repackagers

The third form of supplier (and the smallest source of approved finished-dosage-form drugs) is the *repackager.*[4] Repackagers are of two major types: (1) a repackager that also markets what it repackages as though the product was its own, and (2) a repackager that keeps the drug's identity and label the same on repackaged products.

The first type of repackager also has an FDA labeler license that allows it to repackage from one size to another, then label and market the new package as though it were its own product. For example, a repackager may obtain the right to purchase an analgesic in packages of 5,000 each, then repackage them into bottles of fifty and relabel them with its own name and identifying numbers. Although a repackaged product can be marketed under a new identity, current federal regulations require that the original, actual manufacturer also be identified on the label.

The second kind of repackager does nothing else but repackages from one size to another. The purpose is to take advantage of savings in buying larger sizes. The label on the repackaged container maintains the same information as the original package.[5] Such repackagers may operate within a larger context, e.g., a repackaging department within a large hospital chain, or as independent operators, e.g., a repackager that supplies customers or does contract repackaging work for specific clients.

Suppliers also can be characterized on the basis of the types of products marketed, although the lines of demarcation are largely blurred in today's marketplace.

Brand-Name Manufacturers

Brand-name manufacturers, also known as research-based pharmaceutical manufacturers, tend to focus on developing and commercializing unique NCEs that can be protected by patents and trademarks (including process trademarks). Once approved for marketing in the United States by the FDA, a brand-name manufacturer that has patented the drug has exclusive rights to market it for seventeen years *from the time the patent was filed*.[6] During this period, such manufacturers attempt to recover R&D costs of the brand-name drug (and numerous other chemical entities that it researched but failed to have approved) and to produce a return on stockholder investments. As such, brand-name drugs are priced well above their cost of production.

Other manufacturers are known as *generic drug suppliers*. A generic drug is one without a brand name or trademark. In terms of marketing, any company that files an application and obtains FDA approval can market such a drug in the United States.[7] Generic drugs tend to be priced lower than brand-name drugs.

Branded Generics

Some manufacturers market a hybrid type of pharmaceutical known as *branded generics*. These are pharmaceutical products that do not have patent protection but are marketed on the basis of brand name. Branded generics are often products that were once patented. The manufacturer of such products positions them similar to a brand-name drug and tends to price them at an intermediate level.

Although suppliers are often known as brand-name or generic companies, most brand-name suppliers also sell generic drugs and more generic manufacturers than ever are developing branded items.

Comarketers

Now a number of companies comarket the same drug. Sometimes the same brand name is used by two different manufacturers; in other cases, different brand names are applied to the same drug. The practice is best understood by comparing it to the way different divisions of General Motors (and others) market the same vehicle by "rebadging," i.e., changing the package (the vehicle body) and brand name (vehicle name). The intention is the same—to increase the number of choices consumers have.

WHOLESALE DISTRIBUTORS

Wholesale distributors, known for many years as *drug wholesalers* and, before that, *middlemen* and *jobbers,* are a sometimes overlooked, but vital, link in the channel of distribution. As independent market specialists, wholesale distributors are positioned in the channel between suppliers and pharmacies. The tasks of wholesale distributors are to supply the right quantity of products at the right time to their customers and to provide services needed by their customers.

Breadth of Product Line

A strong majority of wholesale distributors are *full-line* wholesalers, meaning that they stock and deliver virtually any drug, health care, and health and beauty aid product that a pharmacy or clinic needs. *Limited-line* or *short-line* wholesale distributors are exactly what their name implies— distributors that do not stock a full line of products. "Short-line houses," as they were known in the 1940s to 1970s, are becoming less prevalent because pharmacies rely so heavily on wholesale distributors to supply everything on what amounts to a just-in-time basis.

Scope of Services

Most wholesale distributors offer a wide range of customer support services and are described as *full-service* wholesalers. Support services are described as *value added* in that they provide substantive value above and beyond the value of distribution itself, which in general is evolving into a commodity business in terms of pricing and margins. Wholesale distributors also can be *limited-service* wholesale distributors. Few, if any, examples of limited-service wholesale distributors exist today (except as secondary suppliers or discrepancy specialists, described later).

Specialty Wholesalers

One of the few growth segments in wholesale distribution in terms of the number of companies in the marketplace is the *specialty wholesaler.* Unlike full-line, full-service wholesale distributors, specialty wholesalers focus on a particular segment of the market. Some distribute a special class of drugs, e.g., oncology wholesalers, parenteral wholesalers, and biotechnology wholesalers, or even a single drug, e.g., Methadone wholesalers. Other specialty wholesalers focus on a particular type of customer, e.g., clinics, prisons, or free-standing surgery centers.

Secondary Suppliers

For the past quarter century, the drug market has experienced continual price increases. Suppliers often raise prices more than once a year and on a fairly predictable basis. Price increases represent short-term profit potential to any down-channel customer that can afford to buy extra before prices increase and then immediately raise its own prices following the increase. The problem, of course, is that buying and holding extra inventory is not free. Inventory holding costs are significant and can quickly "eat up" profit opportunities from buying extra before prices increase.

Not surprisingly, a market specialist developed to address the need. *Secondary suppliers* are market specialists that *forward buy* large quantities of products that are available "on sale" (less than normal) or at today's price (when the price is going up). They then sell quantities to other channel members, such as wholesale distributors, chain warehouses, and pharmacies, in amounts they can realistically use at the time.

Discrepancy Specialists

Beginning in the mid-1990s, it became increasingly difficult for wholesale distributors to sell pharmaceuticals with less than six months unexpired dating left to pharmacies. At about the same time, a number of (and very quickly most) hospital supply bid-quote requests started to require twelve months of dating on all drugs supplied under contract. It was during the same period that the World Health Organization (WHO) adopted and promoted a requirement that all drugs donated to needy countries and peoples must have at least twelve months of dating left to be accepted. It was not long before wholesale distributors were saddled with significant inventory that was in date (based on FDA and supplier requirements), but effectively unsalable and not returnable.

A related phenomenon began to occur at the pharmacy level when state boards and drug programs changed longtime dispensing rules and practices regarding product dating. Previously, it was acceptable to dispense a drug if it was in date at the time it was dispensed. Thinking changed to require that pharmacists not dispense any drug product if it would go out of date before the patient ran out or stopped using it. This seemingly minor change—and the fact that many state boards of pharmacy and drug plan participation requirements started to require pharmacists to place product expiration dates on prescription labels—greatly exacerbated the unsalable-product problem in pharmacies.

Whenever a market need arises and becomes significant, marketers will address it, and the short-dating, unsalable-products issue was no exception. With the help of the Internet and models such as e-Bay, a new type of market specialist is evolving to address the issue of short-dated, unsalable drugs.

These *discrepancy specialists* attempt to correct the mismatches involving short-dated products languishing on shelves and market specialists that could sell products with less than six to twelve months until expiration.

CHAIN WAREHOUSES

Chain warehouses have the general look and feel of wholesale distributors, except that they are operated to serve a chain's own stores, e.g., drugstores, grocery stores, mass merchandisers, and buying clubs. They tend to stock fewer products—especially prescription items—they offer a narrower range of services, and they deliver orders less frequently than wholesale distributors. Chain warehouses buy primarily from suppliers and wholesale distributors and then resell to company-owned stores.

PHARMACIES—THE PATIENT-PHARMACIST INTERFACE

Pharmacies are where pharmacists serve the public and the predominant source of pharmaceutical supplies. They vary in size, character, and environment but exist for the same purposes. By maintaining significant inventories of pharmaceuticals in local communities, pharmacies provide ready availability of a wide range of drug treatment options for prescribers. Long hours of operation and walk-in access mean convenience and quality care for consumers.

Pharmacists, because of their specialized knowledge and demonstrated judgment, are given certain rights by law and through regulations to handle, compound, and dispense prescription drugs. These activities are carried out in a pharmacy—a term that is defined in law and restricted to particular places that are licensed by a state to store, compound, dispense, and sell drugs and medicines, specifically prescription drugs.[8]

Attempting to describe contemporary pharmacies concisely is akin to trying to depict the "average American consumer." For purposes of discussion, however, pharmacies may be categorized as one of five types:

1. Community
2. Mail order
3. Institutional
4. Specialty
5. Government

Not all pharmacies fall neatly into one category or another, and one pharmacy may simultaneously operate as more than one type, but the designations are sufficient to differentiate pharmacies in meaningful ways.

Community Pharmacy

The most common type of pharmacy is a *community pharmacy*. These are pharmacies located "in the community," in terms of having signed store-fronts and being visible and readily accessible to consumers. Subtypes include the following:

1. *Independent:* Although commonly thought of as three or fewer community pharmacies operated under single ownership, mostly an independent pharmacy refers to a single pharmacy operated by a single owner or a small group of partners. Independent pharmacies that are part of a group of three or fewer may have different, related, or the same names.
2. *Chain stores:* Four or more (often hundreds and in some cases thousands of) community pharmacies are operated under a single-ownership (often a large corporate) structure. Chain stores are operated under a single identity, though in some cases chain units (within a single company) are operated under a separate name or "banner" (usually for historical or identity reasons).
3. *Freestanding:* This type is a chain pharmacy, also known as a chain drugstore.
4. *Food store-affiliated:* This is a chain pharmacy operated by a grocery store (usually as a department within, or adjoined to, a larger food store).
5. *Mass merchandiser:* This is a chain pharmacy operated by a mass merchandiser (usually as a department within a larger mass merchandise store).
6. *Buying club:* This is a chain pharmacy operated by a buying club (usually as a department within a larger buying club store).
7. *Hybrid site:* A small number of community pharmacies are conveniently described as hybrid community pharmacies. Such a pharmacy is physically located and operates within a larger store environment, but most often it is owned or managed separately, essentially as a separate "store within a store."
8. *Leased department:* This is a community pharmacy located within a larger store, such as a food store or office building, but is owned and managed separately. It is often an independent pharmacy operator located within a larger context.
9. *Convenience store:* This type typically involves a leased department located and operated within a larger convenience store, e.g., 7-Eleven, Circle K, White Pantry.

10. *Service station:* This type typically involves a leased department located and operated within a service station, usually a larger "travel" or "minimart" service station.

Institutional Pharmacies

The second most prevalent type of pharmacy in terms of number and volume is an *institutional pharmacy.* In most cases, "institutional" refers to serving inpatients (hospital), residents (long-term care and assisted living), or terminally ill patients (hospice), though exceptions exist.

Hospital pharmacies are prevalent throughout the U.S. market and are located within hospitals that vary greatly in size and scope of services. Most hospital pharmacies exist to serve inpatient hospital populations only, although a growing number also operate outpatient services, i.e., separate pharmacies serving people who have stayed recently in the hospital or require continuing services from the hospital. Most hospital pharmacies are part of, and operated by, the hospital, although more are operated under contract by outside pharmacy service companies.

The second most prevalent type of institutional pharmacy is only rarely located within a health care institution but serves people who are residents of nursing homes and various types (levels) of assisted-living and care facilities. This type is generally called a *long-term care (LTC) pharmacy* because it serves defined populations that are expected to be "in residence" for longer periods.

The origins of long-term care pharmacies can be found among independent community pharmacy operators who were asked (in the 1970s) to provide dispensing services to local nursing homes. As long-term care pharmacies grew, and a new type of pharmacist practitioner known as a consulting pharmacist changed the basis and emphasis of LTC pharmacy, they migrated out of the back room and basements of community pharmacies (both independent and chain) and established themselves as unique types of pharmacies in separate locations and with special clients.

A small number of pharmacies provide pharmaceutical services to hospices (for people who are terminally ill) as a primary or exclusive focus. Most hospice pharmacy services are operated within the context of a community pharmacy. And although most hospice patients are maintained at home (with intermittent hospitalizations), *hospice pharmacies* tend to have the look and feel of institutional pharmacies.

A special category of pharmacy that is part community, part institutional, and part mail-order pharmacy is the *HMO* or *managed care pharmacy.* Pharmacy services are available as part of a coordinated medical and preventive service that is available to a defined population of subscribers (those who purchase the service) or beneficiaries (those who receive the benefit as part of their current or prior employment). Such pharmacies are not available to the general public, but they are handling geometric increases in prescription volume. Until the end of the last decade, managed care pharmacies were providing Medicaid dispensing services to the majority of state programs.

Mail-Order Pharmacies

Mail-order pharmacies are those which dispense prescriptions just as any other pharmacy would but then mail them to customers located all over the country. Such pharmacies have very few, if any, walk-in customers and tend to be high-volume operations that employ extensive information and material-handling technologies.

Specialty Practice

The fourth type of pharmacy may be described as a *specialty pharmacy*, because of how it operates or what types of prescriptions it handles. A small number of pharmacies are known as *nuclear pharmacies* because they specialize in handling compounds that are radioactive, i.e., intended for chemotherapy. Another type of specialty pharmacy is known as either a *parenteral* or *home infusion pharmacy*. Also few in number, home infusion pharmacies specialize in filling intravenous (and other parenteral) prescriptions intended to be administered to patients in their homes.

A limited, but growing, number of pharmacies specialize in compounding prescriptions. Their involvement in compounding goes well beyond what is typically seen in a community pharmacy, and *compounding pharmacies* may be freestanding or practice specialties situated within another type of pharmacy, e.g., a traditional community pharmacy.

The newest type of specialty pharmacy is an *Internet pharmacy*. Internet pharmacies are those which maintain a site on the World Wide Web and interact with customers primarily or exclusively via e-mail (as opposed to other types of pharmacies that have a Web site in addition to providing goods and services directly [independent or chain community pharmacy], by mail [mail-order pharmacy], or to an enrolled recipient group [HMO pharmacy]).[9]

Government Pharmacies

The fifth type of pharmacy is a *government pharmacy*. Federal, state, and local governments operate pharmacies and dispensaries for defined populations. The largest is operated by the U.S. Department of Defense (DOD) for active military personnel and their dependents. Both military and civilian pharmacists work in DOD pharmacies.

The Veterans Administration (VA) operates a network of hospitals and clinics that dispense and administer pharmaceuticals. The VA also has an extensive mail-order pharmacy service for veterans. The U.S. Public Health Service (PHS), including the Bureau of Indian Affairs, dispenses and administers pharmaceuticals to a number of different defined populations.

Pharmaceuticals are dispensed and administered to inmates in federal, state, and local prisons and jails, drug treatment centers, and public health clinics.

RETURN SPECIALISTS—REVERSE DISTRIBUTORS, RECLAMATION SPECIALISTS, AND DISPOSERS

A relatively new type of drug industry market specialist focuses on handling products that are returned by customers for credit to their immediate suppliers, e.g., an outdated trade package of antibiotics that "Able Pharmacy" returns for credit to its own warehouse, to a wholesale distributor, or to the drug's manufacturer. Return specialists also address returns sent by chain warehouses and wholesale distributors to drug manufacturers.

Aside from obvious ordering and shipping errors, which are handled on a routine basis as part of the order fulfillment process, approximately 1.5 to 2 percent of pharmaceutical sales are returned for credit to an up-channel supplier. Products are returned for a number of reasons, the most prevalent being these:

1. Expired date
2. Recalled by the manufacturer/labeler
3. Withdrawn from the market by the manufacturer/labeler
4. Damaged, defaced, or soiled

Less common reasons include these:

1. Changes to manufacturer/labeler product, package, or NDC number
2. Discontinuation by manufacturer/labeler
3. Change in buying group contract supplier or product of choice
4. Patent expiration, leading to generic introduction and reduced demand
5. Short-dated, i.e., less than six or twelve months
6. Overstock from forward (speculative) buying or warehouse closure
7. Slow demand, e.g., unusually slow flu season

The prevailing wisdom is that unsalables and returns are increasing throughout the channel. Further, the growing consensus is that returns processing is very costly to everyone involved. Such thinking has given rise to the first type of return specialist, the *reverse distributor*. About thirty reverse distributors now process returns from pharmacies, wholesaler distributors, and chain warehouses and seek credit from suppliers.

Another type of return specialist is a *reclamation specialist*. Reclamation is an effort to recover returned products that are otherwise salable (either to other customers or in secondary outlets at lower prices) and involves the reclaiming of nonprescription drugs only.

Changes in official policy, enforcement of environmental protection laws, and increasing recognition of substantive liability forced the industry (in the past decade) to stop flushing (in a commode), pouring (in sinks and into streams and lakes), and dumping (in trash cans, dumpsters, and landfills) pharmaceutical waste. Today, more and more pharmaceutical waste is being handled by *disposers*. Such specialists follow detailed guidelines in disposing of pharmaceutical waste in an environmentally responsible way.

CLINICS, SURGERY CENTERS, DIALYSIS CENTERS, LABORATORIES, AND PLANNED PARENTHOOD

Pharmaceuticals, especially vaccines, medical-surgical drugs and aids, diagnostic products, and birth control drugs, are increasingly distributed to medical clinics, freestanding surgery centers, dialysis centers, laboratories, and Planned Parenthood offices. Most of these products are used or administered by health care personnel, although birth control drugs are routinely dispensed with no pharmacist (or other health care oversight) on site.

PHARMACEUTICAL SAMPLING

A remarkable amount of brand-name pharmaceuticals, especially new and expensive drugs, reach the consumer through pharmaceutical sampling—and the practice is growing robustly. Drug sampling is regulated by the FDA under the Prescription Drug Marketing Act of 1987 and involves under what terms a pharmaceutical supplier can distribute drug samples to prescribers (physicians, dentists, and, in some states, physician's assistants and nurse practitioners). Pharmacies and pharmacists are not permitted to possess or distribute drug samples.

INSTITUTIONAL (HOSPITAL) MARKETING

Despite a virtual absence of economic and operational logic, manufacturers historically sold pharmaceuticals directly to hospitals (pharmacies).

In the mid-1970s, however, wholesale distributors were searching for a way to increase their market share, i.e., the percentage of drugs distributed by drug wholesalers, by finding new sources of business, and hospital pharmacy buying practices were a longtime concern.

At the time, hospital pharmacies purchased a very high percentage of pharmaceuticals directly from manufacturers in order to obtain major discounts. Such discounts were based on bids and contracts. The only business given to wholesale distributors involved small, infrequent "fill in" orders when direct shipments were delayed, the manufacturer could not supply an item, or a manufacturer was too small, i.e., had too few items, to justify opening and maintaining a direct account.

Because of ordering "direct," hospital pharmacies spent a great deal of time monitoring inventories, then creating and sending orders to a hundred or more different suppliers. Because of order minimums (by suppliers) and longer order cycles (typically four to eight days), hospitals stocked thousands of dollars of extra inventory, called "cushion stock."

To service hospital pharmacies, drug manufacturers had to establish and maintain more than 10,000 separate accounts and process tens of thousands of small orders. They had to create, mail, and follow up on even more invoices, statements, and credit memos. Hospital pharmacies tended to place smaller orders and to order more frequently. On a direct-order basis, they had higher than average order claim levels and returns. Worse yet, they tended to pay slower than average.

Wholesale distributors looked at the situation—where essentially no one was satisfied—then created a way to improve service to both hospitals and manufacturers, while generating entirely new business and improving market share. The system that emerged came to be known as *institutional marketing,* more informally called the *hospital charge-back system.* It is based on leaving the buyer-seller relationship between hospital pharmacies and drug manufacturers intact, while introducing wholesaler distributors into the mix to handle distribution.

Hospital pharmacies or, more correctly, hospital *buying groups,*[10] still issue requests for quotes (RFQ) to pharmaceutical manufacturers, which in turn prepare and submit written bids that specify

1. which drugs they are willing to sell, at
2. what heavily reduced price, for
3. what period of time, and to
4. which members of the buying group.

If accepted, the "contract" would be awarded to a "prime vendor" wholesaler, which would then supply products at the contract price plus a service fee.

In this manner, the fundamental business relationship between the hospital pharmacy and a successful (awarded a bid) drug manufacturer remained intact. Hospitals could still buy on the basis of bid prices and manufacturers were still able to bid products directly to individual hospitals or groups of hospitals, i.e., buying groups. Everyone benefited!

- Wholesale distributors acquired substantial new business volume (they were the best qualified to handle it).
- Hospitals got much faster (overnight to a few hours) and better (higher percentage of invoice lines filled) service and reduced their costs.
- Drug manufacturers eliminated thousands of slow-paying, high-service cost accounts in favor of fewer than 200 wholesale distributors that placed much larger orders (reduced handling costs) and paid on time (reduced carrying costs).

The key to making the institutional marketing system work is the origin of the term *charge back*. To avoid having to maintain two different inventories—one for pharmacies and one for contract hospital pharmacies—wholesale distributors, in collaboration with drug manufacturers, created the hospital charge-back system. In simplest terms, a charge-back is a type of rebate. Wholesale distributors continued to purchase pharmaceuticals in the same way and at the same cost as before. When they sold a contract item to a hospital pharmacy, it was priced according to the contract between the hospital and the manufacturer (a price materially less than the rest of the market paid). That created a difference between what the wholesale distributor originally paid for the product and the cost basis of the hospital contract. The difference was *charged back* to the manufacturer by the wholesale distributor to recover the shortfall.

Determining a Charge Back

Assume that a wholesale distributor ("Fast-Serv") purchases "Effecta-Mycin" for $150 per 100 tablets from "Effecta-Labs." Also, the manufacturer has a contract to sell Effecta-Mycin to a local hospital buying group for $80. Assume that a hospital pharmacy orders a bottle of Effecta-Mycin. Fast-Serv checks its records and determines that the hospital pharmacy is a current member of the local hospital buying group that has the $80 contract price. The sale is made at $80, plus the wholesale distributor's service fee (a matter between the hospital pharmacy and the wholesale distributor). That leaves the wholesale distributor "out" $70, i.e., $150 less $80. This is the amount that Fast-Serv charges back to the drug manufacturer.

WHOLESALE DISTRIBUTION

Approximately fifty wholesale distributors operate about 230 distribution centers throughout the U.S. market. Wholesale distributors provide five (or more) days of delivery each week of more than 250,000 different kinds of pharmaceuticals, nonprescription drugs, and health and beauty aids to more than 100,000 customer locations.

At one time, some industry members believed that the only thing drug wholesalers did was add inefficiency and cost to the distribution channel. That belief has disappeared, because it was shortsighted, misguided, and completely wrong!

Examples of U.S. Wholesale Distributors

AmeriSource Corporation	J. J. Balan, Inc.
Barnes Wholesdale Drug, Inc.	King Drug Company
Bellco Health	Kinray, Inc.
Bergen Brunswig Drug Company	McKesson HBOC
Bindley Western Drug Company	Miami-Luken, Inc.
Burlington Drug Company	Morris & Dickson Company, Ltd.
Capital Wholesale Drug Company	M. Sobol, Inc.
Cardinal Health, Inc.	N. C. Mutual Wholesale Drug Company
C. D. Smith Healthcare, Inc.	Penner & Welsch, Inc.
D&K Healthcare Resources, Inc.	Prescription Supply, Inc.
Dik Drug	Quality King distributors
Diversified Healthcare, Inc.	Rebel Distributors Corporation
Dixon-Shane Drug Company	Remo Drug Corporation
The F. Dohmen Company	Rochester Drug Cooperative
FMC Distributors, Inc.	Smith Drug Company
General Drug Company	Valley Drug Company
Goodwin Drug Company	Valley Wholesale Drug Company
Harvard Drug Group	Value Drug Company
H. D. Smith Wholesale Drug Company	Walsh Distribution
Jewett Drug Company	

Note: Mergers result in regular changes to company names.

In fact, just the opposite is true. Without wholesale distributors, the U.S. drug industry would be nowhere near as effective or efficient as it is today. Without wholesale distributors as essential channel intermediaries, each of more than 1,000 pharmaceutical producers would have to maintain accounts and service at least 100,000 customer accounts, including wholesale distributors, chain warehouses, pharmacies, government agencies, clinics and laboratories, and reverse distributors. Most of these accounts—at least 75 percent!—would order infrequently, in very small amounts, and then be slow in paying their bills.

Because of the distances involved, delivery uncertainties, and order minimums, pharmacies and others would be forced to order, store, and finance much more inventory than operationally warranted. Manufacturer order minimums alone would effectively preclude most customers from even ordering a manufacturer's line at all. Communicating with 100,000-plus customers, which wholesale distributors do routinely, would be a costly and time-consuming hurdle that only the largest manufacturers could undertake effectively. The cost and time required for drug recalls and withdrawals, product and promotional information, and new product introductions would be substantially higher absent wholesale distributors in the drug distribution channel.

Life without wholesale distributors would be much different for pharmacies, pharmacists, and everyone else involved in health care, including 281 million consumers. Pharmacies would be forced to interact with hundreds of suppliers on a routine basis. Each pharmacy, HMO, clinic, or lab, no matter how small or understaffed, would have to track drug usage and needs by manufacturer line and place individual orders to each one.

Wholesale distributors provide *better and faster delivery service* than direct distribution (buying directly from drug manufacturers) and *reduce the cost of order fulfillment, delivery, and shipping for their suppliers* (manufacturers) and customers. Wholesale distributors are in fact the *vital link* in the drug distribution channel in that they also

- finance manufacturer inventory;
- maintain accessible inventory close to dispensing points;
- shorten the time between order and delivery;
- furnish twenty-four-hour emergency supply service;
- provide essential trade credit;
- operate an effective new-product introduction pipeline;
- act as an essential backup supply of critical medicines during a national emergency;
- offer effective returns good processing;
- support manufacturer drug withdrawals and recalls;
- act as an efficient order conduit to other products not stocked;

- provide product and promotional information; and
- supply a wide range of customer critical support products and services.

Examples of common value-added services include private-label programs, special handling services—including vaccines, frozen products, and orphan drugs—generic source programs, pharmacy computer systems, third-party claims processing, zone pricing systems, point-of-sale systems, product and shelf stickers, and product movement reports.

These efforts have propelled wholesale distributors into a recognized leadership position in distribution efficiency. Wholesale distributors have continually reduced their operating costs and prices to the point that their customers routinely buy pharmaceuticals for the same or lower prices than they can get directly from the actual manufacturers. Best price and an impressive array of value-added services have reduced drug distribution costs, and therefore the nation's health care bill, by tens of billions of dollars—and wholesale distributors continue to play an ever more vital role in drug distribution.

SECTION V: PROMOTION

Chapter 13

Principles

Mickey Smith

INTRODUCTION

The four Ps that are used as the framework for much of this book are a convenient way of categorizing the functions of marketing, but they are not without problems as a framework. *Promotion* is one "P" with a bit of a problem. Promotion sounds like what many, if not most, laypeople believe marketing to be—efforts to sell things that one may or may not need at a price one may or may not be able to afford. This is really unfortunate, inasmuch as promotion, at least in the context of *this* book, is communication. Perhaps the "P" in this case should be *professional* communication or *pharmaceutical* communication or *people* communication.

In any case, the promotion of pharmaceutical products is the linchpin of the marketing mix. Promotion is the vehicle by which the product, its price, and methods of distribution should be described to the firm's audiences in a way that is both coherent and persuasive. The definition, then, is "what and how markets are informed of the firm's product, place, and price."

Promotion, especially advertising, tends to have more glamour than do the other mix components. It is certainly more visible and often appears to be more creative. The other elements of the marketing mix are of little value unless their advantages are communicated to those who need to know. On the other hand, promotion cannot long succeed if one or more of the other elements of the marketing mix are unsatisfactory.

Promotion can sell a good product or service, but it cannot take the place of quality or sustain poor products or services for long. (Some of the finest television advertising is for franchised goods and services. Do you see much resemblance between the television McDonald's or Century 21 or Midas Muffler and your local version? It is long way from Madison Avenue to Main Street, USA).

Portions of this chapter are updated and adapted from material appearing in Chapter 11 of an earlier work by Mickey C. Smith, *Pharmaceutical Marketing: Strategy and Cases* (Binghamton, NY: The Haworth Press, 1991), pp. 326-394.

In this chapter we will examine several issues relating to principles of promotion. The first is what to say. In essence, this means how best to explain to the customers and physicians what the company wants them to know about its goods and services. The next question addressed is who should receive these messages. This is followed by descriptions of the various media available to accomplish this communication. In a subsequent chapter we will discuss some of the technical aspects of promotion.

It is difficult to make any quantitative assessments of the information required by the categories of people who need to use or have access to such information. It has been suggested that, in terms of typewritten pages, the information required by the various categories would probably be of the following orders of magnitude:

1. The pharmaceutical industry—4,000 pages (but see Chapter 5)
2. The regulatory agency—200 pages
3. Academic investigators—500 pages
4. Prescribers—20 pages
5. Patients—2 pages[1]

Faced with some of the restrictions described in the next chapter, one might expect those in charge of pharmaceutical promotion to be reduced to staid, colorless, industrial messages. On the contrary, the challenge of regulation seems to have engendered an extraordinary level of creativity in writing, illustration, and media.

For prescription drugs the most frequent target for promotion is still the physician, and we will use the physician as our main example in this section.

Copy refers to the content of an advertisement. In the advertising industry, the term is sometimes used in a broad sense to include the words, pictures, symbols, colors, layout, and other ingredients of an ad. Copywriting is a creative job, and its quality depends to a large extent on the creative ability of the writers in the advertising agency or the company. However, creativity alone may not produce good ad copy. In the book *Medicine Avenue*, which will be quoted elsewhere in this book, Frank Hughes states:

> The art of writing medical advertising requires knowledge about the product and the science behind it as well as ability to give life to the data that renders an argument for the product both compelling and *luminous* [editor's emphasis], with words that are fresh and memorable. The art of writing medical advertising is especially difficult, given the medicine. Unlike consumer advertising where you might be writing the only ad for a fountain pen in a magazine carrying ads for perfume, cars, food, and clothes, in medical advertising we are often writing an ad for an antihypertensive to appear in a cardiology book (magazine), in which most of the ads are for antihypertensives.[2]

A marketing strategist needs to have his or her own perspectives incorporated in the copy and needs to furnish information on ad objectives, product, target customers, competitive activity, and ethical and legal considerations. The creative person will carry on from there. In brief, although copywriting may be the outcome of a flash of inspiration on the part of an advertising genius, it must rest on a systematic, logical, step-by-step presentation of idea, especially with pharmaceuticals.

Physicians *tend* to be more rational in their decision making than do ultimate consumers. They prescribe to fit the needs of their patients, and these needs normally are of a practical nature. It should not be forgotten, however, that these physicians are individuals having personal needs, which sometimes become enmeshed in their roles as decision makers for their patients. Thus, even choice of a prescription drug may be made on bases that are nonrational or emotional. The advertisers have recognized the various factors that influence prescribing decisions and have structured their advertising appeals toward these factors. Table 13.1 contains a list of types of appeals used to influence prescription drug decisions.

The advertising objectives could be any one or all of the following:

1. To generate product awareness—*recall*
2. To communicate new information—*communication*
3. To increase interest or product usage—*persuasion*
4. To generate positive convictions about products—*persuasion*

Effective advertising of any product depends on a chain of events similar to this: attention → interest → consumption (of the message) → motivation → action. Appeals, as presented, are most active (or inactive if unsuccessful) in the first two or three steps, but they are a part of the entire process. The last step, however, is the key to the sequence. If there is no action, the advertisement is a failure.

The function of the advertising, as all marketing people know but sometimes ignore, is to communicate effectively information preplanned to encourage directly or indirectly the purchase of goods or services. For pharmaceutical advertising, the same function includes three parts:

1. To secure a greater part of an existing market
2. To broaden the range of indications
3. To expand the total market

Any advertiser attempts to relate the specific benefits of the product to the specific needs of the consumer of the advertising message. Varying advertising appeals are merely reflections of varying needs of the advertising target as determined by the advertiser. This is true for any advertising. Pre-

TABLE 13.1. A Typology of Pharmaceutical Advertising Appeals

Rational Appeals	Nonrational Appeals

Product-related appeals
  Economy
  Degree of innovation
  Differentiation/position
  Packaging
  Dosage form/taste
	Empathy
	Humor
	Sex
	Curiosity
	Fear
	Unusual nonclinical illustration

Physician-related appeals
  Peer/specialist approval
  P&T committee approval
  Therapeutic aid in practice
	Ego gratifying
	Anger/defensiveness
	Patriotism

Clinical use appeals
  Dependability
  Safety
  Clinical illustration
  Effectiveness
  Reminder	

Patient-related appeals
  Compliance
  Quality of life
  Patient acceptance/preference	

Manufacturer-related appeals
  Experience
  Service
  Special expertise	

scription drug advertising is a special case, however. Some of the distinctive characteristics of this market are listed here:

1. The consumer of the advertising is often not the consumer of the product.
2. Institutional advertising (designed to enhance the firm's image rather than promote a specific product) is of greater importance here than in many other markets.
3. Because of the nature of the products, advertising and scientific communication tend to be confused. On one hand, advertising may disseminate research results. On the other, favorable scientific reports in reputable journals may stimulate the sale of products. Some claim, with justification, that pharmaceutical advertising at times is

educational in character, since the information it contains may constitute a valuable aid to therapy. It is certainly true that physicians and pharmacists read advertising.

4. The plethora of information on prescribing physicians and purchasing pharmacists in the United States practically fixes the population of the market and allows for more exhaustive analysis. Theoretically, this should mean that it is easier to tailor the advertising message to suit their needs.

5. In theory, the physician is a rational decision maker, somewhat similar to the industrial goods purchaser, so that the emotional appeals of consumer advertising might (again in theory) be inappropriate to the audience. In actual practice, however, it is not at all unusual to see an emotional appeal in prescription drug advertising. Our working hypothesis is that the rational appeal is more useful for primary-demand stimulation, and the emotional appeal for selective-demand simulation.

6. Actual readership seems to depend, in a major way, on the physical characteristics of the advertisements. This, of course, is somewhat the case in any kind of graphic advertising.

7. Readership of an ethical drug advertisement may depend, in large part, on the general readability and reputation of the journal in which the advertisement is published. A favorable attitude toward advertising may be expressed simply because of the confidence in the journal itself. Many journals have screening personnel who disallow the publication of dubious claims or presentation of doubtful products.

8. Readers may be predisposed to confidence in the advertiser, particularly, but not necessarily, large pharmaceutical companies. Product and institutional advertising (or combinations) are important to the pharmaceutical manufacturer trying to establish its brand names. Although straightforward advertisements by unknown manufacturers may be effective under special conditions, they may be viewed with some suspicion by some readers.

9. Pharmaceutical products seem to be adopted in response to the combined stimulus of an unusual number of different forms of promotion (detailing, journal advertising, direct mail, and communication with other physicians and/or pharmacists). The relative influence of each advertising medium in stimulating the *continued* use of a drug product may be entirely different from its relative influence in *introducing* the same product.

10. Drug advertising is unique in presenting both the good and the bad about the product. Although federal regulation plays a large role in

this, few, if any, other industries routinely point out the shortcomings of their products in their advertising.

Appeal Objectives

The appeals that might be used to advertise a given product are as numerous and varied as the motives of those to whom they are directed. The possibilities for verbalizing or symbolizing a given appeal are infinite; however, the appeal objectives of typical pharmaceutical promotion usually fall into one or more of the following categories:

1. Create awareness of the existence of a product or brand
2. Create a brand image
3. Supply information regarding benefits and superior features of the brand, e.g., reduction of side effects, ease in administration
4. Combat or offset competitive claims
5. Build familiarity and easy recognition of package or trademark
6. Build corporate image and favorable attitude toward the company
7. Establish a reputable platform for launching new brands or products
8. Register a unique selling proposition in the minds of the prescriber while stimulating sales

As Table 13.1 shows, we have identified several fairly distinct types of appeals beyond this classification. In general, the major distinction is between appeals to what might be termed rational and nonrational prescribing motives. These might be defined, respectively, as those which involve the process of matching means with ends and those more involved with the emotions and senses. This classification is made with the qualification that the concept of rational versus nonrational behavior is not fully accepted by marketing theorists and that behavior may be *rational*, but *stupid*.

RATIONAL APPEALS

Product-Related Appeals

- *Economy:* In recent years, pharmaceutical advertising has greatly increased this type of appeal.
- *Innovation:* Innovation is a traditional part of the development of the pharmaceutical industry. New products are the staff of life to the industry. As a consequence, the word "new" appears with sufficient frequency in drug advertising to lose some of its effect. Nevertheless, the

effect of a message that a significant medical advance has appeared may be powerful.

- *Differentiation:* It is sound marketing policy to attempt in some way to differentiate a product from the otherwise similar products of the competition. Flavors, dosage forms, and unique packaging are methods of accomplishing this.
- *Mode of action or use:* This is one of the most rational of appeals. In this case, the doctor is told what the product is good for or how it works. Particularly when the physician has or recently has had a patient requiring this activity, interest is aroused.

Physician-Related Appeals

- *Approval of peers:* A product gains something in reputation by use among large numbers of physicians, especially specialists.
- *Therapeutic aid to physicians:* In advertisements of this type, it is made very clear that the product is a tool for use by the physician. In this context, the product appears valuable without subtracting from the importance of the physician.

Clinical Use-Related Appeals

- *Product dependability:* The advertisement is designed to capture attention and arouse interest by presenting a claim that is impressive but believable. Copy and layout strategy are designed to inspire confidence by presenting unmistakable evidence of the product's successful use.
- *Safety:* This is a reflection of the medical dictum *Primum non nocere* (first do no harm). Safety is a primary consideration at present, with the continuing interest in adverse drug reactions.
- *Clinical illustration:* In some cases, the quality of the art in the advertisement offers an aid in explanation of the workings of the compound in vitro. The producer of the advertisement is in the position of creating a more believable instrument by illustrating a clinical situation, rather than giving a sterile presentation of facts.
- *Reminder:* The manufacturer orients the pictorial message to the physicians' experience. The advertising message tends to be perishable for two reasons: (1) the physician may forget about products used infrequently, and (2) the products themselves change. For these reasons, the reminder advertisement is important.
- *Patient response:* The principal objective of this type of appeal is to show the actual effect of the drug. The before-and-after illustration is frequently employed in this type of advertisement.

Manufacturer-Related Appeals

In this type of appeal, an effort is made to give a favorable impression of the manufacturer to the physician. Since confidence in the manufacturer is one element in prescribing motivation, such an effort is justified.

NONRATIONAL APPEALS

- *Empathy:* Empathy is the participation in the feelings or ideas of another. As used in the present context, it describes the appeal used in pharmaceutical advertising to project the feelings of the patients into those of their physicians.
- *Humor:* Humorous approaches to the advertising messages are common in both medical and consumer advertising. Marketing people recognize, however, that merely succeeding at being funny is not tantamount to success in conveying the advertising message. The ability to construct an advertisement in which the humor is a natural lead-in to the effective advertising message is rare talent.
- *Sex:* There is a temptation to introduce sexual appeal into advertising products that would not logically lend themselves to this appeal when nothing better can be developed. When this occurs, the result is the irrelevant use of both copy and illustration.
- *Curiosity:* Curiosity seems to be a quality inherent in physicians in even greater quantities than in the rest of the population. As a consequence, it is frequently used as an attention-getting device in the drug advertisement.
- *Illustration layout:* The incongruous, the shocking, and the unusual can be used to advantage in adding attention value to the advertisement. If they are carefully selected so that they are relevant to the rest of the massage, they literally may be "worth a thousand words."
- *Ego gratifying:* This appeal is basic, going to that which is most interesting to anyone—oneself. In advertisements of this type, the physician is primary, the product, secondary.

Since analysis of the advertising content of medical journals shows both rational and nonrational types of appeal, it would seem to follow that the physician may be subject to nonrational motivations in the choice of prescription drugs. How can this be justified in a decision area that seems to demand only rational considerations?

An internal debate is constantly being waged by the physician, who must justify each prescription, relating the decision to a personal value system. Nonrational appeals play a part in this process of justification. The degree of rationality, in the final analysis, is a function of the physician's ability to match ends and means. The theory of cognitive dissonance may help us to understand this.

Cognitive dissonance is a multifaceted research tool that has been used to give further meaning to many types of motivational behavior. Ever since Festinger's theory of dissonance first appeared in 1957, it has at the same time tantalized researchers with its fascinating possibilities and been widely criticized as an oversimplification of a set of factors not readily amenable to such analysis.

Inherent in every decision process is a certain degree of uncertainty. It has been hypothesized that this will lead to psychological discomfort, which Festinger refers to as dissonance. In an effort to *reduce* dissonance, the decision maker will seek positive or favorable elements (i.e., information) that will reinforce his or her choice. These elements may take the form of advertising, irrational or biased thinking, or favorable opinions from supposed authorities.

Physicians constantly receive various kinds of information about pharmaceuticals from colleagues, direct mail advertisements, journal ads, medical journals and texts, sales representatives, and a variety of other sources. According to the theory of cognitive dissonance, physicians would much prefer to have all these bits of information be consistent with one another. If these cognitions are not consistent, the theory holds that physicians will try to reduce the inconsistency (dissonance), and the physicians try to reduce dissonance after making prescribing decisions.

Thus, a doctor who selects Brand A tranquilizer over another brand might experience dissonance because he is aware of the beneficial features of the rejected brand and of the unattractive features of Brand A. One way to reduce dissonance would be to read advertisements of Brand A tranquilizer (the one prescribed) that would reinforce the prescribing decision.

Some of the theory presented in conjunction with consumer research has potential application to the physician-marketing interface. This statement is made even though we recognize that analysis of physician behavior involves many interacting forces, and the postdecision emphasis of dissonance theory represents only one part of a complex problem.

As Table 13.2 shows, one prescribing situation may produce dissonance while another does not. In this table, we have taken some of the dissonance and buying situations from consumer research and applied them to the prescription situation. As this tabulation shows, several factors may be operative at the same time—one may produce dissonance; two others may be dissonance reducing. It is equally true that the dissonance aroused by these differing conditions may be reduced in a variety of ways. The prescriber may change evaluations of the drug, select supporting information about the drug, or ignore (consciously or unconsciously) conflicting information.

TABLE 13.2. Dissonance and Prescribing

Factors Affecting	Prescribing	High Dissonance	Low Dissonance
Attractiveness of rejected alternative	Doctor must choose between four tranquilizers.	Three are proven to be effective.	One is clearly superior.
Negative factors in chosen alternative	Doctor chooses between two similar drugs.	Chosen drug has desired action but is habit forming.	Chosen one has desired action but is not habit forming.
Number of alternatives	Doctor wants to prescribe a diuretic.	There are eight brands to choose from.	There are only two to choose from.
Cognitive overlap	Doctor prescribes cough medicine.	Both choices have codeine; other ingredients vary slightly.	Both choices have codeine; other ingredients differ.
Positive inducement	Doctor prescribes antiobesity preparation.	Patient is three pounds overweight.	Patient is thirty pounds overweight.
Information available	Doctor prescribes for angina pectoris.	Doctor prescribes new pharmaceutical entity—little data available.	Doctor prescribes nitroglycerine.
Anticipated dissonance	Doctor insists on very expensive brand-name drug for hospital patient.	Drug is not on the formulary, but similar drugs are.	Drug is on hospital formulary.

Experimental studies are needed to determine the extent to which cognitive dissonance is a factor in the marketing of prescription drugs. Inventive design of such studies might well point out means of bringing more efficiency to the promotion of these products. Both pharmaceutical marketing and postgraduate medical education stand to benefit from increased knowledge of the psychological factors that influence the choice of drugs and information about drugs.

TO WHOM SHOULD PRODUCTS BE PROMOTED?

Choosing targets for promotion of prescription drug products seems comparatively straightforward. Promotional messages should be sent to those who need information about the firm's price, place, and product and who make or influence decisions concerning product purchase.

Deciding to whom to promote precedes such additional strategic decisions as these:

- What appeal is best?
- What part of your budget should be spent on this promotional target?
- Which promotional method(s) is (are) the best choice?

Clearly, prescribing physicians are a logical target for promotion of prescription drug products. Beyond that, basic decisions involve pharmacists, nurses, administrators, and especially consumers. In addition, the pharmaceutical company is facing new breeds of gatekeepers whose motivations, role, background, education, and title are all markedly different from that of the physicians and even the pharmacists—considered the more traditional decision makers. In many settings, such as managed care organizations and hospital consortia, these new gatekeepers control access to major portions of the marketplace with a single formulary or purchasing decision.

A SPECIAL CASE:
PRESCRIPTION DRUG ADVERTISING TO CONSUMERS

The 1980s saw a revolution of sorts in prescription drug promotion. For virtually the first time, advertisements to the general public alluded to conditions for which the treatments were to be prescription drugs (see Table 13.3).

The strategies, concerns, and expectations that led to some of the earliest experiments in direct-to-consumer (DTC) prescription drug advertising are illuminating. In a 1986 symposium jointly sponsored by the American Medical Writers Association and the Pharmaceutical Advertising Council, the views of some of the early practitioners were expressed and included those of Elizabeth Moench, who described some of the strategic considerations of DTC at Boots.[3]

In 1969 the Boots Company, a British-based $3 billion company, licensed to the Upjohn Company for the U.S. market a product called "ibuprofen." Upjohn has been marketing ibuprofen under the brand name of Motrin since 1974. Boots, at the time of the licensing arrangements, made it clear that, at some time in the foreseeable future, as and when Boots established a presence in the States, Boots would market its own version of ibuprofen. With the acquisition of Rucker Pharmacal in Shreveport, Louisiana, in 1977, Boots established its base and introduced Rufen in September of 1981.

TABLE 13.3. "Genealogy" of Direct-to-Consumer Advertising

Year	Product/Indication	Company
1981	Pneumonia vaccine	Merck
1982	Hepatitis B vaccine	Merck
	Consumer program	Pfizer
1983	Rufen versus Motrin	Boots
1983-1985	FDA moratorium on DTC advertising by product name	
1984	Menstrual cramps	Syntex
	Smoking cessation	Merrell Dow
1985	Painful leg cramps	Hoechst Roussel
	Quality of life	Squibb
1986	Genital herpes	Burroughs Wellcome
	Allergy sufferers	Merrell Dow
1987	Diabetes/recipes	Roerig Pfizer
	Arthritis/angina	Pfizer
	Tavist-1	Sandoz
1988	Ulcers	Smith Kline French
	High cholesterol	Merck

Source: Kathleen McRoberts, "Direct to Consumer: New Route for Ethical Drug Marketers," in *Pharmaceutical Executive* November, 8(11): 48-52, 1988.

Boots faced many difficulties in marketing Rufen, unique to Boots, and also to the industry. Boots was to compete against its licensee Motrin, which was the brand leader.

Boots had only 110 sales representatives, against 5,164 representatives at the time in the nonsteroidal anti-inflammatory market. In the United States, Boots was virtually unknown and the company had to convince both pharmacists and physicians that Rufen was not a generic, but that Boots was both the patent holder and developer of ibuprofen.

Due to patent expiration in 1985, Boots had a limited time in which to establish Rufen in the marketplace. The only selling message that Boots had was the "Rufen was the same as Motrin but costs less." The cost-benefit advantage was to be the marketing approach in detailing Rufen to physicians. This posed a final dilemma. How could Boots assure the doctor that patients would indeed receive Rufen at a lower price? The answer was the introduction of the $1.50 rebate coupon, and a 25-cent contribution to arthritis research for every coupon redeemed. This marked also the first time price, rather than a product's clinical and therapeutic advantages, have been detailed to physicians, and the first test of consumers' response to price.

The $1.50 rebate program became the catalyst for Boots' direct-to-consumer advertising program for Rufen.

In preparing for the direct-to-consumer approach, it was necessary first to conduct market research with consumers, then with physicians and pharmacists. The consumer research was done in three waves.

First, consumer knowledge and understanding about arthritis and prescription drugs was determined. Second, price-advertising concepts were tested in order to measure reaction and comprehension. The third wave of testing was the television commercial itself. From the market research the target audience was identified and a strategy was designed to test the advertising concepts.

Boots would advertise in two markets (Tampa, with Miami as the control, and Oklahoma City, with a control of Tulsa). In the selection of the test market many factors were considered, including population demographics, third-party pay/Medicaid reimbursement, and advertising costs. The test would be for six months, during which time independent market research and research by Boots' own market research team would be conducted.

Prior to the launch of the consumer program, it was essential to test physician response to the television commercial in the Tampa area, and to inform them of the program.

If you are asked to give your opinion on direct-to-consumer advertising for a prescription drug, what comes to mind? Would you be in favor or adamantly opposed to the concept? When physicians were asked to picture a prescription drug being advertised to consumers they were principally opposed, having nothing to compare the commercials to other than those already on television for OTC products. It is human nature to assume the worst, and when physicians were surveyed by asking to give their views as to "Should prescription drugs be advertised directly to the public?" the answer is almost always "No!"

This brings me to the point of emphasizing that Boots felt, during this time, there was a need for more in-depth market research, for specific commercials out of the laboratory setting, and that they be implemented by both industry and the FDA in order to evaluate the merits of direct-to-consumer advertising and in formulation of policy. In comparing the Boots' Rufen commercial to other OTC medications which make veiled promises to rheumatic patients, I would ask you to make your own decision as to merits. The physicians sampled in Florida were highly in favor of the Rufen commercial. Information kits about the consumer program were sent to all health care professionals in the Tampa area.

With the additional data regarding physician acceptance, the first commercial was launched on May 19. Boots' President John Bryer appeared on the *Today Show* with Commissioner Hayes, and on the afternoon of May 23, the FDA held their first consumer exchange meeting in Washington, where the consumer ad was discussed. The commercial was withdrawn and a letter sent to the FDA rebutting all the comments made in their letter, especially since Boots felt the advertisement, composed mostly by attorneys, complied with all existing regulations.

The FDA was then provided with this alternate commercial, which was then approved May 24. The newspaper advertisement was delayed for several weeks since it was revised to adhere to all the points raised in the regulatory letter.

I should point out that the consumer advertising program was not just a television commercial and newspaper advertisement but included patient information, physician information, and a new magazine called *Go!* specifically designed for arthritis patients, with $1 from each subscription to be given to the Arthritis Foundation.

The public relations campaign was highly successful; press kits containing full information were sent to all major media. The launch of the consumer program was planned for May 19 to coincide with the article in *The Wall Street Journal.* In one day Boots talked to over thirty reporters and held a press conference in New York, the same week Cable Health Network announced FDA approval for the advertising of prescription drugs.

Boots viewed the FDA's action to approve Cable Health Network (Lifetime) as somewhat hypocritical. On the one hand they had requested a moratorium on direct-to-consumer advertising other than price, yet they permitted advertisements to air on a consumer network whereby the FDA publicly stated they could expect "eavesdroppers" with demographics of "8.5 million consumers, and 40,000 physicians" (at that time).

Following the launch of the first direct-to-consumer advertising program for Rufen, I spoke at the FDLI (Food and Drug Law Institute) meeting and stated:

> This is the first time a marketing plan has been devised where the consumer is the central core: in other words, we have responded to the needs of consumers without impairing Boots' relationship with doctors, and what we have done must surely be a sign for what is yet to come.

On February 26, 1986, Zenith announced a consumer program for tolazamide modeled after the Rufen $1.50 rebate coupon. The company has also announced that more innovative programs are yet to be launched. Many other companies have come close to a direct-to-consumer approach, but none have taken the quantum jump.

Direct-to-consumer advertising can, and will, only succeed when the profile of the respective patient can be clearly defined, understood, and a marketing program narrowly tailored to the particular audience. I also believe that products for long-term chronic use will be the products most conducive to direct-to-consumer advertising. But as Milton Friedman recently wrote in *Newsweek*—"Be wary of the self-proclaimed 'experts' and an expert on predicting the future I am not, only a speculator!"

Kirk Schueler, then an award-winning marketer at Merrell Dow, described their approach differently.[4]

OTC drugs are advertised directly to consumers, and appropriately so, since in order to qualify for over-the-counter status a product is supposed to be (1) for a condition which is easily self-diagnosed, (2) can be reasonably self-treated, (3) with a modest or reasonable level of information necessary regarding proper use. The product itself is one for which (4) there is a substantial amount of experience and (5) general recognition of safety and effectiveness.

Rx drugs differ from OTC drugs on one or more and sometimes all of the above criteria. They can be for (1) difficult to diagnose conditions, (2) which require professional treatment decisions and monitoring, (3) with a more in-depth level of information required regarding proper use. Rx products may have (4) a limited amount of usage experience, and (5) a still developing safety and/or efficacy profile.

These distinctions mandate a different method of distribution, the requirement of the involvement of a physician, and a different mode of promotion. It is, in our opinion, unacceptable to advertise prescription drugs in a manner similar to OTC drugs.

What factors, then, lead us to favor direct-to-consumer promotion? By definition, we are excluding product-specific ads. The promotion we are including is disease-oriented advertising and there are many factors which favor such promotion:

1. Consumers desire more in-depth information on health issues. A better informed consumer is generally a healthier consumer. Pharmaceutical manufacturers can help consumers become better informed about important health issues.
2. Consumers are generally more oriented to self-treatment than ever before. While this is beneficial to them in some circumstances, it can be detrimental in others. Direct-to-consumer promotion can help consumers identify appropriate times and circumstances where a physician's guidance can be beneficial.
3. Our medical knowledge and the availability of treatment alternatives are expanding. Direct-to-consumer promotion can help consumers be more aware of this information and thereby use it to their advantage.
4. Drugs are often used incorrectly. Compliance might be improved through direct-to-consumer promotion. Greater communication between patients and health care professionals can also be fostered regarding proper use and potential side effects of medications.

These direct-to-consumer promotional efforts can have a favorable impact on the sales of specific products, but without a brand-name orientation within the promotion. So, what's wrong with brand-name focus? Why do we oppose prescription drug advertising to the consumer? There are several important reasons:

1. Product-specific ads will result in product-specific requests from consumers to physicians. As we've discussed, if a product is on prescription status, it requires a physician's expertise. That expertise may be essential for proper diagnosis, proper treatment selection, and proper usage instructions. Drug manufacturers should be preserving and indeed building the doctor-patient relationship, not eroding or circumventing it.
2. Product-specific ads that result in physicians prescribing products based on patient requests would increase the drug manufacturer's liability since the learned intermediary role of the physician is compromised. Primary responsibility of communicating precautionary information to the patient would now fall on the manufacturer rather than the physician. We certainly can't want to increase liability issues.
3. Adequate precautionary information would be extremely difficult to provide in prescription drug advertising to the consumer. Attempts to provide that information would also add considerably to the cost of such advertising due to the air time and publication space needed for that information.
4. Multiple product-specific ads within individual therapeutic categories would be likely to result in considerable consumer confusion and a general

increase in health care promotion costs. To speak to the confusion issue, let's take the antihypertensive market as a hypothetical example. Imagine one manufacturer of an alpha-blocker promoting the "alpha advantage," another manufacturer the beta difference; a third emphasizes the importance of once-a-day dosing, and a fourth says a major factor in hypertension is fluid retention and our product is the "most potent diuretic or fluid reducer on the market." How is a consumer supposed to sort out these messages? Imagine further that a consumer found the "alpha advantage" message very convincing and went to his or her doctor asking the physician to "give me the alpha advantage." The patient-product match may not be appropriate. The physician is then placed in the position of either talking the patient out of the "alpha advantage" or possibly risking losing the patient to another physician who would honor the patient's request. If the doctor succumbs to the pressure and prescribes the product for fear of losing the patient from the practice, then we run into the problems we talked about with increased manufacturer liability and deterioration of the doctor-patient relationship. I don't think that's the kind of health care system any of us want.

In summary, prescription drug advertising to the consumer could result in improper matches of product and patient, insufficient precautionary information for patients, a deterioration in the doctor-patient relationship, increased liability for the manufacturer, and escalated health care promotion costs.

Direct-to-consumer advertising would seem to make sense only when certain conditions exists:

- The consumer can be taught to identify the condition the product treats.
- The consumer can be convinced to visit a physician for help.
- The physician will have only that product available.
- The physician will prescribe it.

Clearly, the marketing equation for the pharmaceutical industry has changed. Pharmaceutical marketers must identify and investigate the new target audiences and add them to the marketing equation. Regardless of the marketing issue a pharmaceutical company is facing, it must first determine the participants in the decision-making process and the roles they play.

WHERE TO PROMOTE:
STRATEGIC CHOICES AMONG MEDIA

Strategic decisions in the area of promotion concern the allocation of effort among the different methods of promotion (media). For prescription drugs the broad classes of media available are

1. advertising—journals, direct mail, and other;
2. personal selling (detailing)—in person, by telephone, at conventions, etc.;
3. sampling;
4. sales promotions, giveaways, calendars, pens, other product reminders; and
5. news media—television, radio, computers, and the "Web."

A critical need exists for developing a conceptual framework to make promotion mix decisions. A variety of factors may be considered to determine the appropriate promotion mix in a particular product/market situation. These may be categorized as product factors, market factors, customer factors, budget factors, and marketing-mix factors, as outlined in Table 13.4. This section discusses the significance of each of these categories in determining the promotion mix.

Product Factors

Factors in this category relate principally to the way in which the product is prescribed, used, bought, consumed, and perceived. The perceived risk of

TABLE 13.4. Sample Criteria for Determining Promotion Mix

Category	Factor
Product	Nature of product Risk-benefit relationship Degree of exploration required for successful use Potential for demonstration Potential for OTC switch
Market	Position in its life cycle Market share Industry concentration Intensity of competition Demand perspectives Generic competition
Customer	Hospital or drugstore Customer power Physical distribution considerations
Environment	Regulatory controls Social climate
Budget	Financial resources of the organization Traditional promotional perspectives
Marketing mix	Relative price/relative quality Distribution strategy

a decision is another variable here. Generally speaking, the more risk a prescriber perceives to be associated with prescribing a particular product, the higher will be the importance of personal selling over advertising. The prescriber generally desires specific information on the product when the perceived risk is high, and this necessitates an emphasis on personal selling. Personal selling is also important in delivery of messages of unusual or complicated product benefits.

Market Factors

The first market factor is the position of a product in its life cycle. The creation of primary demand, hitherto nonexistent, is the primary task during the introductory stage; therefore, a high level of promotion effort is needed to explain a new product to potential customers or prescribers. This is often the logical time to use samples.

In the maturity phase, competition becomes intense, and advertising, along with sales promotion, is required to differentiate the product from competitive brands. During the decline phase, the promotional effort does not vary much initially from that during the maturity phase, except that the intensity of promotion declines. Later on, as price competition becomes keen and demand continues to decline, overall promotional perspectives are reduced.

For a given product class, if market share is high, both advertising and personal selling are used. If the market share is low, the emphasis is placed on either personal selling or advertising. If a market is concentrated among a few firms, advertising will achieve additional significance for two reasons: (1) heavy advertising may help discourage other firms from entering the field and (2) sustain a desired position for the product in the market. Heavy advertising constitutes an implied warranty of product performance and perhaps decreases the uncertainty associated with new products. In this way, new competition is discouraged and existing positions are reinforced. Intensity of competition tends to affect promotional blending in the same way that market share does. When competition is keen, all types of promotion are needed to sustain the product's position in the market. This is because promotion is needed to inform, remind, and persuade. On the other hand, if competitive activity is limited, the major function of promotion is to inform and perhaps remind about the product.

Hypothetically, advertising is more suited for products that have relatively latent demand. This is because advertising investment would open new opportunities in the long run, and if the carryover effect is counted, expenditure per sales dollar would be more beneficial. If demand is limited and new demand is not expected to be created, advertising outlay would be uneconomical. Thus, future potential becomes a significant factor in determining the role of advertising.

Customer Factors

Certainly the choice of promotion mix will be determined by the customers. Selling in a multimillion-dollar bid situation certainly requires personal presence and the facility for give and take. On the other hand, promotion of a seasonal cold remedy deal may be accomplished as well through a journal ad.

Environmental Factors

We will describe in the next chapter the stringent controls on prescription drug promotion imposed by the FDA. There are social considerations, as well. Major television networks, for example, have been reluctant to accept ads for contraceptive products such as condoms. The drug diversion problems that reached a peak in the 1980s resulted in both regulatory controls on samples and some professional distaste for the sampling procedure itself.

Budget Factors

Ideally the budget should be based on the promotional tasks to be performed. However, intuitively and traditionally, companies place an upper limit on the amount that they will spend on promotion. Such a limit may influence the type of promotion that may be undertaken. Budget factors affect the promotional blend in two ways. First, a financially weak company will be constrained in undertaking certain types of promotion. Second, in many companies the advertising budget has been traditionally linked to revenues as a percentage. This method of allocation continues to be used so that expected revenues will indicate how much might be spent on advertising in the future. The allocated funds then automatically determine the role of advertising.

Marketing-Mix Factors

The promotion decision should be made in the context of other aspects of the marketing mix. The price and quality of a product relative to competition affect the nature of its promotional perspectives. Higher prices must be justified by actual or presumed product superiority. Thus, in the case of a product that is priced substantially higher, advertising achieves significance in communicating and establishing the product's superior quality.

The promotion mix is also influenced by the distribution structure employed for the product. If the product is distributed directly, the sales force will largely be counted on to promote the product. Indirect distribution, on the other hand, requires greater emphasis on advertising, since the sales force push is limited.

MEDIA TYPES

In this section* we will touch briefly on the major promotional media available for use by the prescription drug industry. Specifically,

- space media (journals, magazines, newspapers),
- direct mail,
- personal selling (detailing, conventions and meetings, telemarketing),
- samples, and
- sales promotions, as well as electronic and "other" media.

Space Media

Space expenditures represent the amount of money spent for advertising in journals, magazines, and newspapers.

Distinction is made between journals, magazines, and newspapers, with the difference between them being in the editorial content. Journals, for the most part, offer technical information relating to an individual's professional practice. *The Journal of the American Medical Association, Archives of Internal Medicine, GP,* and the *Journal of the American Pharmaceutical Association* are examples of professional journals. *Medical Economics* and *Dental Management* are in the magazine category because their editorial content is not specifically devoted to the scientific aspects of the reader's training, but it is nonetheless important to the business side of professional practice. Newspapers require no definition and include publications such as *Medical Tribune* and *Family Practice News.*

Another distinction involves the matter of payment. Physicians may subscribe to individual publications (e.g., *New England Journal of Medicine*), they may pay for it as part of a professional membership (e.g., *Journal of the American Medical Association*), or they may receive it without charge, so-called "controlled circulation."

Among other methods by which space media may be distinguished are the following:

- Circulation, general/specialty/mixed
- Advertising-editorial ratio
- Readership studies
- Physical placement of ads (e.g., throughout or only at beginning and end sections)

---

*Dr. Max A. Ferm contributed materials for this section in a previous work edited by Mickey Smith, *Principles of Pharmaceutical Marketing,* Third Edition (Binghamton, NY: The Haworth Press, 1988), pp. 369-399.

- Whether press releases are accepted
- Presence of advertisers' index
- Frequency of publication

There are, literally, hundreds of different publications from which the advertiser may choose. Some deal only with matters of clinical interest. Some cover aspects of practice such as politics and economics (*Medical Economics* is a perennial leader in advertising revenues). Others, although they contain drug ads, feature editorial content on such subjects as travel, financial planning, and leisure activities.

Among other options are single-sponsor publications and "house organs." A single-sponsor publication is independently published and has just a single advertiser-supporter rather than many advertisers. In most other ways—purpose, audience, editorial content—it is about the same as an open-advertising publication. It is not a house organ, which traditionally reflects the views and activities of the company that sponsors it. The content of the single-sponsor publication is divorced from the sponsoring company.

Direct Mail

The use of direct mail has a distinct advantage over space advertising in that it can be directed to specific individuals rather than groups of individuals. A premium is paid for this advantage because, on a per-contact basis, direct mail is more costly. It is, however, a separate medium and requires understanding of the facilities available to be employed properly.

The AMA, for the most part, provides basic lists used in medical promotion to franchised mailing houses, from whom they are available. An AMA royalty fee is included in the mailing charge each time the list is used. Lists are supplied by computer and are frequently revised because inaccurate lists give rise to undelivered mail, which adds a heavy burden to the cost of this medium.

Lists are available in almost any manner desired. One can purchase the use of physicians' names by specialty, age, type of practice, state or county of practice, and other statistics.

Direct mail, in addition to its selectivity, permits the use of promotional techniques not readily available in space media. For example, past experience has shown that physicians are not easily motivated by coupon insertions in journals, while product requests from the physicians can be obtained in the form of self-addressed business reply cards included with direct mail promotional material. This is an important consideration because it establishes a relationship between manufacturer and physician that can be measured and utilized.

When a campaign is developed, various types of mailing pieces are employed by manufacturers. Some of these are in the form of self-mailers, envelope mailers, letters, or box mailings. The least expensive is the self-mailer, which requires no envelope and is usually prepared as a jumbo card (two sides) or four-page mailer. A mixture might include all or several of these types, each one printed in sufficient quantity to be used more that once. For example, one might select three individual pieces, each mailed three times, for a total of nine mailings.

Studies with business reply cards as the measurement have focused upon the difference in response that can be obtained by altering such factors as the introduction of a letter, the use of postage stamps instead of printed indicia, personalization, and other variations.

Although direct mail is a desirable medium, it has a major disadvantage. Unlike journals, which offer an editorial environment designed to appeal to the physician's need to improve clinically, economically, or culturally, the average mailing piece is obviously promotional in design. The challenge is to create interest while delivering a selling message.

One device employed to overcome this drawback is the preparation of a manufacturer-sponsored journal, or house organ. This provides the advantage of both types of media by offering an interesting editorial format with direct mail specificity. It is an expensive means of promotion that has found favor among advertisers. The preparation of editorial matter incurs the majority of cost because it requires additional staff not required for advertising needs. For this reason companies have been formed to gather the editorial material. By specializing in one area—such as news or clinical abstracts—a single staff of writers can be employed for the preparation of several house organ magazines appealing to different physician specialties.

Personal Selling/Detailing

Done well, detailing is generally accepted to be the most effective form of pharmaceutical promotion. Comparisons and contrasts between this form of promotion and print advertising are shown in Table 13.5, while the nature of sales training is reported in Table 13.6.

Although practices vary, companies tend to limit their advertising departments to space media and direct mail media, while the balance of promotional expenditure is usually administered by the sales promotion department. The distinction between the responsibilities of the advertising department and those of the sales promotion department can best be described by their different methods of communicating the selling message—the advertising department primarily employs written or visual messages, while the sales promotion department primarily relies upon the use of sales personnel in personal, primarily oral, presentations.

As noted earlier, personal selling is expensive. Two methods of retaining some of the benefits of personal selling are convention exhibits (manned by sales staff) and telemarketing.

TABLE 13.5. Advertising and Detailing: Similarities and Contrasts

Characteristics	Advertising Differences	Similarities	Detailing Differences
Functional	One-way communication. Abundant "noise" in the communication channel. Relatively inflexible. Good control over the message. Almost impossible for physician to avoid some exposure to the message.	Both must be understandable, interesting, believable, persuasive.	Two-way communication. Some control over "noise." Can be tailored to the situation. Difficult to maintain company control of the message. Physician may refuse to see.
Perceptual	Difficult to reinforce the message during the course of presentation.	Both must penetrate sensory mechanisms of the physician, with careful selection of stimuli necessary.	May stimulate all five senses as well as vary them selectively. May reinforce and repeat in a single call.
Cognitive	Works primarily by suggestion. Primarily an interest-arousing technique.	Both attempt to present firm and product as different and better than competition.	May carry physician through reasoning process. May be a problem-solving technique.
Feeling state	Single message may elicit varying feelings. No possibility to adapt.	Both attempt to induce favorable feelings.	May evaluate and take advantage of either favorable or unfavorable feelings.
Transactional	Primarily pretransactional, with posttransactional activity primarily limited to dissonance reduction.	Both important as reminders to continue use.	May also effect a prescription as a direct result of sales call. Possible to supply sample for patient in the office at the time.

TABLE 13.6. Emphasis Placed on Training Topics

	Average Score (1 = no emphasis; 5 = maximum emphasis)		
Subject	Initial training	New product training	Retraining/ CE* Programs
Company mission and goals	3.86	3.78	3.22
Verbal communication skills	4.47	4.18	4.14
Writing skills	1.86	1.70	1.97
Product knowledge			
Anatomy	4.07	3.78	3.11
Physiology	4.26	3.89	3.30
Pharmacology	4.02	4.02	3.44
Biochemistry	2.86	2.94	2.52
Microbiology	2.81	2.77	2.34
Medical terms	4.43	4.16	3.45
Clinical drug interactions	3.81	4.00	3.57
Government regulations	3.23	2.97	3.02
Ethics	4.39	3.55	3.75
Comparative analysis of competitors'			
Products	4.55	4.71	4.30
Pricing	3.45	3.97	3.28
Distribution	3.23	3.34	2.77
Promotion	4.05	4.34	3.74
Sales force	3.18	3.39	2.82
Communication skills with			
Physicians	4.89	4.38	4.80
Pharmacists	4.34	4.36	4.11
Nurses	4.08	3.94	3.88
Drug wholesalers	3.37	3.43	3.26

Source: S. Kodiyalam, R. Segal, and D. S. Pathak, "Anatomy of Today's Sales Training Programs," *Medical Marketing and Media*, March 1, 23: 8-12, 1988.
*Continuing education

Convention exhibits combine some of the qualities of advertising (the physical display) and personal selling and, because of their hybrid nature, bring their own strategic decisions. Douden suggests seven steps in a marketing approach to exhibit planning.[5] These steps are elaborated on here:

1. *Careful evaluation of upcoming show, on a twelve-month basis.* From other marketing plans you already know target markets. Each medical spe-

cialty, however, has a long list of state, regional, national, and international meetings, workshops, conventions, and symposia that allow exhibitor participation.

2. *Development of specific objectives for each show considered on the upcoming year's schedule.* One strategy would be to use the year's exhibit schedule to introduce and demonstrate a new product to various segments of the market. Firms with no new products can take advantage of trade show opportunities by gathering marketing and product R&D data from booth visitors or by providing additional product information.

3. *Determination of budget funds available and allocation of them among the desired shows.* Trade show participation is expensive, but studies have indicated that the cost per visitor for a presentation can be far lower than a trip to the person's individual office. So exhibit expenses should be viewed as a necessary marketing "background" expense that often sets up such other activities as direct mail and office visits. Studies also show that firms which do not cut back on their trade show exposure during difficult economic times make speedier sales recoveries when more prosperous times return because they have maintained their market visibility. So exhibiting also has some long-term marketing investment factors to consider.

4. *Decision on how best to carry out the above objectives, in terms of exhibit design, production, scheduling, shipping, and return.* If detailed one-on-one marketing messages are planned, one may want to design screened-off quiet areas; if it is to be an educational audiovisual display, make it the focal point. Whatever the purpose, be sure the final physical design uses modular pieces that can be adapted to fit various booth sizes and can be modified to meet other objectives as they change during the three- to five-year life of a booth.

Some booths have only a logo and no marketing copy; others have so many signs that the passerby does not know where to start. To avoid the pitfalls of supplying too much or too little information, think of the booth as a billboard and reduce the message to a simple statement of an exclusive feature or the overriding product benefit. As a guideline for determining the content, go back and review your exhibiting objectives. The aim is to give visitors a quick message about who you are and what they will find in the booth.

5. *Careful planning of backup materials and facilities, including invitations, special registration, hospitality rooms, and special events during the show.*

6. *Firm plans for participation by the right personnel, given thorough orientation on conduct and objectives.* The actors on the stage of the booth can make or break the performance, so representatives need to be taught the difference between making an everyday office call and conducting a trade show exhibit "encounter."

Thus, the purpose of talking to a booth visitor is to qualify the person quickly and to determine the proper follow-up activity. That is really about all the time one can spend with each visitor, and probably all the time that each one will linger in the booth. The staff person who becomes involved in an extended conversation with one person is wasting valuable time that could be spent meeting other equally qualified people.

Also consider including in the booth people who are not detail staff. Perhaps someone from the lab or R&D department could be on hand to help the representatives answer questions. In addition, invite important clients to stop by the booth and then introduce them to other visitors and encourage them to tell in their own words the benefits they have enjoyed with your product. Moreover, other members of the marketing team, such as the advertising director and customer service people, could use the exposure to update their knowledge of the "climate" of the marketplace.

7. *Development of a built-in system for measuring results from participation in each show.* All the lead cards collected at the booth should go to the home office after each show. There, make photocopies, add the names to your centralized prospect mailing list, and send out the appropriate follow-up literature, as noted on each card, along with thank-you letters. Then mail the original cards in batches to the proper sales representative for further follow-up.

Telemarketing

Telemarketing is sales promotion via telephone. Certainly many of the advantages of in-person communication are lost (eye contact, body language, demonstration), as is what is often a personal relationship of some standing. Nevertheless, this technique retains the advantage of give-and-take and is certainly less expensive than in-person calls.

Most telemarketing is conducted by specialists in the field on assignment from the drug manufacturer. Telemarketing salespeople need special training and skills that are usually easier to give on an as-needed basis rather than to develop the in-house capabilities to perform this function. Examples of some of the uses of telemarketing are to

- generate sales leads,
- supplement/follow up field staff,
- detail products not normally supported in the field,
- reach physicians who refuse to see detail staff, and
- reach physicians in specialties not usually detailed.

Sampling

The use of samples is, in some ways, the most rational of promotional methods. If a medicine is effective, what better way to demonstrate this than by actual use by a patient? Each physician, after all, must ultimately conduct a personal "clinical trial" with each new product prescribed. Nevertheless, sampling practices have long been controversial, and as a result of the Prescription Drug Marketing Act of 1987, it is much more difficult to do.

In a study conducted for the Pharmaceutical Manufacturers Association (now PhARMA) by National Analysts in 1986,[6] sampling was found to be generally well received by physicians. Among the conclusions of the study were these:

1. Physician use of drug samples appears restrained; four out of five patients seen in a typical week of practice receive no sample of prescription medication.
2. Samples do not appear to divert substantial revenue from retail pharmacies. When used to provide immediate therapy in the doctor's office, they serve a function for which a retail pharmacy's inventory cannot substitute. Moreover, the vast majority of samples are accompanied by a prescription that must be filled at a pharmacy.
3. Physician familiarity with many of the medications that they provide as samples should not be misinterpreted to show that samples serve no trial function. Prescription samples are frequently used in a "test mode," especially by internists; familiarity with the product in general does not imply familiarity with its activity in any given patient. The data make it clear that physicians attach greater importance to assessing efficacy and side effects when the drug is new to the patient, rather than new to the doctor.
4. Samples play an important direct therapeutic role, particularly for pediatricians, and when pharmacies are closed or not easily accessible, they may be the only resource at hand. Any modification of existing sampling procedures would need to address this time-critical function in some way.
5. Among the various alternatives to sampling, rejection of a proposed substitution by coupons is overwhelming. Even though economic reasons are frequently cited as a basis for using samples, they are not sufficient to allow approval for a procedure that would address economic but not medical (e.g., immediate medication, assessing patient tolerance) concerns.
6. It is likely that a coupon system will impede physician use of new pharmaceutical products. Those who have used coupons can be regarded as "expert witnesses" on how the system works; their general agreement with nonuser physicians that the coupon system is inferior to the current system of distributing pharmaceutical samples, and that it will delay adoption of new medications, is significant because of the experience base that underlies it.

7. A policy of requiring a written request for pharmaceutical samples, although not eliciting as strong a reaction as coupons, also appears to have potential for retarding the trial of new products, since these physicians indicate less likelihood of requesting unfamiliar drugs, compared to products that they have used frequently.

8. Requiring physicians to sign receipts for packages of medication samples arouses the least opposition among the possible modifications to the current system of sample distribution. Although over one-third of physicians view it as inferior to the current system, three-quarters would have obtained the most recently sampled medication had such a requirement been in effect.

In spite of the results just reported, it was the view of Congress, translated into law, that the "existing system of providing drug samples to physicians through manufacturers' representatives has been abused for decades and has resulted in the sale to consumers of misbranded, expired, and adulterated pharmaceuticals." The resulting amendment to the Food, Drug, and Cosmetic Act included the following provisions:

- Requires state licensing of wholesale distributors under federal guidelines that include minimum standards for storage, handling, and record keeping
- Bans the reimportation of drugs produced in the United States, except when reimported by the manufacturer or for emergency use
- Bans the sale, trade, or purchase of drug samples
- Bans trafficking in or counterfeiting of drug coupons
- Requires practitioners to ask for drug samples in writing
- Prohibits, with certain exceptions, the resale of drugs purchased by hospitals or health care facilities
- Sets forth criminal penalties for the violation of these provisions

The essence of the requirements on sampling was spelled out in the FDA's letter:

> The manufacturer or distributor of a prescription drug may distribute samples to a licensed practitioner—or to a pharmacy of a hospital or other health care entity at the request of a licensed practitioner—by mail or common carrier, provided the licensed practitioner submits a written request setting forth certain specified information and the recipient of the drug sample executes a written receipt upon its delivery and returns the receipt to the manufacturer or distributor.

In other words, sales staff would not be able to drop off unsolicited samples anymore. A detailer could deliver a sample in response to a written request but must get a signed receipt.

The FDA will permit firms to distribute preprinted request forms for practitioners to send to the companies to obtain samples. These forms must contain all required information identifying the requester, the name of the drug, the amount wanted, the name of the manufacturer or distributor, and the date of the request. "FDA requests that separate written requests be made for each sample or group of samples and that open-ended or 'standing' requests not be used to order drug samples," the agency's letter stated.

The requirement for written requests may be the least burdensome of the new rules. There appears to be no bar to an almost instantaneous exchange of requests and samples between practitioner and detailer.

Where the burden is felt is in the storage, distribution, and record-keeping requirements that the new law imposes. The FDA's interim policy statement requires, among others, the following:

- *Proper storage of drug samples:* All drug samples have to be stored under conditions that will maintain their stability, integrity, and effectiveness.
- *Inventories of company representatives:* Drug manufacturers have to conduct complete inventories of all drug samples in the possession of the representatives.
- *List of representatives:* Drug manufacturers have to maintain lists of the name and address of each of their representatives who distribute drug samples and the sites where the samples are stored.

Alternate Media

The combination of new technology, competitive pressure, "clutter" in the traditional media, and changing characteristics of promotional targets has resulted in the development of a collection of promotional techniques that, because the phrase seems to have found common usage, we will call "alternate media." These media are too diverse to be covered here in detail, and certainly it is impossible to weigh their relative merits here.

MEDIA SELECTION PROCEDURE

Media selection calls for two decisions: (1) which medium to use and (2) with a given medium, which specific vehicles to choose. For example, if magazines are to be used, in which particular ones should ads be placed? The following two approaches can be used in media selection: (1) cost-per-thousand-contacts comparison and (2) matching of audience and medium characteristics.

Cost-per-Thousand-Contacts Comparison

Traditionally, the cost-per-thousand-contacts comparison has been the most popular method of media selection. Although simple to apply, the cost-per-thousand method leaves much to be desired. Basing media selection entirely on the number of contacts to be reached ignores the quality of contacts made.

Further, the cost-per-thousand method can be highly misleading if one considers the way in which advertisers define the term exposure. According to the media definition, exposure occurs as soon as an ad is inserted in the magazine. Whether the exposure actually occurs is never considered. This method also fails to consider editorial images and the impact power of different channels of a medium.

Matching of Audience and Media Characteristics

An alternative approach to media selection is to specify the target audience and match their characteristics with those of the medium.

Medium selection, even just among print media in journals, is a complex, multivariate exercise. There are more than 400 publications just for physicians. Each must be evaluated on such criteria as

- editorial climate of the journal,
- the frequency of publication,
- amount of paid circulation,
- stacking of ads,
- availability of special issues,
- closing dates, and
- market and audience profiles.

Pharmaceutical media specialist Georgiana Papazian provided excellent guidance for this process:[7]

> Media selection is a direct extension of the marketing plan; the journal is one marketing tool that a product or service may use to help accomplish its marketing goals. Good marketing/media input derived from the marketing plan, therefore, is the key to developing the journal program.*

*This excerpt is reproduced with permission from *Pharmaceutical Executive*, March 1985, p. 50. Copyright 2001 Advanstar Communications Inc. Advanstar Communications Inc. retains all rights to this material.

The journal budget, target audiences, and advertising strategy are no longer enough to formulate a journal schedule. In today's climate, other questions must be asked—and answered—and other issues addressed to provide data that will help in the journal selection process. Some of those questions and issues are:

- What is the therapeutic class and what are the major competitive products within the class?
- What is the advertising period? This should be explicit to give the planner good insight into how to place the ads.
- Into which market sector should advertising be concentrated: office-based, hospital-based, or both? Should equal target weighting be assigned the physician specialties in each of the marketing areas?
- Should special consideration be given to reinforcing the coverage and awareness in markets with upward sales trends or, conversely, to markets on a downward trend?
- Are any nonphysician audiences being targeted? What is the time frame for this advertising? The advertising strategy? Is this part of the promotion included within the overall budget?

Although some planners are more comfortable compiling journal schedules manually, the proliferation of journals, with its attendant confusion, has fostered increased use of computers to compile publication schedules. Computer capabilities permit merging the target audience with valid and tested audience research and other variables to develop a quantitative analysis. Journal ranking and target specialty breakdowns for specific journal groupings primary to the product's promotion are recalled, examined, and reexamined. Different programs are tested on the computer until the right journal combination evolves—one that closely matches the target goals.

Industry, as a rule, views journal media as conveyors of advertising messages. The number of exposure opportunities offered by a single publication or the journal schedule customarily is not analyzed per se; but these opportunities now can be subdivided into reach and frequency, and their cost efficiency analyzed.

Reach is best defined as the number of different readers exposed to one publication or schedule within a given time period. Frequency is the average number of times each person is exposed to one publication or schedule during the same time frame.

Considering reach and frequency when compiling a program ensures that the advertised message gets wide exposure and is not restricted to a limited target audience.

DECIDING HOW MUCH TO SPEND

The amount that a company may spend on its total promotional effort, which consists of advertising, personal selling, and sales promotion, is not easy to determine. No unvarying standards indicate how much should be spent on promotion in a given product/market situation. This is so because the decision on promotion expenditure is influenced by a complex set of circumstances.

Promotion expenditure makes up part of the total marketing budget. Thus, the allocation of funds to one department, such as advertising, will affect the level of expenditure elsewhere within the marketing function. For example, it may be debated whether additional expenditures on advertising are more desirable than a new package design. In addition, the perspectives of promotion expenditure must be examined in the context of pricing strategy. A higher price obviously provides more funds for promotion than does a lower price. The amount set aside for promotion expenditure is also affected by the sales response of the product, which is very difficult to estimate accurately. A related matter here is the question of the cumulative effect of promotion. The major emphasis of research in this area, even where the issue is far from being resolved, has been on the duration of advertising effects. Although it is generally accepted that advertising effects, and maybe those of other forms of promotion as well, may last over a long period, there is no certainty about the duration of these benefits.

Promotion induces competitors to react, and there is no way to anticipate accurately competitive response and thus decide on a budget.

Despite the difficulties involved, practitioners have developed rules of thumb for determining promotion expenditures that are strategically sound. These rules of thumb may be distinguished as being of two types: breakdown methods and the buildup method. Before discussing these methods, however, it will be worthwhile to review briefly the application of marginal analysis to the promotion expenditure decision.

The marginal approach was the earliest organized framework for developing a promotion budget. With this approach, the expenditure on each ingredient of promotion should be made so that marginal revenue is equal to marginal cost. For example, the outlay on advertising should be incurred to the point where it just equals the incremental profit earned on the additional business generated by advertising. Similarly, the expenditure on personal selling should be equal to the profit on sales generated by the sales force. For the communication mix as a whole, the optimum budget should be set so that the marginal revenues per dollar of costs from advertising, personal selling, and sales promotion are equal. In other words, the appropriation for each of the ingredients of promotion should be increased or decreased until marginal revenues are equal.

Theoretically, the approach appears sound. However, measurement of marginal costs and revenues poses a difficult problem. Even if margins can be estimated, the marginal approach may not be feasible. For example, no firm may want to hire and fire salespeople in an attempt to reach the optimum point at which marginal cost is equal to marginal revenue. Besides, what if the margin is reached at three-fourths of a salesperson? Likewise, in advertising, either one places an ad in a magazine or one does not advertise in a magazine at all.

The question of the carryover effect of advertising is a complex one, and there is no agreement on how long advertising affects sales. Traditionally, it has been held that advertising's effects on sales last several years. Some work in the area, however, suggests that the effects of advertising on sales are a short-term phenomenon, lasting between three and fifteen months. In brief, then, although the marginal approach for allocating promotional expenditures provides a good theoretical framework, its practical use is limited.

Breakdown Methods

A number of breakdown methods can be helpful in determining promotion expenditures. Under the percentage-of-sales approach, promotion expenditure is a specified percentage of the previous year's or predicted future sales. Initially this percentage is arrived at by estimate. Later on, historical information is used to decide what percentage of sales should be allocated for promotion expenditure. The rationale behind the use of this approach is that expenditure on promotion must be justified by sales. This approach is followed by many companies because it is simple, is easy to understand, and gives managers the flexibility to cut corners during periods of economic slowdown. Among its flaws is the fact that basing promotion appropriation on sales puts the chicken before the egg. Further, the logic of this approach fails to consider the cumulative effect of promotion. This approach, then, considers promotion a necessary expenditure that must be apportioned from sales revenue without considering the relationship of promotion to competitors' activities or its influence on sales revenues.

Another approach for allocating promotion expenditure is to spend as much as can be afforded. In this approach, the availability of funds or liquid resources is the main consideration in making the decision on promotion expenditure. In other words, even if a company's sales expectations are high, the level of promotion will be kept low if its cash position is tight. This approach can be questioned on several grounds. It makes promotion expenditure dependent on the company's liquid resources, when in fact the best move for a cash-short company may be to spend more on promotion with the hope of improving sales. Further, this approach involves an element of risk. At a time when the market is tight and sales are slow, a company may spend more on promotion if it happens to have the resources available. This approach does, however, consider the fact that promotion outlays have long-term value, i.e., the cumulative effect of advertising. Also, under conditions of complete uncertainty, this approach is a cautious one.

The competitive-parity approach assumes that promotion expenditure is directly related to market share. The promotion expenditure of a firm should therefore be in proportion to those of competitors in order to maintain its position in the market. Thus, if the leader in the industry allocates 2 percent of its sales revenue to advertising, other members of the industry should spend about the same percentage of their sales on advertising. Considering the competitive nature of the industry, this seems a reasonable approach. There are, however, a number of limitations. First, the approach requires a knowledge of competitors' perspectives on promotion, and this information may not always be available. For example, the market leader may have decided to put its emphasis not on promotion per se but on reducing prices. Following the firm's lead in advertising expenditures without reference to its prices would be an unreliable guide. Second, one firm may get more for its promotion dollar through judicious selection of media, timing of advertising, skillful preparation of ads, a good sales supervision program, etc. Thus, it can realize the same result as another firm that has twice as much to spend. Since promotion is just one of the variables affecting market performance, simply maintaining promotional parity with competitors may not be enough for a firm to preserve its market share.

Buildup Method

Many companies have advertising, sales, and sales promotion (merchandising) managers who report to the marketing manager. The marketing manager specifies the objectives of promotion separately for the advertising, personal selling, and sales promotion of each product line.

In practice, it may not always be easy to pinpoint the separate roles of advertising, personal selling, and sales promotion, since the three methods of promotion usually overlap to some degree. Each company must work out its own rules for a promotion mix. Once the tasks to be performed by each method of promotion have been designated, they may be defined formally as objectives and communicated to the respective managers. On the basis of these objectives, each promotion manager will probably redefine his or her own goals in more operational terms. These redefined objectives then become the modus operandi of each department.

Once departmental objectives have been defined, each area works out a detailed budget, pricing each item required to accomplish the objectives of the program. As each department prepares its own budget, the marketing manager may also prepare a summary budget for each of them, simply listing the major expenditures in light of overall marketing strategy.

The buildup method forces managers to analyze the role they expect promotion to play and the contribution it can make toward achieving marketing objectives. It also helps maintain control over promotion expenditure and avoid the frustrations often faced by promotion managers as a result of cuts in promotion appropriations due to economic slowdown.

CONCLUSION

The promotion mix consists of advertising, personal selling, sales promotion, and publicity. Objectives should be established in each of these areas, and the objectives established for each element of the promotion mix should collectively reflect the objective established for the promotion function. Likewise, the objectives established for the promotion function should, in conjunction with those established for the other elements of the marketing mix (product, price, and place), reflect the objectives established for the marketing function, and so on.

When sales objectives are established for advertising, they are usually *marketing* objectives. Despite the likely assumption that sales increases occur because of the marketing manager responsible for developing the strategy, to produce an increase in sales uses every tool in the marketing mix. Such sales increases that take place may be due to a reduction in price, a change in channels of distribution, a change in the product (or package), or a faster method of delivering the product (logistics)—all in addition to, or instead of, advertising. Thus, it would be difficult, it not impossible, to identify any one tool as the only factor producing the sales increase.

If one of the reasons for establishing objectives is to facilitate measurement of performance, how can the effectiveness of advertising be determined if its contribution to the sales increase cannot be isolated? If, after an advertising campaign, sales did in fact increase by 10 percent, how much of that increase was due to advertising alone? Continuing research can help.

John Palshaw has described the sequence of events in a marketing communications cycle as follows:[8]

- Review of a marketing problem or opportunity
- Market satisfaction study*
- Decisions on positioning, market segment of opportunity
- Benchmark research versus key competition*
- Application of findings to campaign planning, goal setting
- Quantitative concept testing of claims or features*
- Input to the creative team, initiate ad development
- Qualitative prescreening of ad roughs*

---

*Research procedure is needed.

- Decisions on ad production following sifting
- Quantitative, diagnostic, and predictive pretesting*
- Final creative decisions, fine-tuning, and production
- Campaign appearance in the media
- Posttest evaluations of per-unit ad performance*
- Tracking of overall campaign impact*
- Recycle

Ultimately, promotion and its effects move along a hierarchy as follows:

- Awareness
- Knowledge
- Liking
- Preference
- Conviction
- Prescription purchase

Chapter 14

Environment

Mickey Smith

The single most important environmental factor in the promotion of pharmaceuticals (see Figure 2.1 in Chapter 2) is legal/regulatory. Although all promotion must conform to the Federal Trade Commission regulations regarding false and/or misleading advertising, the promotion of legal prescription medications is subject to the additional regulations of the Food and Drug Administration. Indeed, the FTC and the FDA maintain separate jurisdictions in this regard—even separate philosophies.

LEGAL/REGULATORY

The FDA

The so-called 1962 drug amendments empowered the FDA with jurisdiction over the labeling of prescription medications. The FDA interpreted "labeling" to include not only printed promotion but also the verbal promotion by salespersons in physicians' offices—and virtually everything else.

In contrast to almost any other commodity, a prescription medication may be promoted—in any medium—only if it is totally consistent with an FDA-approved package insert (discussed shortly), only if it contains a "fair balance" of the good and potential ill effects of the medication, and only if it offers full disclosure of these effects. Incidentally, the FDA requires that print advertising for prescription medications by brand name include the generic name in type at least one half as large as the brand name. (This is not, in the author's opinion, part of the FDA mandate.)

Well, what does all this mean?

Let us start with the package insert, which is, typically, a piece of paper about one and one-half inches wide and often two to three feet in length that provides the official (i.e., FDA approved) labeling for a prescription medication. It is called a package insert because every package of prescription medication is required by FDA regulation to contain or have attached to it this printed information. Designed, one believes, to provide vital information to the prescriber, the leaflet in fact is typically discarded, unread, by the pharmacists at the time of dispensing. The package insert (or at least its contents) is nevertheless vitally important to the promotion of prescription pharmaceuticals, as the information contained therein is the standard against which promotional information is measured—which leads to another important linkage.

The information contained in the package insert (or approved labeling) is entirely dependent upon the NDA as approved by the FDA. Thus, the activities in the R&D process lead to the contents of the NDA that, in turn, form the basis for the content of promotional messages. Thus, promotion begins, in fact, in the structure and success of clinical trials, or at least it should. A medication never tested on, for example, females over the age of sixty will probably not be permitted to use promotional illustrations showing patients of this gender and age, hence the importance of involving marketing throughout the R&D process.

The FDA, and the pharmaceutical industry, faced a special challenge in direct-to-consumer advertising of prescription-only medications. Some of the rules were comparatively easy to follow (name of the generic in half-size type). But how to and why provide the consumer, especially in television ads, with the small-print information required by the FDA in ads to prescribers? An uneasy compromise has consisted of referring television viewers, after a condensed version of warnings, to print versions in one or more consumer magazines.

An article in the April 2000 issue of *Pharmaceutical Executive* underscored the economic significance of FDA regulations and failure to adhere to them. The authors, after analyzing some 376 "Notices of Violation" and twenty "Warning Letters" concluded that "noncompliance with FDA (promotional) regulation is expensive."[1] How expensive? If the FDA requires corrective action, here are some of the possible costs:

- Advertisements in journals can be costly, e.g., a one-page ad and a one-page summary in the *Journal of the American Medical Association* costs nearly $15,000.
- "Dear Doctor" letters, according to the authors, and depending on the number of physicians involved, may cost $15,000 to $130,000.
- All sorts of sales support materials may be required to be destroyed or revised. Some of the more elaborate items may cost as much as $20 each.
- The personal sales force probably will require remedial sessions that could cost $400 to $500 per representative plus travel and lodging expenses.
- Intangible costs accrue as well, as the company is forced to announce publicly, "What we've been telling you is in some way not correct by FDA standards."

How can one avoid these and other costs and problems? Do it right the first time! The authors of this article suggest these kinds of "avoidance tactics":

- Advertising and promotional programs balance the presentation of efficacy claims with appropriate safety information.
- Comparative claims and quality-of-life claims are based on adequate and well-controlled data.
- Materials avoid promoting products and new indications before they receive FDA approval.
- Materials avoid promotion of investigational medications until the FDA has reviewed the supporting data and granted an authorization to market—even though IND regulations permit "full exchange of scientific information" in "scientific or lay media."
- Company regulatory affairs and legal departments have reviewed promotional materials to ensure that they comply with the most current interpretations of FDA requirements.
- Company and contract personnel involved in the development or use of advertising and promotional materials receive clear, realistic guidance on what they can and cannot do to promote the company's products.[2]

Nonprescription medications are the regulatory responsibility of the FTC and have always been. Interestingly, when a medication is "switched" from Rx to OTC, it is also switched to a different federal regulatory agency, an agency whose standards regarding false and misleading advertising apply equally to mousetraps or medicines.

The FDA had little experience with consumer advertising when DTC began and at the turn of this century was still struggling with this new-for-them environment.

ETHICAL/CULTURAL

The primary ethical/cultural environmental aspects of pharmaceutical promotion center on the targets of OTC promotions and the depiction of patients in prescription drug promotion. In an early paper, "Where Are the Blacks in Prescription Drug Advertising?" we found blacks to be considerably underrepresented in medication advertising illustrations.[3] Much has changed since those observations, but drug advertising particularly still often does not offer in its illustrations a realistic picture of the people in a physician's waiting room.

TECHNICAL

As the century rolled over the biggest technical challenge was how best to use electronic media. Personal selling, mail, print media, sampling, and exhibits had all proven themselves as greater or lesser successes as promotional devices. The incredible technical potential of electronic media, although recognized as such, had yet to be thoroughly researched and harnessed.

Virtually every professional and a very large segment of the lay population had access to and some, or considerable, experience in the use of computers to retrieve information about almost anything, including medications. How much to spend, whom to target, what to say—age-old promotion questions—now had to be applied to new media. The potential is enormous, and the end is not in sight. Neither are the potential hazards.

E-commerce, as this is written, is already having a significant impact on the transfer of information, as well as on the actual sale and delivery of medications. Whereas mail-order prescriptions were already growing in importance for a variety of reasons, the growth of drug distribution through the computer seems likely to far outstrip mail order both in quantity and rate of growth.

ECONOMIC

Medicines cost too much! That will always be the general view because most people would prefer not to buy them. Why do they cost so much? One of the most frequent charges against the industry is that it spends too much money promoting these medicines. Thus, promotional expenditures will always be a target of criticism with regard to pharmaceuticals.

As this was being written, serious discussion, concerning usually an outpatient drug benefit program under Medicare, is underway regarding some sort of price controls on prescription medicines. Such price controls are in place in other countries, but aside from public utility rates and the controls instituted in times of war, the United States has a tradition of free-market economy. If, and nothing is certain, some sort of price controls were to be instituted, companies would be forced to reevaluate their budgets for promotion as well as for other expenses.

SOCIAL

Direct-to-consumer advertising of prescription medicines is the major symptom of changes in the social environment in the twenty-first century. Clearly, consumers want to have greater control over their health, and it appears that they are much more sophisticated (or at least well-read) with regard to their medical therapy than ever before in history. Not only do they know more about their medicines and conditions, but research shows that substantial numbers feel no reluctance to ask their physicians about or for a medication they have learned about on television or elsewhere.

The opinions of physicians, organized and individually, concerning DTC promotion have been variable. On the one hand, a physician can hardly be outraged if a DTC ad sends him or her patients who would not otherwise be in the office, or at least would have shown up later in the course of their disease. Data also shows instances in which patients, encouraged by a DTC ad to visit a physician for one problem, were found to have one or more other conditions in need of treatment. On the other hand, some, perhaps most, physicians see DTC promotion as interference with their practice and decision process.

It is indicative of the change that in the late 1950s to early 1960s some major pharmaceutical firms established separate divisions with different names to separate their OTC from their Rx activities in physicians' minds.

COMPETITIVE

It is the nature of this industry that much is known about what the competition is doing—especially in promotion because it is so visible. Statistics are generally available in such publications as *Medical Marketing and Media* on expenditures by company and by product. Much more detailed information is available on order and for a price from marketing research firms specializing in this kind of market intelligence.

Information about what the competition is saying and where they are saying it, combined with sales data available through various prescription audit services, and with due regard for comparative prices can be combined in models to assist in planning promotional programs. Of course there is an obvious time lag between the time this analysis is done and a program—and often the competition has changed one or many of its activities in the interim.

INTERNAL

Within each company there is competition as well, assuming that the budget for promotion has some limits as to where the money should be spent. DTC promotion is expensive and a fairly recent item in promotional budgets. It could be expected that the sales division, for example, might not appreciate a cut in budget, or at least no increase, so that funds could be funneled into DTC ads. Add to that the possibility that the personal-selling staff received the brunt of physician complaints about DTC ads, and the potential for internal conflict is obvious. It is a test of the skill of marketing directors to keep in balance and to assign reasonable credit for the various components of the promotional plan. We might add that importance must be given to the task of promoting the product to the company's own employees.

INDIVIDUAL PATIENTS/CONSUMERS

Needs, Demands, Knowledge, and Beliefs

As we consider the individual in this chapter on promotion, we should remind ourselves again that although promotion has a persuasion component, its primary function is one of providing information. Reviewing Figure 2.1 one can see some general tasks facing those engaged in pharmaceutical promotions:

- *Knowledge*—This one is easy. Promotion can and should provide the consumer with the information necessary to make informed decisions about his or her health or the health of someone in his or her care. The "knowledge" requires assessment, however. As humorist-philosopher Josh Billings once observed, "It ain't the things people don't know that causes all the trouble in the world; it's the things they know that ain't so."
- *Beliefs*—These are different from knowledge. They may or may not be based on knowledge or the truth. Placebos work on the basis of beliefs—and they often work very well! Promotion can, and should, correct beliefs based on incorrect information—but do so very carefully. It is unusual for a person to appreciate fully an effort to change a closely held belief.
- *Needs*—Matching needs and demands (discussed next) is one of the single most important tools of the health care system—and promotion can play a pivotal role. An obvious example is the role played by the pharmaceutical industry (and many other players) over the years in motivating people to have their blood pressure checked. The need was there for many, but this usually asymptomatic condition (hypertension) rarely urged people to the physician's office (now blood pressure is often assessed by students in shopping malls). Surely, the drug companies, using enlightened self-interest, sold more medicine—"did well by doing good"—but how much less morbidity and mortality would we have experienced without their efforts?
- *Demands*—We return to DTC ads again. A true risk is that patients *will* be swayed by ads to "demand" medications that are inappropriate for them. We would note in this regard that it is the responsibility of

physicians, pharmacists, and other health professionals to serve as guardians. We would add that it is the responsibility of those who promote pharmaceuticals not to limit their cautions to those imposed by the FDA, but to ensure that they have provided adequate warnings against inappropriate demands for, and use of, medications—both Rx and OTC.

THE HUMAN MEDICAL CONDITION

This overriding environmental concern is one of continuing and inevitable change. Indeed, our definition of what are "medical" matters is, and will continue to be, in a state of flux. Is male pattern baldness a "medical condition"? How about erectile dysfunction? Where do unwanted or unplanned pregnancies fit? Are they social issues or medical matters? Each of these is treatable by medicines and by medical personnel. Should we even be worried about defining medical conditions? If the technology to change genetic makeup, to alter thinking patterns, and to affect growth patterns exists, should we not "let the chips fall where they may" and let society define and redefine what are the provinces of Medicine (consciously capitalized)? And what have these rhetorical questions to do with promotion?

CONCLUSION

Knowledge is power, so goes the adage. Promotion provides knowledge—sometimes in a blatant effort to convince the customer to buy, sometimes to inform customers that a medical solution to their problem may exist, sometimes to alert them to a problem about which they may not even be aware. There is power in this function, and as environmental influences change in character, as they most assuredly will, it will be a challenge to those who make their careers in pharmaceutical promotion to change as well.

Chapter 15

Practices

Mickey Smith

In light of the environmental factors described in the previous chapter (and many others that it has been impossible to include) what have those charged with the promotion of medications done to fulfill their responsibility—let us face it—to sell medications?

In this chapter we will highlight some of the promotional strategies and tactics employed by professionals in one of the most challenging of all markets. After a bit of history we will examine promotional practices in terms of targets, messages, life cycle considerations, product issues, blending the promotional mix, and budgets, concluding with some of the industry's views of its own practices.

Before doing all of that, let us take a mini case look at the product chosen by *Med Ad News* (see May 2000) as the brand of the year for the last year of the twentieth century—Celebrex. Celebrex generated $2.5 billion in sales in its first year on the market. How did this happen? Using the chapter outline, here is a glimpse.

- *Targets:* A strong introduction to certain prescribers was followed by an aggressive direct-to-consumer program.
- *Messages:* Claims of once-a-day relief from pain and lack of gastrointestinal problems helped compliance.
- *Life cycle considerations:* This was the first of an entirely new class of drugs and an extension of indications under way.
- *Product considerations:* Novelty, safety, and a unique mechanism of action (at the time of launch) were highlighted.
- *Blending the promotion mix:* Some 3,000 Searle/Pfizer sales representatives were involved. Searle was strong with rheumatologists and orthopedists, Pfizer with primary care physicians. This was supplemented by an aggressive advertising campaign to prescribers and consumers. The novelty of the drug also generated substantial media news coverage.
- *Competition:* At the time of launch no other COX-2 inhibitors were on the market, but Vioxx and Mobic soon appeared, with the latter using

price difference as an appeal. As this was written, it appeared that expansion of indications and second-generation products would be among the Celebrex responses to competition.

- *Budgets:* According to a Searle official, "We almost doubled the amount of resources that Searle puts forward into the marketplace for other products."

So, on to the practices.

A BIT OF HISTORY

In 1999 the medical advertising Hall of Fame published *Medicine Avenue,* subtitled *The Story of Medical Advertising in America.* This beautifully illustrated text is highly recommended for its readability, attractiveness, and personal account of medical advertising since the end of World War II. Frank Hughes and John Kallir write, "Together with our clients, we have captured the imagination of physicians and turned an [sic] nascent industry into one of the most successful businesses in the world today."[1]

Similar histories have not been written about the other components of the promotional mix, but some texts, e.g., *One for a Man, Two for a Horse,*[2] provide accounts of the rather sordid history of promotion prior to the modern era. The term "snake oil salesman" (there really was a "snake oil" product) arose from that era, and at least some residue still effects the skepticism plaguing modern promotion, in spite of the strong regulatory forces described in the previous chapter.

A kind of dynamic tension has existed, especially since 1962, between the FDA and the pharmaceutical industry regarding regulation of promotion. A quasi-system of checks and balances exists in which the FDA issues frequent "thou shalt nots" and industry professionals attempt to, and often do, find ways to effect change in the FDA's stance. Not too surprisingly, those whose profession is creating promotion are often a bit ahead of those whose job is to regulate it.

TARGETS OF PROMOTION

A recent advertisement for the journal *The Female Patient* featured this headline: "Today, the Real Health Care Decision Makers Are the Female Patient and Her Physicians." Three points stand out in the line. First, it recognizes the increased role of the individual patient in selection of his or her own therapy. Second, the term "decision makers" reflects the certain fact that a *prescription* may not necessarily be the final step in a successful promotional plan. Finally, it recognizes that a patient, in this era of medical specialization, may seek and use the services of multiple physicians. (The author of the present chapter used the services of a family physician, a cardiologist, an electrophysiologist, and a urologist all in the space of three months.)

Overall the primary target for promotion of prescription (and to some extent nonprescription) medications has been, and for the foreseeable future will continue to be, the prescribing physician. The physician has been joined, however, by a variety of other decision makers, each of whom may need to be considered as targets for the promotion of a given product. Among these are

- pharmacists, especially those influencing formulary makeup and where generic drugs are involved;
- nurses and nurse practitioners;
- other doctors—dentists, veterinarians, optometrists in some states;
- managed care executives;
- policymakers, in and out of legislatures; and
- consumers and their representatives.

Insofar as the prescribing physician is concerned, the industry is notable for its ability to segment the larger target into a plethora of subtargets. It is possible to identify physicians by medical specialty, frequency and nature of drug use, and type of practice (solo, group, hospital, etc.). This information is available for use in direct mail, journal ads, and personal-selling applications and offers the potential for considerable efficiency in promotional spending. The same is true to a lesser extent regarding other health professionals. It is even possible to obtain lists of *consumers* known to be asthmatic, diabetic, or hypertensive for use in DTC promotion.

Other decision makers, including HMO and other managed care executives, are also targets. More than two dozen magazines, such as *Modern Healthcare, Business and Health,* and *Medical Interface,* are used extensively as promotional media. Most of their readers do not themselves prescribe but may have considerable administrative and economic influence over the medication that is ultimately used.

Consumers are obvious targets for promotion of nonprescription medications and have always been. Indeed it has been written that magazines were "invented" so that early patent medicines would have a ready advertising medium. (An interesting parallel is the early commercial-free radio programming designed to encourage consumers to buy radios.)

By the year 2000, it was obvious that the consumer had became a target for *prescription* drug advertising as well. More than $2 billion was spent that year in DTC promotion. This comparatively new phenomenon brings with it certain challenges and opportunities, as two mini cases will illustrate.

In 1991 (then) Ciba-Geigy began an ad campaign in a number of consumer magazines for its product Actigall.

- The ad, titled "Gallbladder Surgery. What If You Can't or Won't Have It?," suggests that your doctor "may prescribe Actigall, ursodial" if he or she has "told you that you to need surgery, and you can't or won't have it." Noting that not all gallstone patients need treatment, the ad states that "patients with mild symptoms might just be watched by their doctor to see if there are further developments."
- In the ad Actigall is described as a gallstone-dissolving agent, with diarrhea mentioned as the most common side effect of the drug. "Recurrence of gallstones within five years of complete dissolution has been observed in up to 50 percent of patients," the ad advises. The "Ask your doctor" phrase is included at the end of the copy, and a brief labeling summary appears at the bottom of the ad.

In preparation for the consumer ad, Ciba-Geigy ran in medical journals a two-page ad that included the consumer ad and a sidebar explanation for physicians of the consumer ad strategy in the form of fictional dialogue between company executives.

- The professional spread ran in January and February issues of magazines and journals directed at physicians, including the *Journal of the American Medical Association, American Family Physician, American Medical News, Internal Medicine News,* and *Medical Economics.* The ad also ran in several pharmacy publications, such as *Drug Topics, Pharmacy Times,* and *American Druggist.* In addition, the 500-member sales force detailing Actigall distributed 1.4 million copies of the consumer ad in brochure form to physicians and pharmacists.

The professional campaign was designed to meet the challenge of physician resistance to the DTC program.

In 1992 a (then Marion Merrell Dow) consumer ad told patients taking Cardizem about the new Cardizem CD.

- New Cardizem CD:
- Should be more economical
- Is easier to take
- Ask your doctor if Cardizem CD is right for you

The same ad included a toll-free number that the patient could call for a free subscription to *CardiSense,* "a newsletter on healthy living."

This ad was aimed at three opportunities:

- With the patient's help, it acted as another reminder to the physician of the new product.
- For every patient switch, generic substitution could be avoided, as there was no generic equivalent. (See the Life Cycle Considerations section.)
- Subscribers to CardiSense became a mailing list.

MESSAGES

In Chapter 13 we listed a typology of appeals used ⬚
cation advertising. They constitute part of the promoti⬚
that consists of one of three objectives.

Informing

These messages are educational in nature:

1. We are new and we are available.
2. We have changed.
3. This is how to use our product successfully.
4. These are some applications you may have overlooked. For example, an ad for Berocca Plus tablets described for the physician some types of "Candidates for Nutritional Therapy":
   * 10,000,000 alcoholics
   * 25,500,000 geriatric patients
   * 23,500,000 surgical patients
   * 5,000,000 hospital patients with infections
   * Incalculable millions on calorie-reduced diets

   Buttressed by photos of illustrative patients the ad clearly was informative.

Persuading

Much of promotion is persuasive in nature: "Choose this product and here are the reasons why." The appeals in Table 13.1 (Chapter 13) are designed to be persuasive, and all are used in various combinations in the industry and in all promotional media.

Reminding

Perhaps there is little new to say, but one does not shut off the engines at 40,000 feet because the plane is going along well. An ad with a picture of an apple occupied the back of the *Journal of the American Medical Association* for years. It stated simply, "Rocephin Once a Day."

LIFE CYCLE CONSIDERATIONS

As noted earlier, Celebrex was named brand of the year because of the success of its launch in 1999. In 1995 the *Med Ad News* brand of the year was Premarin, a product that was then fifty-two years old! In a list of reasons for its selection by the editors were the following:

MESSAGES

In Chapter 13 we listed a typology of appeals used in prescription medication advertising. They constitute part of the promotional message system that consists of one of three objectives.

Informing

These messages are educational in nature:

1. We are new and we are available.
2. We have changed.
3. This is how to use our product successfully.
4. These are some applications you may have overlooked. For example, an ad for Berocca Plus tablets described for the physician some types of "Candidates for Nutritional Therapy":
   - 10,000,000 alcoholics
   - 25,500,000 geriatric patients
   - 23,500,000 surgical patients
   - 5,000,000 hospital patients with infections
   - Incalculable millions on calorie-reduced diets

   Buttressed by photos of illustrative patients the ad clearly was informative.

Persuading

Much of promotion is persuasive in nature: "Choose this product and here are the reasons why." The appeals in Table 13.1 (Chapter 13) are designed to be persuasive, and all are used in various combinations in the industry and in all promotional media.

Reminding

Perhaps there is little new to say, but one does not shut off the engines at 40,000 feet because the plane is going along well. An ad with a picture of an apple occupied the back of the *Journal of the American Medical Association* for years. It stated simply, "Rocephin Once a Day."

LIFE CYCLE CONSIDERATIONS

As noted earlier, Celebrex was named brand of the year because of the success of its launch in 1999. In 1995 the *Med Ad News* brand of the year was Premarin, a product that was then fifty-two years old! In a list of reasons for its selection by the editors were the following:

- Strength in consistent growth
- Strength in multiple indications
- Strength in surviving patent expiration
- Strength in holding the trust of physicians and patients

Wyeth Ayerst headlined in its ads, "Nothing else is Premarin."

From Celebrex to Premarin, products go through various stages of a product life cycle, and one of the challenges of the promotion function is to adapt to and sometimes influence each stage.

In the *introductory* stage, marketing must *inform* of availability and sometimes, as in the case of Celebrex, create *primary* demand by explaining a new class of drugs. The first entrant thus does some work for those who follow. (It was far easier for Merck to say that Vioxx was a COX-2 inhibitor.) (See Table 15.1.)

In the *growth* stage, promoters are charged with establishing that "our brand is best"—stimulating *selective* demand. Comparative promotion based on price, safety, efficiency, ease of use, and other factors is often used in this stage.

In the market *maturity* stage, when there may be many competitors, promotion must work even harder, and often spend even more, to maintain market share. For firms with consistently high market share, "reminder" promotions may be a comparatively less expensive way to say, "Our brand is better, really."

In the sales *decline* stage, promotion usually decreases, although targeted efforts may be directed toward those known to continue to prefer the product.

It should be noted that the length of the stages will vary. Further, working with R&D in introducing new indications, new dosage forms, new packages, and the like can give promotion new messages to deliver and prolong or even change the stage. The product Hytrin, for example, experienced *two* introductory stages, first for hypertension and again for treatment of benign prostatic hyperplasia (BPH).

PRODUCT CONSIDERATIONS

The nature of the product (and the conditions it treats) affects the nature of the promotion. Some products require considerable instruction for effective use—personal selling may predominate in such cases. Other products may perform differently than products in the same class. The actual physical appearance is often important. For a variety of reasons, prescribers may need to know what the product looks or tastes like. The naming of the product can be important. Serious therapeutic misadventures have been caused

TABLE 15.1. Launch Activities

Advertising	Marketing	Sales
Determine literature and promotion costs	*Marketing services*	*Sales promotion*
Determine direct-mail costs	Collect and analyze marketing data	Assign detailing positions
Contact advertising agency	Prepare initial market plan	Develop selling sheet
Develop graphic concepts and strategy	Conduct focus group interview(s)	Develop preliminary launch plan and schedule
Prepare preliminary journal costs	Request works cost analysis	Schedule conventions
Submit journal schedule	Conduct initial market forecast	Develop convention panels for exhibit
Submit journal advertising proposal	Request stability studies	Develop and produce slide, tape, or video programs
Develop and route direct mail/promotion copy	Issue NDA packaging specifications	Draft launch and selling plan
Test and approve journal advertisement	Determine product and package cost	Send selling sheet to advertising
Prepare convention panel (mechanicals)	Conduct focus group data analysis	Route convention panels
Develop promotional layout	Issue product and package pricing	Review launch and selling plan
Prepare advertising film	Develop final sample package	Produce convention panels
Review and approve journal schedule	Develop and route package mechanicals	Print launch and selling plan
Route and approve promotional material specifications	Issue packaging particulars	Send final insert copy to staff
Prepare and award promotional material bid	Issue packaging specifications request	Ship convention panels
Print direct mail and promotional material	Issue budget	Send staff launch and selling plan
Have advertising agency send insert order to journal(s)	Issue production order	Advise staff of final NDA approval
Develop press release	*Marketing product planner*	Present slide, tape, or video program to staff
Issue press release to trade journal(s)	Finalize market plan	
Mail promotional material	Submit market plan to management	*Sales training*
	Contact wholesale services	Initiate assessment by training department
	Contact sales promotion	Prepare disease and product learning unit
	Contact government services	Issue disease unit to test staff
	Contact hospital services	Issue product unit to test staff
	Contact convention department	Send final training unit to staff
	Contact retail services	Revise training unit with approved label
	Prepare initial market forecast	
	Prepare preliminary product report	
	Prepare unit forecast	
	Propose budget	
	Request works cost analysis	
	Finalize	

Source: Adapted from Bert Spilker, *Multinational Pharmaceutical Companies* (Philadelphia, PA: Lippincott-Raven), p. 362.

because of confusion between names—and prescribers should not be troubled by learning to pronounce the name of a product.

Can the product be taken successfully once a day? Will children tolerate it? Is it truly unique?

In the March 1999 issue of *R & D Directions,* some forty-six newly approved medicines were identified, each with one or more unique characteristics and offering opportunities for promotion.[3] A few examples:

- Celebrex, described earlier
- Paxil, treatment of obsessive-compulsive disorders and "social anxiety"—a new indication
- Zofran-ODT, a new formulation for cancer patients unable to use suppositories or tablets
- Combipatch, the first combination hormone replacement therapy in patch form
- Preven, the first emergency contraceptive kit for use up to seventy-two hours after sexual intercourse

These and the many other examples in the article provide a multitude of opportunities for promotional progress.

After studying and understanding the market environment, the first and most critical strategic decision to be made is the choice of the target product benefit segment. Once this segment has been chosen, the market management team must determine the product's competitive positioning.

What Is Positioning?

According to Ries and Trout,

> Positioning is not what you do to the mind of the prospect. That is, you position the product in the mind of the prospect. The basic approach of positioning is not to create something new and different, but to manipulate what's already up there in the mind, to retie the connections that already exist.[4]

Positioning Notes

- Positioning starts by segmenting the market based on the different benefits that each target group seeks from the product.
- Positioning is often intuitive.
- Positioning helps to develop a mental map of where the competitors are in terms of determining factors such as benefits and quality features.

- A positioning map can be used to identify opportunities and to specify the current and desired position of the product.
- The goal is to develop a differentiated product that creates a unique mind share, particularly in the target market segment.
- Positioning involves careful thinking about all of the products in a company's line.
- Positions are best attacked by focusing resources and promotion on a particular positioning or quality feature.
- Positions are best defended by an aggressive, mobile counterattack involving repositioning existing products and introducing new products.
- When designing the product, make sure that quality is incorporated into the features that most affect the desired competitive positioning of the product.

Types of Positioning Strategy

1. Attribute positioning
2. Price/quality positioning
3. Use/application positioning
4. User positioning
5. Product class positioning
6. Competition positioning

Zoloft (sertraline HCL)
Manufacturer: Pfizer
Type of positioning: Attribute

Zoloft is indicated for the treatment of depression. Prozac might be a main competitor. Zoloft is trying to position the image to physicians that it gives patients a happier life through the continuing change of titles and pictures in its ads.

Pravachol (pravastatin sodium)
Manufacturer: Bristol-Myers Squibb
 (origin: Sankyo Japan ¥133.5 billion)
Type of·positioning: Use/application
                       Competition

Zocor (simvastatin)
Manufacturer: Merck
Type of positioning: Use/application
                       Competition

Both of these products are classified as antihypercholesterolemic agents, which have same mode of action (HMG-CoA reductase inhibitor). They differentiate from each other, however, by focusing on their exclusive indications related to heart failure. While Pravachol positioned itself to the *specific patient risk* to emphasize reducing the risk of a first *myocardial infarction* (MI), Zocor positioned itself to more broad aspects of patient risk to emphasize reducing the risk of *total mortality* by reducing coronary death, nonfatal MI, and myocardial revascularization procedures.

Allegra (active metabolite of terfenadine)
Manufacturer: Hoechst Marion Roussel
Type of positioning: Attribute
                      Price/quality

Allegra is an antiallergic agent, and the company is trying to switch its drug Seldane to this new product. To differentiate from the former drug, Allegra positioned itself to the mind of the prospect as a "nonsedating" antiallergic agent that is a better therapeutic option for the physicians and a cost benefit compared to Seldane and any other nonsedating antihistamines.

Kytril (granisetron HCI)
Manufacturer: SmithKline Beecham
Type of positioning: Price/quality

Kytril is classified as an antiemetic and used for the prevention of nausea and vomiting caused by cancer chemotherapy. Kytril positioned itself to the economies of cost compared to main competitor Zofran and its parenteral form.

Tylenol (acetaminophen)
Manufacturer: McNeil
Type of positioning: Use/application
                      Competition

Tylenol positioned itself to specific symptoms by matching the seasonal changes in disease patterns. Furthermore, it differentiates itself from the other pain relievers that have gastrointestinal (GI) side effects, which exacerbate colds and the flu.

Naldecon (phenylpropanolamine, chlorpheniramine,
    phenyltoloxamine, phenylephrine)
Manufacturer: Apothecon (BMS)
Type of positioning: User

Naldecon is a drug for the treatment of cough and cold. It has four different formulations, from senior to pediatric drops: senior, adult, children, and infant formulations. Naldecon positioned itself to users of all ages with its different formulations.

> Nyquil Cold Medicine (doxylamine succinate, dextromethorphan Hbr,
> acetaminophen, pseudoephedrine HCI)
> Manufacturer: Procter & Gamble
> Type of positioning: Use/application

Nyquil is a drug for the treatment of cold and flu symptoms. Since those symptoms are worse at night, Nyquil positioned itself to the relief of those symptoms at night. Among many kinds of cold and flu symptom relievers, Nyquil has very unique positioning and appeal in consumers' minds. It is a classic example of successful positioning.

BLENDING THE PROMOTIONAL MIX

The list of promotional media available for use is extensive. The traditional four—personal selling, journal advertising, direct mail, and samples—have been joined by a plethora of other methods of promotional, from coffee cups to the Internet. How best to use all of these?

The two biggest challenges in blending the promotional mix are *consistency/coherence* of the promotional messages and *budgets,* which are discussed in the next section. Sample, but not exhaustive, criteria for determining the promotional mix were listed in Table 13.4 (Chapter 13).

The complexity of the blending process is illustrated by the items in Table 15.1, covering only some of the planning activities required to launch a new medication.

Ultimately, the "buck" for coordinating all of these and other activities stops in the marketing department, even though different functions are designed and coordinated by various subdepartments or divisions. Further, some of what must be considered as promotion is treated in other ways (e.g., medical education) within the company. Finding the proper blend is usually more art than science, although the tools for division do exist.

BUDGETS

Consider the vice president of sales who has just been informed that her sales *budget* be cut (but not her sales *quota*) to allow for DTC. Such spending conflicts are frequent when financial resources are—always—limited.

The industry publishes little information on the size and distribution of their promotional budgets. We can learn, for example, that Schering-Plough spent $223 million in 1999 on consumer advertising, but *not* how much was spent in personal selling.

One hopes that the promotional budgeting process is more often a result of careful, quantitative planning then of internal battles over dollars. Tools are available to make these decisions.

In the December 1993 issue of *Product Management Today*, Robert Girondi described one method of applying a logical system to promotional planning.[5]

"Applying Relative Media Values to the Pharmaceutical Promotion Planning Process"

The promotion planning process is more important than ever. Never before has so much attention been paid to return-on-promotional investment (ROPI). Advertising agencies and the product teams they serve are asking the same question in many different ways, but always with the same thought in mind: *What measurable return can I expect from the promotion plan under consideration?*

During the course of nearly every business day, we make qualitative judgments and related decisions based on the value of media exposures that are more frequent and have less impact versus exposures that are less frequent and have greater impact. We are forced to make specific-ROPI-related decisions, such as whether to use telephone message pads, journal advertising, detailing, or patient record forms to communicate a message—all of these decisions are usually based on judgments that consider relative costs, personal experience, sales presentations, and so forth. Until recently, there has not been any alternative method to consider.

Complexity of the Message

The answers to the above considerations really depend on the complexity of the message to be delivered and the ability of the available, affordable media to achieve the exposure goal. This goal is defined as providing a contact in advance of each and every opportunity the target physician has to prescribe your product. In the end, some media mix is necessary to do the job. This leads to the more important question: What are the relative values for each of the various dissimilar media under consideration?

Intuitively, we understand that the impact of an exposure provided by telephone message pads is less than that provided by a detail, but it is more difficult to know how much less, when one considers the potential of the former to provide a dramatically greater frequency of exposure than the latter.

To provide an answer to this important issue, and to document actual "relative values" for the various media available to the pharmaceutical marketer, HCI Inc. conducted more than 260 controlled tests among more than 12,000 physicians over the past five years. The results of this promotion research provide specifics needed to address relative values of dissimilar media at a time when maximum effect at minimum costs is the only acceptable way of doing business [Table 15.2].

It is important to understand that the concept of "relative values" is not based on sales response, but on the relative ability of the next exposure provided by a medium to communicate a message as part of a normal media mix for an ongoing program. With this information, it is possible to appropriately weight and merge journal and nonjournal media, including promotion such as detailing, conventions, dinners, etc.

Application of Relative Values to the Promotion Planning Process

In order to address the question of maximizing ROPI most efficiently, several steps in a very logical process should be addressed:

1. By combining prescribing cycle needs (how often a particular target must be contacted each week to produce a memorable, actionable effect), the number of working weeks a product is to be promoted, and the target audience definition, the product team can calculate the total number of exposures needed to provide the required impact [see A in Table 15.3].
2. The remaining exposures required are then allocated to nonpersonal media in the ration appropriate to the requirements dictated by the product's position in its lifecycle [see B and C in Table 15.3]. For example, a product in the initial stage of its lifecycle would need to establish its position in the minds of its target audience, to build brand and benefit awareness, and to obtain adoption by target market innovators. Because research shows that journal advertising is the medium that can best provide the broad-based,

TABLE 15.2. Results of Research on Relative Values

Promotion Method	Relative Value to Journal Ad
Dinner meetings	5.00
Symposia/conventions	4.66
Detail with sales aid (primary)	3.33
Detail with sales aid (secondary)	2.33
Medical television	2.00
Convention detail	1.66
Direct mail	1.17
Reminder detail	1.00
Journal Ad	**1.00**
Reference publications	0.66
Rx pads	0.33
Other office forms/scratch pads/pens	0.16

Source: Data from HCI, Inc., Princeton, New Jersey.

TABLE 15.3. Exposure Goals: Antihypertensives—Equivalent Values Adjustment

	Beginning of Product Life Cycle	Adjusted for Equivalent Value	Resultant Print Budget
Purchasing cycle	3	3	
Working weeks	× 50	× 50	
Target audience	× 122,000	× 122,000	
Exposure goal **A**	18,300,000	18,300,000	
Detailing exposures **B**	366,000 **D × 3.3**	1,207,800	
Exposures needed	17,934,000	17,092,200	$7,435,107 **E**
Journal exposures	13,450,500	12,819,150	$4,871,277 **E**
Nonjournal media exposures	4,483,500 **C***	4,273,050 **C***	$2,563,830 **E**
Exposures achieved	18,300,000	18,300,000	

*3:1 ratio between journal and nonjournal media

high-reach, high-frequency, low-cost means needed to meet these promotion objectives most efficiently, this medium is selected to deliver 75 percent of the required exposures, with the balance allocated to nonjournal print media (prescription pads, compendia, etc.). The remaining 25 percent are needed to cover the top quartile of prescribers more frequently and routinely than can be provided using journals alone.

The relative values discussed above can now be applied to this process. Returning to our example [see D in Table 15.3], because the relative value of a primary detail using a sales aid is 3.3 times that of a journal ad in its ability to convey a message as part of an ongoing process, the value of the exposures provided by detailing is increased from 366,000 to 1,207,800 (366,00 × 3.3). This reduces the number of additional exposures needed from nonpersonal print promotion media to 17,092,000, which are reapportioned using the 3:1 journal-to-nonjournal media ratio previously determined to be the most appropriate for the product where it exists in its lifecycle.

3. In combination with known media costs, prescribing cycle requirement, and the number of working weeks in the promotion cycle under consideration, target audience definition and frequency-based exposure goals can be converted into the dollar equivalents needed to complete marketing plans.

4. To satisfy the inevitable need to establish promotion budget levels for overall return-on-investment (ROI) planning and tactical implementation, the exposure allocations can be converted to dollar budgets simply by multiplying them by their respective average costs [see E in Table 15.3]. In this case the following holds true:

- 12.8 million journal exposures at $0.38 each = $4.9 million
- 4.3 million nonjournal media exposures at $0.60 each = $2.6 million
- Total print budget needed to achieve objectives = $7.5 million

This "grass roots" zero-base budget may be refined further to more closely reflect competitive spend levels or to reflect response model norms if either is deemed more appropriate. It even may be appropriate to adopt a spend level that represents an average of all three of these varied approaches.

Developing the Media Schedule

Once specific dollar amounts have been agreed upon, the usual media schedule can be developed up to these levels. It is at this stage that the individual relative values for each of the many varied media options are applied (a fertile area for discussion but not the subject of this article).

A little experimentation with this process can be rewarding, especially in its ability to enable "what if" scenarios to be considered. Among its many other benefits is a comfort level for the promotion planner—a degree of credibility that can serve the planning team well in defending its proposed spend levels. There is nothing like research-based numbers to enhance acceptability.

The benefits of applying the research-based relative values of the media available for pharmaceutical promotion are many and obvious. But none is so obvious and more important than providing the ability to unite detailing with the other elements of the promotion mix in a way that synergistically enhances the impact of each of the elements and ensures the most efficient ROPI. [Reprinted with permission from *Product Management Today*, December 1993.]

CONCLUSION

As the most important of the four Ps, promotion bears the responsibility of both informing and persuading. The responsibility is discharged relatively effectively, if not always efficiently. The necessarily creative nature of promotion *can* lead to more attention to creativity than to results.

The "Manny" Awards for the Advertising Agency of the Year, published annually by *Med Ad News*, use the following criteria in selecting winners:

- Management ability
- Income growth
- Creative marketing ability
- New accounts
- Lost accounts
- Ability to attract, develop, and keep people[6]

Although all of these are important in the success of those involved in advertising and other media of promotion, the need remains to measure and reward the ability to inform and to persuade.

SECTION VI:
CONCLUSION

Chapter 16

Prospects: Linking Therapy to Patient Needs

Mickey Smith

In this final chapter we will reflect on what has gone before in this text. We will examine the premise that good pharmaceutical marketing is good medicine and review some aspects of the four Ps in this context.

PUBLIC PERCEPTIONS OF PHARMACEUTICAL MARKETING

Few industries have been criticized more often, more inaccurately, and more unfairly for their marketing activities than the pharmaceutical industry. The term "marketing" is often used imprecisely, and in a disparaging sense. Critics commonly hold one or more of the following *negative* opinions and appear to be unaware of the positive benefits of pharmaceutical marketing.

Inaccurate Negative Opinions

- Pharmaceutical product development is not based on the needs of patients or payers, and marketing is used to sell useless, costly, or redundant medicines invented by out-of-touch researchers.
- Promotion is unnecessary. Good products with important benefits will always find users. Doctors always know what is new and good.

Much of the material in this chapter is taken from a monograph, "Pharmaceutical Marketing: Linking Therapy to Patient Needs," written by Dr. Richard Levy, Vice President of the National Pharmaceutical Council, and Mickey Smith. The monograph was published in 1993 by the National Pharmaceutical Council and the materials are used with permission of the Council. Representing our best thinking when originally published, this chapter identifies and projects a number of marketing trends just beginning at the time. In the interim, many of these trends have come to pass, most notably the need for pharmaceutical companies to show the economic value of medicines and to communicate with patients directly. Increasing activity in these areas over the past several years shows this is indeed taking place.

Promotion is biased to such an extent that it is not credible or useful to doctors.

- Companies spend too much money on marketing, especially on promotion and advertising.
- Marketing drives up the cost of medicine.
- Pharmaceutical marketing is mostly promotion. Other, less visible functions of marketing, such as maintenance of efficient distribution channels, are not significant features.
- Stimulation of demand for medicines is inappropriate and encourages unnecessary spending.

In short, critics believe that marketing adds little value to pharmaceutical products. These opinions, which are often strongly held, indicate a great need for clarification of the role of marketing in the pharmaceutical industry and for a description of the substantial value it adds to products. Of course, that is one of the goals of this text.

WHAT PHARMACEUTICAL MARKETING IS AND DOES

There is obvious added value in having medicines available in convenient dosage forms, palatable flavors, and efficient packaging. Marketing, however, adds many other, more profound values to pharmaceutical products, but most of these values are less obvious and are generally not understood.

The fundamental role of pharmaceutical marketing is technology transfer. A medication has value only if it is available when and where it is needed. The essence of pharmaceutical R&D is assembling information about how chemical compounds work in the body. The essence of pharmaceutical marketing is communicating this information to providers and consumers. Thus, research, development, and marketing are elements of an information continuum, whereby research concepts are transformed into practical therapeutic tools and information is progressively layered and made more useful to the health care system. Transmitting information to end users through marketing is a crucial element of pharmaceutical innovation. Unless physicians are informed about the treatment opportunities offered by new medicines, there is effectively no innovation.[1]

The thread of marketing is woven throughout the fabric of the pharmaceutical industry. It binds together the many aspects of this complex industry and underlies the business operations of all successful pharmaceutical companies. At a time when there is serious talk of strict governmental regulation of health care, policymakers and the public must recognize that marketing by the pharmaceutical and other health care industries is, and must be, an integral part of any system that evolves. A more complete understanding of pharmaceutical marketing is required to recognize that, not only is marketing a necessary business function, but it is vital to the nation's health. The following concepts are central to this understanding.

WHAT DRIVES PRODUCT DEVELOPMENT?

Companies are increasingly organized to reflect the fact that R&D and customer needs must be closely linked for commercial success. The involvement of marketing personnel on product development teams provides the perspectives of the patient, physician, and payer.

Medicines themselves have little appeal; what is desired is their beneficial effects on patients' lives and on health care costs. Accordingly, the perceptions and needs of end users guide product development. Marketing identifies needs, refines the product to meet them, and communicates the availability of the product and its characteristics to doctors, patients, and payers. Thus, pharmaceutical development is "customer driven"; marketing links user needs with appropriate products and is essential at each stage in the creation of a medicine.

Product development is a cycle that starts with the patient, is guided by the patient, and ends with the patient. Marketing transmits information at each stage of the process. Marketing sequentially

1. guides the creation of medicines, based on an assessment of patient needs;
2. communicates to physicians the availability and attributes of medicines; and
3. encourages patients in their proper use.

Marketing moves us from a general condition of unmet patient needs to a stage at which many of those needs are fulfilled by new therapies. The cycle begins again as marketing reveals product shortcomings.

Marketing does not force products on the medical profession; rather, it provides doctors with an informed choice of carefully characterized agents to fit the specific needs of individual patients. The therapeutic requirements of patients vary widely, based on the nature of the disease and symptoms, concurrent diseases, concurrent medicines, tolerance to specific side effects, age, gender, ethnic and racial background, previous experience with medicines, allergies, and many other factors. A broad choice of available agents enables the precise tailoring of therapy. Marketing enables health care professionals to make informed choices by educating them about the attributes of individual products.

Market research seeks out commercial opportunities in the form of unmet patient needs. For example, although there is a clear need for better cancer therapy, research is required to determine specific gaps in existing therapy, troublesome side effects that could be eliminated, and compliance problems that warrant correction. Marketing identifies such potential and supplies this information to the R&D team.

Marketing must take its cues from the patient and the physician. Products designed to meet nonexistent needs will fail, despite the vigor of the sales force. Market failures are expensive, and ultimately this cost is passed along to the consumer. Marketing helps hold costs down by weeding out those candidates destined to fail commercially.

Some products are discontinued during development, and others are repositioned. A small market size per se, however, will not necessarily kill a product; that "orphan" drugs are developed by the pharmaceutical industry is evidence of a firm's willingness to meet a real medical need with little chance of substantial economic gain. Commercial success is maximized through the development of a product that is "user friendly," i.e., with optimal dosing, dosage form, flavor, ease of use, tolerance, and packaging. Development rarely ends with approval by the FDA; it simply takes a new direction, largely determined by marketing considerations. Typical developments after introduction include the following:

- Lower dosage formulations for use by the elderly and other patient groups
- Additional indications
- Long-acting delivery system to reduce dose frequency
- Improved flavor and packaging
- Further definition and quantification of adverse reactions

In addition to its primary job of determining and satisfying the needs of patients, marketing now has the added challenge of demonstrating the economic value of products to payers. Governments, managed care organizations, employers, and other purchasers of health care are now scrutinizing the price and value of all components, including pharmaceuticals.

In the 1980s, pharmaceutical firms began to respond positively to these new market demands. They began to regard technology assessment as a new "playing field," and demonstrating value became a new way to compete. The major firms began to supply the techniques of cost-effectiveness analysis in the (correct) belief that these studies would be increasingly required by the marketplace.[2]

Pharmaceutical companies have played a large role in the establishment, funding, and refinement of the exciting new field of pharmacoeconomics. The seminal and influential effort in this field, dating back at least to 1977, was the demonstration by Smith, Kline & French of the dramatic economic benefit realized from the use of cimetidine as an alternative to ulcer surgery. In 1981, Duncan Neuhauser, professor of epidemiology and community health at Case Western Reserve University, reviewed the body of economic research sponsored by this company, judged it an important contribution, and advocated such analysis "for a wide range of medical interventions."[3]

Additional developments in pharmacoeconomics have continued, and the research literature now abounds with comparisons of alternate drug therapies, drug therapy with other treatments, and assessments of a medication's value as opposed to its price.

These initiatives have become a driving force in the marketplace. The number of published health economic evaluations of pharmaceuticals has exploded in recent years. Studies have expanded into such areas as quality-of-life assessment, outcomes measurement, and decision analysis. Companies are paying particular attention to making pharmacoeconomic studies an informative and scientifically valid component of product marketing strategies. The techniques they pioneered are now used as serious tools for decision making by formulary committees, third-party administrators, and government policymakers.

MARKETING EXERTS DOWNWARD PRESSURE ON THE PRICE OF MEDICINES

A unique problem for the pharmaceutical industry is the public's often negative perception of its products. Everyone wants quick symptom relief or effective cures, but few can fully appreciate the value of products that accomplish these apparently simple objectives. Patients having diseases without symptoms often resent an expense that shows no immediate or visible benefit and would prefer instead to purchase something with clear value— new clothes, a movie ticket, or dinner at a restaurant. The purchase of medications by a sicker or chronically ill patient is complicated by the emotions secondary to illness. Last, medications are often paid for up-front and out of pocket, whereas other, often more expensive health care components have the financial cushion of primary insurance coverage. These factors combine to make medicines unpopular—and their prices even more unpopular. There is no right price—only a "too high" price.

Marketing does help, however, in controlling the price of pharmaceuticals, as companies compete for market share. The entire generic pharmaceutical industry is based on competition focused on pricing, but price competition is also ongoing among different branded products in the same therapeutic class. Although different products are rarely therapeutically equivalent, a rough substitute can often be found. Thus, an overpriced product, resulting from poor market analysis, will find few buyers.

In addition to the mechanism of price competition, marketing also reduces the price of medicines by expanding the customer base. Pricing is, in part, based on the estimated size of the market, and stimulation of appropriate demand through promotion is essential to reach that potential. Wide use of a medication can enable economies of scale and reduced price. R&D costs and manufacturing are amortized over a wider base, so unit costs are held down. That is why widely used medicines for chronic conditions, such as arthritis and hypertension, are priced much lower than those used by relatively smaller numbers of patients, such as oncology products.

COST SAVINGS THROUGH EFFICIENT DISTRIBUTION: A KEY ELEMENT OF MARKETING

Pharmaceutical products do not automatically find their way to pharmacy·shelves. A vital, but seldom discussed, function of pharmaceutical marketing is the development and maintenance of a system for the physical distribution of medicines. Marketing has created in the United States one of the most efficient and cost-effective medication distribution systems in the world.   ·

This system allows for the rapid distribution of lifesaving new medicines immediately after they are approved for marketing. Following FDA approval, the availability of an important new medicine can be communicated immediately to all practicing physicians in the United States, and the product shipped to every pharmacy in the country within forty-eight hours.

This distribution system also enables a rapid, corrective response to bad news, by informing doctors and pharmacists about important, newly discovered adverse effects. If quality control or tampering problems are discovered, batch destinations can be quickly traced to locate and recall products from individual pharmacies.

The availability of virtually any prescription medicine in any town in America documents the success of this effort. This distribution system was developed mutually by the manufacturing, wholesaling, and retailing segments of the pharmaceutical industry. This system is virtually invisible to consumers.

Manufacturers are just one element of the complex pharmaceutical industry, and many other components play important roles in providing access to medicines. The successful establishment of an efficient interface between manufacturers and customers required the creation of complex distribution channels that include independent and chain pharmacies, mail-order services, physician-dispensers, wholesalers, retailers, hospitals, clinics, and government installations. The selection of a given channel is determined by the situation, needs, and desires of different patients. The geographic location of the patients and the establishments in the distribution channels affect plant location, warehousing, development of sales territories, and transportation of the product.

The thousands of retail pharmacy outlets are themselves part of the pharmaceutical industry. Many provide home delivery—the ultimate in convenience. Product accessibility to consumers is facilitated by manufacturers' liberal return-goods policies, which enable pharmacists to stock many products. Other "back office" marketing activities link producers to distributors to help ensure product availability. Liberal credit policies, efficient invoicing, and good communications regarding the availability and nature of the company's products ensure that the patient actually takes title to the medicine.

The wholesaler segment of the pharmaceutical industry makes a special contribution to efficiency and cost savings. Wholesalers select, purchase, and store goods in close proximity to pharmacies. Wholesalers provide economic savings by concentrating goods, dispersing them in economic quantities, and then transporting these goods to pharmacies. This sorting function reduces the number of transactions required, thereby saving the system considerable costs.

The National Wholesale Druggists' Association estimates that the total number of annual transactions using wholesalers is 40.3 million (7.8 million manufacturer-to-wholesaler transactions and 32.5 million wholesaler-to-pharmacy transactions).[4] This compares favorably with 439.2 million transactions if all products were distributed directly from manufacturers to pharmacies. Thus, wholesaler operations reduce the total number of pharmaceutical transactions in the United States by 90.8 percent. *This translates to a savings of more than $10 billion annually in the cost of distributing pharmaceuticals.*

COMMUNICATING WITH PHYSICIANS: LINKING PRODUCTS TO PATIENT NEEDS

Pharmaceutical companies would prefer not to spend money on promotion; they would rather use the money for operations or pass it along to shareholders. Unfortunately, however, although marketing may succeed in providing the right product, at the right price, the product will fail in the marketplace without a strong communications link with prescribers and dispensers. Promotion is the vehicle for such communication.

Certainly, one objective of promotion is to drive sales. The marketing communications activities of the industry, however, are primarily informational and serve to educate the medical profession regarding how to use a medicine, when to use it, and when not to use it. These are among the most important activities of the industry. At its core, this research-intensive, high-technology industry is also an information service industry.

Marketing communication is a frequent target of criticism, much of which reflects an incomplete understanding of

1. the need for communications activity, over and above noncommercial sources of information;
2. the accuracy and usefulness of promotional materials; and
3. the role and relative importance of advertising.

Why the Medical Literature Is Not Enough

> In nearly all health care settings—from those involving a village healer to those involving a Western subspecialist—essentially no mechanisms exist that require health care providers to remain at all current with the developments in pharmacology that have occurred since the completion of their training.[5]

At present, the marketing communications activities of the pharmaceutical industry represent the major organized and comprehensive effort to update physicians and other decision makers about the availability, safety, efficacy, hazards, and techniques of using medicines. Medical schools, hospitals, and medical societies acknowledge the educational contributions of the industry and recognize that they do not have the personnel or funds to support medical education at current levels if the industry were to withdraw its support. The American Medical Association believes that industry support of medical education is "a critically important part of the health care system,"[6] and then FDA Commissioner Kessler has stated that "the FDA has long realized that industry-sponsored presentations by physician researchers can play an important part in informing and educating health care professionals."[7]

If a ban were suddenly placed on all promotion of medicines, the effect on the knowledge levels of prescribers, barring the introduction of some new information source, would be immediate and negative. Accordingly, responsible critics of this essential source of information must offer an alternative. Any alternative information system must be measured against the present one in terms of scope, objectivity, timeliness of information, effectiveness of communication, and cost. The relative importance of these factors to providers, payers, and patients may differ, and a given alternative may be less acceptable to many than the current system of company-based promotion. One scholar proposed replacing commercial information with a program to be conducted by a National Drug Education Foundation. This hypothetical program would have cost an estimated $167 million annually in 1976 dollars,[8] which was almost certainly an underestimate.

Marketing communications by pharmaceutical companies are a key channel through which physicians obtain information about medicines. In contrast with the training and formal continuing education programs available to most doctors, marketing communications from pharmaceutical companies present information about their products that is timely and dynamic.

The basic piece of information that must be communicated about a product is its availability. Before physicians can prescribe a product, they must know it exists. The physician engages in a "vicarious search" on behalf of the patient; that is, knowing the needs of the patient, the physician searches the characteristics of available products. Although the search is active and educated, the physician is unlikely to become aware of a product unless someone, usually the manufacturer, has made a formal and systematic effort to communicate its availability.

The medical literature is extensive, but access to it in the real world of medical practice is difficult. From the doctor's perspective, the pharmaceutical sales force represents an extremely efficient and effective means of obtaining information. By investing five or ten minutes, and without traveling to a medical library, practicing physicians who have little time to read the enormous amount of literature on drug therapy can obtain the specific information they need. Sales calls are expensive for the company but are a valued service to doctors, providing them with an enormous savings in time that can be devoted to patient care.

The relative importance of company-sponsored information in physician education regarding a given product depends on where that product is in its life cycle. For newly launched products, the commercial sponsor is the primary source of information, since at this time very few articles on the product have appeared in the medical literature. The sponsor, however, is in possession of considerable information about the product, developed in support of its application to the FDA for marketing approval. Thus, commercial materials are particularly important in educating physicians about new pharmaceutical technology and in helping patients to benefit early from these developments. (From a business perspective, intensive distribution of product information at launch is required to establish the product, and overall economic success depends heavily on success in the initial years of a product's life cycle.) As the product matures, reports in the published literature become more numerous, and the burden of product education is taken up by official medical texts, compendia, review articles, and other published sources.

Successful pharmaceutical promotion relies on physician understanding of the condition being treated and the mechanism of action of the medication being offered. For example, one of the tasks of those companies introducing the first beta-blocker, the first oral antidiabetic agent, was to review the physiologic principles underlying the drug's action. Considerable educational value accrues from this activity.

Educational activities directed at physician prescribing must sometimes be preceded by efforts to assist the physician in the diagnosis. An example is the condition of ulcerative colitis. Research in the early 1960s showed that primary care physicians were slow to reach the diagnosis of this condition. This often resulted in delays in selecting effective therapy, sometimes with tragic results. Educational efforts by the manufacturer of the leading medication were targeted at improved diagnosis. These efforts certainly helped sales but also resulted in more prompt patient care.

Some believe that promotion is biased and therefore of dubious value as a source of information. Although information coming from a commercial source does present the product in the best possible light, physicians are well aware of this bias and correct for it. Moreover, the credibility of the sales representative, in an ongoing relationship with the doctor, depends on the veracity of the information. Sales representatives are most effective when they have created an atmosphere of trust, based on a foundation of accurate, noninflated claims of approved indications. Representatives who stray from the truth quickly undermine their credibility.

Competition exposes physicians to multiple biases and multiple facets of the story, as each company promotes the advantages of its own product and compares it to the alternatives. This exposure to different perspectives enables physicians to make a more informed choice of the best medicine for the individual patient.

The regulation of pharmaceutical promotion has created a level playing field. FDA regulations clearly circumscribe what companies can and cannot communicate about a medicine. Communication is limited to the essential advantages of the product, such as efficacy, improved dosage form, lower cost, or fewer interactions with other medications. Also, sales representatives are not allowed to draw physicians' attention to uses that are not included in a product's official labeling, even if substantial clinical evidence supports such off-label indications.

Advertising in Perspective

Advertising is what many people mean when they speak of promotion, although advertising is only a small part of promotion. Relatively little is spent on the high-profile activities visible to the general public.

Across the industry, less than 10 percent of marketing budgets is allocated to journal advertising, and an estimated 20 percent of that amount is spent on the brief summary mandated by the FDA.[9]

The main purpose of advertising in medical journals is not to convince the doctor to prescribe a product or to provide comprehensive information, but rather to establish or reinforce the image of the product or the company. Advertising is a cost-effective mechanism for creating awareness about new products, approved new uses for existing products, new formulations, and new adverse effects. Advertising stimulates doctors' interest in receiving more information from sales representatives or from journal articles. Advertising is not intended as a major route of information transfer; it merely seeks to capture the product's essential differences from competing products.

Although many advertisements are for new products, many others are for established medicines. These serve to remind the physician of alternatives to therapy and that the newest is not necessarily the best for an individual patient. The mix of advertisements for new and existing products helps physicians maintain awareness of the elements of a "balanced portfolio" of choices in treating a given disease.

Pharmaceutical product advertising in medical journals is different from consumer product advertising; it is technical and scientific, and what can be said about a medication is strictly regulated by the FDA and is restricted to the approved labeling. Since FDA punishments for transgressions are costly, embarrassing, and damaging to a firm's reputation, companies make serious attempts to avoid advertising that may be considered false or misleading. Self-regulation is provided by policymaking bodies of advertisers (Association of National Advertisers) and advertising agencies (American Association of Advertising Agencies).

The FDA has a legislative mandate to ensure that prescription advertising and labeling is accurate, truthful, and balanced; that labeling contains the latest information for safe, effective use of medicines; and that labels are presented and distributed in the most effective way.

Companies must submit to the FDA all proposed labeling, advertising, and promotional materials (printed, audio, and visual) at the time they are disseminated to the public. Launch campaigns for new prescription products are also reviewed for compliance with regulations. In addition, companies can ask the FDA to review a competitor's promotional materials, if they believe such materials are in violation of regulations.

Although advertising is not a major expenditure for marketing departments, it does play a major role in supporting the flow of medical information in noncommercial channels. Advertising revenues enable medical publishers and professional societies to lower the cost of medical journals for researchers, doctors, and libraries. The journals' advertising and editorial departments are kept strictly separate, and advertising dollars cannot influence the selection or content of medical reports.

COST SAVINGS THROUGH MARKETING DIRECTLY TO PATIENTS

Despite the failures mentioned previously, the extensive marketing effort directed at physicians does reflect the industry's understanding of the need to communicate effectively with prescribers. One great omission in pharmaceutical marketing, however, has been the absence of a major effort in the last, crucial step in the information continuum—communication with the ultimate end user, the patient. Increased spending on marketing to consumers would have beneficial economic and clinical effects. Medications would be used more appropriately and consistently by patients, and as a result, overall health care costs would most likely decrease.

Leading pharmaceutical firms have become sensitized to this failure of information "throughput" to the ultimate consumer and are beginning to mount serious patient- and provider-directed compliance education programs. Research confirms that these marketing efforts aimed at improving compliance with medication regimens can be effective in lowering overall treatment costs.

The major responsibility for the proper use of pharmaceutical products resides with the firms that manufacture them. Those firms which have committed marketing resources to improved compliance with medications have "taken the bull by the horns"; they realize that although prescribers and dispensers have a role in compliance education, they cannot be expected to assume the point position. It is the companies themselves who must spearhead efforts to educate consumers about medicines and to educate providers in effective techniques for talking to patients about medicines. The companies must shoulder the additional marketing costs associated with these activities.

In the past two decades, pharmaceutical marketers have begun to focus some marketing effort directly on consumers. Although controversial, these programs have probably resulted in greater public awareness of disease risks; in earlier treatment of hypertension, ulcers, smoking, menopause, and depression; and in improved management of contraception.

Paul Rubin, a former senior economist with the Federal Trade Commission, noted that "[a]dvertising and promotion of prescription drugs is beneficial to consumers because of the information provided. Deception in this market—of physicians or consumers—is particularly improbable."[10]

Rubin further asserts that direct promotion of pharmaceuticals to consumers is likely to result in lower prices:

> If there is any harmful effect of advertising to professionals, it is that such advertising might lead to increased market power and thus increased prices. The most efficient way to reduce this effect is to allow increased direct advertising because consumers have the strongest interest in price reductions. Increasing regulation of advertising to professionals would be harmful and would not generate benefits.[11]

Masson and Rubin have argued that the price of medicines would probably fall if DTC advertising provided four types of information:

- *Existence of a disease*—i.e., a person should have assistance in recognizing symptoms of a treatable problem.

- *Availability of treatment*—learning of the existence of a new treatment for an already diagnosed condition may induce a person to return to a physician for treatment.
- *Side effects*—knowing that more tolerable treatment is available may move a patient to discuss it with the physician, with a probable increase in compliance.
- *Risk*—one cannot assess the risk of a therapy without information about that therapy.[12]

PHARMACEUTICAL MARKETING STIMULATES DEMAND: GOOD FOR THE HEALTH CARE SYSTEM

Stimulating demand for pharmaceuticals through marketing contributes to a sound market, and attempts to manage demand, by controlling the flow of information through restrictions on marketing, will create an inefficient market.

The free flow of information is essential to our market-directed economy, the basic purpose of which is to satisfy consumer needs. In the health care arena, patients, providers, and payers have somewhat different needs and make choices of goods and services based on their own objectives, economic situations, and values. To make informed choices, each of these players requires good information regarding the availability, cost, and quality of competing products and services.

In an efficient health care market, the supply-demand relationship is continuously tuned through the flow of information—and that information flow is facilitated by vigorous marketing. This is the classic role of marketing in an economic system. There is some concern, however, that marketing, by stimulating demand for products and services, drives up health care costs by forcing upon the system goods that are unnecessary or overused. These value judgments, however, are best made by the consumers, who know their individual needs and can make a good cost benefit decision—if they have relevant, high-quality information.

The system is not perfect, however, and medicines sometimes are overused, but their underuse through poor compliance and underprescribing is more common and represents a greater cost to society. Compared with other forms of treatment, medicines are usually the cheapest route to an effective outcome, and their underuse results in increased treatment costs and represents a burden to the economy.

Although information about medicines is needed for the operation of a sound market, it is also important that marketing practices be appropriate and that the information be accurate. Examples of inappropriate pharmaceutical marketing practices include misinformation, unsubstantiated claims, or bribery—subtle or overt. Thus, the quality of the information should be controlled, but not the quantity.

It is especially important that any changes in the market for pharmaceuticals be carefully thought out, since an effective and efficient market currently exists, having evolved over the past several decades. The greatest shortcoming of our present health care marketing system is in the area of fair allocation of goods and services, including pharmaceuticals. The policy challenge is to provide fair access to pharmaceuticals without destroying the effectiveness, efficiency, and research incentives that characterize our present system.

Appendix

Resources

BOOKS

Basara, L. and Montague, M. *Searching for Magic Bullets*. Binghamton, NY: The Haworth Press, 1994.

Bonk, R. *Pharmaceutical Economics in Perspective*. Binghamton, NY: The Haworth Press, 1999.

Corstjens, M. *Marketing Strategy in the Pharmaceutical Industry*. New York: Chapman and Hall, 1991.

Dubos, R. *Mirage of Health*. Piscataway, NJ: Rutgers University Press, 1987.

Huttin, C. and Bosanquet, N. *The Prescription Drug Market*. New York: North-Holland, 1992.

Kolassa, M. *Elements of Pharmaceutical Pricing*. Binghamton, NY: Pharmaceutical Products Press, 1997.

Kotler, P., Ferrell, O.C., and Lamb, C. *Cases and Readings for Marketing for Nonprofit Organizations*. Englewood Cliffs, NJ: Prentice-Hall, 1983. (Any text by Philip Kotler is a good resource.)

Levitt, T. *The Marketing Imagination*. New York: The Free Press, 1986. (Any text by Theodore Levitt is a good resource.)

Lidstone, J. *Marketing Planning for the Pharmaceutical Industry*. Aldershot, UK: Gower Publishing, 1987.

Mintz, M. *The Therapeutic Nightmare*. New York: Houghton Mifflin, 1965.

Pelton, L., Strutton, D., and Lumpkin, J. *Marketing Channels*. Chicago: Irwin, 1997.

Silverman, M. and Lee, P. *Pills, Profits and Politics*. Berkeley: University of California Press, 1974.

Smith, M.C. *Pharmaceutical Marketing: Strategy and Cases*. Binghamton, NY: The Haworth Press, 1991.

Smith, M.C. (Ed.). *Pharmaceutical Marketing in the 21st Century.* Binghamton, NY: The Haworth Press, 1996.

Smith, M.C. (Ed.) *Studies in Pharmaceutical Economics.* Binghamton, NY: The Haworth Press, 1996.

Spilker, B. *Multinational Pharmaceutical Companies,* Second Edition. New York: Raven Press, 1994.

Werth, B. *Billion-Dollar Molecule.* New York: Simon and Schuster, 1994.

PERIODICALS

American Journal of Health-System Pharmacy
American Society of Health-System Pharmacists
7272 Wisconsin Avenue
Bethesda, MD 20814

American Journal of Pharmaceutical Education
American Association of Colleges of Pharmacy
School of Pharmacy
University of North Carolina
Chapel Hill, NC 27599-7360

Business & Health
Medical Economics Company, Inc.
5 Paragon Drive
Montvale, NJ 07645-1742

The Consultant Pharmacist
American Society of Consultant Pharmacists
1321 Duke Street
Alexandria, VA 22314-3463

Drug Topics
Medical Economics Company, Inc.
5 Paragon Drive
Montvale, NJ 07645-1742

Health Affairs
Project HOPE
7500 Old Georgetown Road, Suite 600
Bethesda, MD 20814-6133

Healthcare Distributor
E.L.F. Publications

5285 W. Louisiana Ave., Suite 112
Denver, CO 80232

Inquiry: Journal of Health Care Organization, Provision, and Financing
P.O. Box 25399
Rochester, NY 14625

Journal of the American Pharmaceutical Association
American Pharmaceutical Association
2215 Constitution Avenue, NW
Washington, DC 20037

Journal of Managed Care Pharmacy
Academy of Managed Care Pharmacy
P.O. Box 6565
Athens, GA 30604

Journal of Pharmaceutical Marketing and Management
The Haworth Press, Inc.
10 Alice Street
Binghamton, NY 13904

Journal of Pharmacy & Law
The Pharmacy-Law Institute
Ohio Northern University
Robertson-Evans Building
Ada, OH 45810

Journal of Research in Pharmaceutical Economics
The Haworth Press, Inc.
10 Alice Street
Binghamton, NY 13904

Managed Healthcare
ADVANSTAR Communications, Inc.
7500 Old Oak Boulevard
Cleveland, OH 44130-3369

MedAd News
Engle Publishing Partners
820 Bear Tavern Road
West Trenton, NJ 08628

Medical Marketing & Media
CPS Communications, Inc.
7200 W. Camino Real, Suite 215
Boca Raton, FL 33433

Pharmaceutical Executive
ADVANSTAR Communications, Inc.
859 Williamette Street
Eugene, OR 97401-6806

Scrip Magazine
PJB Publications, Ltd.
1775 Broadway, Suite 511
New York, NY 10019

Scrip World Pharmaceutical News
PJB Publications, Ltd.
1775 Broadway, Suite 511
New York, NY 10019

Notes

Chapter 1

1. American Marketing Association. 1985. *Marketing News,* March. p.1.
2. Quoted in E.J. McCarthy. 1981. *Basic marketing.* Burr Ridge, IL: Irwin, p. 10.
3. Ibid.
4. E.J. McCarthy and W.D. Perreault. 1984. *Basic marketing.* Burr Ridge, IL: Irwin, p. 11.
5. T. Levitt. 1986. *The marketing imagination.* New York: Free Press, pp. 5-6.
6. G. Sonnedecker. 1986. *Kremers and Urdang's history of pharmacy,* Fourth edition. Madison, WI: American Institute of the History of Pharmacy.
7. Quoted in McCarthy, *Basic marketing,* p. 12.
8. Levitt, *The marketing imagination,* p. 6.
9. W. Alderson. 1965. *Dynamic marketing behavior.* Burr Ridge, IL: Irwin, p. 186.
10. Levitt, *The marketing imagination,* p. 19.

Chapter 2

1. T. Levitt. 1986. *The marketing imagination.* New York: Free Press, p. 139.
2. A. Maslow. 1943. A theory of human motivation. *Psychological Review* 7(43), pp. 70-78.
3. New era of lifestyle drugs. 1998. *Business Week,* May 11, pp. 54-57.
4. A.C. Twaddle and R.M. Hester. 1977. *A sociology of health.* St. Louis, MO: C.V. Mosby.
5. D. Mechanic. 1968. *Medical sociology.* New York: The Free Press.
6. D. Stimson. 1979. *Journal of the Royal College of General Practitioners.*
7. H. Rappoport. 1976. *Journal of the Royal College of General Practitioners.*
8. M.C. Smith. 1991. *Pharmaceutical marketing: Strategy and cases.* Binghamton, NY: The Haworth Press, p. 103.
9. R. Dubos. 1987. *Mirage of health.* Piscataway, NJ: Rutgers University Press, p. 196.
10. Dubos, *Mirage of health,* pp. 142-143.
11. P. Stolley, 1971. "Cultural lag in health care." *Inquiry,* VIII(3). p. 223.
12. Dubos, *Mirage of health,* pp. 130-131.
13. Ibid., p. 134.
14. F. Lewis. 1971. *Tufts Medical Alumni Bulletin,* 30(1), pp. 5-8.
15. E. Freidson. 1970. *Profession of medicine.* New York: Dodd Mead, p. 224.

16. Ibid., p. 235.

17. G. Dukes. 1997. Editorial. *International Journal of Risk and Safety in Medicine*, 10, p. 62.

18. Ibid.

19. R. Dubos, *Mirage of health*, p. 126.

20. R.N. Wilson. 1970. *Sociology of health*. New York: Random House, p. 116.

21. Dubos, *Mirage of health*, p. 161.

22. M. Gross. 1966. *The doctors*. New York: Random House, p. 27.

23. Dubos, *Mirage of health*, p. 166.

24. Ibid., p. 123.

25. Ibid., p. 144.

26. Editorial. 1997. *The Wall Street Journal*, July 21, p. 47.

27. L. Garrett. 1994. *The coming plague*. New York: Penguin Books.

28. Dubos, *Mirage of health*, p. 172.

29. Ibid., p. 156.

30. M.E. Porter. 1980. *Competitive strategy*. New York: The Free Press.

31. W. Alderson. 1965. *Dynamic marketing behavior*. Burr Ridge, IL: Irwin, p. 207.

32. J.T. Connor. 1964. *Drugs in our society*. New York: Free Press, p. 122.

33. Levitt, *The marketing imagination*, p. 140.

Chapter 3

1. S.C. Jain. 1993. *Marketing planning and strategy*, Fourth edition. Dallas, TX: Southwestern Publishing, p. 2.

2. T. Levitt. 1986. *The marketing imagination*. New York: Free Press.

3. Jain, *Marketing planning and strategy*, pp. 156-157.

4. Ibid., pp. 167-168.

5. Ibid., p. 246.

6. B. Henderson, Boston Consulting Group, personal communication, 1981.

7. T. Dao, personal communication, 1992.

8. W. Koberstein. 1998. Pharma mergers—Point/counterpoint: A conversation with Frederick Frank of Lehman Brothers. *Pharmaceutical Executive*, 18(16), pp. 78-86.

Chapter 4

1. National Pharmaceutical Council. 1990. *Pharmaceutical research: Therapeutic and economic value of incremental improvements*. Reston, VA: Author.

2. CNNfn. 1999. Drug firms post healthy 4Q. Available: <http://www.cnnfn.com/1999/01/26/companies/drugs> (accessed May 19, 2000).

3. Minnesota Mining and Manufacturing Company. 1998. 3M reports first-quarter 1998 sales and profits. St. Paul, MN: Author. Available: <http://www.mmm.com/front/1qtr98> (accessed May 19, 2000). Copyright 1997-1999 3M.

4. Yahoo Search Engine: Gentech List Archive. 1997. Monsanto to spin off chemical business (September 3) (accessed May 19, 2000).

5. Novartis press release. 1997. Novartis starts with strong growth in first quarter (April 17).

6. Warner-Lambert. 2000. Warner-Lambert reports first quarter sales and earnings results. Business Wire, press release (April 19). Document ID 20000419050000074.

7. Mergers and new products dominate. 1995. *Chemical & Industry New,* 21(November 6), p. 861. Available: <http://ci.mond.org/9521/952109html> (accessed May 19, 2000).

8. J.G. Perkins. 1999. *Remembrance of FEDs past: A reflection of the effective enhancement of an established allergy/cold product at Wellcome; 1976-1984.* Paper presented at University of Mississippi, April 5.

9. J.D. Reiff. 1984. Actifed—Flying high in the OTC market. *Pharmaceutical Executive,* 4(11), pp. 46-47.

10. SWITCH FORECAST. 1999. Available: <http://www.rxtootcswitch.com/trends/difore.html>.

11. R.P. Juhl. 1998. Prescription to over-the-counter switch: A regulatory perspective. *Clinical Therapy,* 20(Supplement C), pp. 111-117.

12. SWITCH FORECAST.

13. Juhl, Prescription to over-the-counter switch.

14. M.C. Smith. 1998. Rx-to-OTC switches: Reflection and projections. *Drug Topics,* 142(July 20), pp. 70-79.

15. U.S. Food and Drug Administration. 2000. IVD OTC List (March 10). Washington, DC: Center for Devices and Radiological Health.

Chapter 5

1. H. Schwartz. 2000. Parting shots. *Pharmaceutical Executive,* 20(8), p. 18.

2. M. Angell. 2000. The pharmaceutical industry—To whom is it accountable? *New England Journal of Medicine,* 342(25), p. 1902.

3. Adapted from *PhRMA Industry Profile,* 1999.

4. Angell, The pharmaceutical industry, p. 1902.

5. K. Levit, C. Cowen, H. Lazenby, A. Sensenig, and P. McDonnell. 2000. Health spending in 1998: Signals of change. *Health Affairs (Milwood),* 19(January/February), p. 124.

6. S. Murray and L. Lagnado. 2000. Drug companies face assault in prices. *The Wall Street Journal,* May 11, p. B1.

7. *Tufts Center for the Study of Drug Development Impact Report,* 1999.

8. P.E. Barrat. 1996. *20 years of pharmaceutical results throughout the world.* Rhone-Poulonc Rover Foundation.

9. A.T. Kearney. 1997. *Maximizing health in the next millennium: A prescription for increased shareholder value.* Chicago, IL: Author, p. 1.

10. H.G. Grabowski and J.M. Vernon. 1994. Return to R&D in new drug introductions in the 1980s. *Journal of Health Economics* 13, pp. 384-406.

11. Ibid.

12. Kearney, *Maximizing health in the next millennium,* p. 6.

13. *Tufts Center for the Study of Development Impact Report.*

14. Barrat, *20 years of pharmaceutical results.*

15. S. Gardner and R. Hamer. 2000. Informatics magic—How to turn data into knowledge. *Pharmaceutical Executive,* 20(12), p. 62-67.

16. D. Kniaz. 2000. Drug discovery adopts factory method. *Modern Drug Discovery,* 3(5), pp. 67-72.

17. N. Sleep. 2000. Sorting out combinatorial chaos. *Modern Drug Discovery,* 3(7/8), p. 37.

18. Kniaz, Drug discovery adopts factory method, p. 67.

19. K. Andrews-Cramer. 2000. Molecular informatics and the drug discovery factory. *Pharmaceutical Visions,* Spring, p. 62.

20. K. Pal. 2000. The keys to chemical genomics. *Modern Drug Discovery,* 3(9), p. 47.

21. E.K. Wilson. 2000. Gearing up for genomics' protein avalanche. *Chemical and Engineering News,* September 25, p. 41.

22. J. Craig Venter et al. 2001. The sequence of the human genome. *Science,* February 16, p. 1304.

23. E.S. Razvi and L.L. Leytes. 2000. Genomics: How SNP genotyping will affect the pharmaceutical industry. *Modern Drug Discovery,* 3(5), pp. 41-42.

24. L. Peltmen and V.A. McKusick. 2001. Dissecting human disease in the postgenomic era. *Science,* 291(5507), pp. 1224-1227, 1229.

25. M. Liebman. 1999. Competing drug companies cooperate in a bold race for gene therapies. *Medical Marketing and Media,* 34(8), pp. 68-73.

26. Ibid.

27. A.M. Edwards, C.H. Arrowsmith, and B. Des Pallieres. 2000. Proteomics: New tools for a new era. *Modern Drug Discovery,* 3(9), pp. 35-44.

28. L.J. Lesko et al. 2000. Optimizing the science of drug development: Opportunities for better candidate selection and accelerated evaluation in humans. *Journal of Clinical Pharmacology,* 40, p. 804.

29. A. Clemento. 1999. New and integrated approaches to successful accelerated drug development. *Drug Information Journal,* 33, p. 709.

30. Ibid., p. 708.

31. K.A. Getz and A. deBruin. 2000. Speed demons of drug development. *Pharmaceutical Executive,* 20(7), pp. 78-84.

32. Ibid., p. 79.

33. Ibid., p. 82.

34. Ibid.

35. M.B. Brennan. 2000. Drug discovery: Filtering out failures early in the game. *Clinical and Engineering News,* June 5, p. 63.

36. Ibid.

37. P. Pigache. 2000. Beyond the mouse. *Pharmaceutical Visions,* Spring, pp. 67-71.

38. Ibid., p. 68.

39. Brennan, Drug discovery, p. 72.

40. Lesko et al., Optimizing the science of drug development, p. 806.

41. Brennan, Drug discovery, p. 69.

42. Ibid., p. 72.

43. S. Tasher. 2000. Web-based clinical trials: How electronic report forms can speed trials and offer other advantages over paper forms. *Modern Drug Discovery,* 3(9), pp. 89-90.

44. C.R. Schoenberger. 2000. An Alzheimer's drug goes on trial. *Forbes,* March 20, p. 94.

45. G. Curtis et al. 2000. Use early drug development to understand NMEs for faster drug development. *Applied Clinical Trials,* 9(7), pp. 52-55.

46. P. Banerjee and F. Skirrow. 2000. R&D.Com—Research to revenue. *Pharmaceutical Executive Supplement,* December, p. 28.

47. Ibid., p. 30.

48. Ibid., p. 32.

49. G. Harris. 2001. The path to a novel painkiller. *The Wall Street Journal,* January 10, p. A1.

50. S.C. Stinson. 2000. Chiral drugs. *Chemical and Engineering News,* October 23, p. 56.

51. Ibid., p. 55.

52. B. Davis. 2000. Particles that deliver drugs by stealth. *Scrip Magazine* No. 90(May), pp. 40-42.

53. A.M. Rouhi. 2001. Simple molecules and drug uptake. *Chemical and Engineering News,* January 15, p. 49.

54. Davis, Particles that deliver drugs by stealth, p. 40.

55. Taren Grom. 2000. Annual report: Drug delivery timed for revival. *Med Ad News,* 19(6), p. 1.

56. Ibid., p. 56.

57. E. Pena. 2000. Special feature: Medicines for the ages. *Med Ad News,* 19(8), p. 36.

58. C. Littlehales. 2000. Paying for the lifestyle drugs. *Modern Drug Discovery,* 3(6), pp. 47-52.

59. Andrews-Cramer, Molecular informatics and the drug discovery factory, p. 61.

60. B. Agnew. 2000. When Pharma merges, R&D is the dowry. *Science,* March 17, p. 1952.

61. Ibid.

62. Ibid.

63. B. James. 2000. Tying the knot. *Pharmaceutical Visions,* Spring, p. 15.

64. W. Koberstein, C. Petersen, and L.J. Sellers. 2000. The mergers: Miracle, madness or mayhem? *Pharmaceutical Executive,* 20(3), pp. 48-64.

65. James, Tying the knot, p. 16.

66. J. Ansell. 2000. The billion dollar pyramid. *Pharmaceutical Executive,* 20(8), pp. 64-70.

67. D. Pilling. 2000. Drugs giant plans radical research move. *Financial Times,* December 11-12, p. 1.

68. Ansell, The billion dollar pyramid, p. 70.

69. James, Tying the knot, p. 16.

Chapter 6

1. D. Kniaz. 2000. Drug discovery adopts factory method. *Modern Drug Discovery,* 3(5), pp. 67-72.

2. Ibid.

3. Ibid.

4. N. Sleep. 2000. Sorting out combinatorial chaos. *Modern Drug Discovery,* 3(7/8), pp. 37-42.

5. B. Agnew. 2000. When Pharma merges. R&D is the dowry. *Science,* March 17.

6. M. Liebman. 1999. Competing drug companies cooperate in a bold race for gene therapies. *Medical Marketing and Media,* 34(8), pp. 68-73.

7. Ibid.

8. M.B. Brennan. 2000. Drug discovery: Filtering out failures early in the game. *Chemical and Engineering News,* June 5, p. 63.

9. Home page of California's twenty-ninth congressional district. Available: <www.house.gov/waxman/pharm/orphan/orphan.html>, p. 2.

10. Ibid., p. 1.

11. Ibid.

12. *PhRMA Industry Profile,* 2000, Chapter 3, p. 10.

13. J.T. Zenne. 2000. Orphan drugs. In *New drug approval process.* New York: Marcel Dekker, Inc., pp. 365-380.

14. Ibid.

15. Ibid.

16. CDER 1999 report to the nation: Improving public health through human drugs, p. 9.

17. AAC Consulting Group, Rockville, Maryland, personal correspondence, August 20, 1999.

18. Pediatric pharmacotherapy. The FDA drug approval process. Available: <www.people.Virginia.edu/~5mb4v/pedpharm/vin11.html>, p. 3.

19. T.R. Beam Jr. 1999. Current U.S. Food and Drug Administration requirements for new drug approval. *Infections in Medicine* 9(Supplement D), p. 16.

20. J.G. Perkins et al. 1990. Utility of Retrovir's phase IV research program from a regulatory perspective. *Drug Information Journal,* 24, p. 598.

21. Ibid., pp. 597-603.

22. M.E. Gosse et al. 1998. Effects of U.S. regulatory policies on the research development and approval of new biotechnology derived biopharmaceuticals: Points to consider for OSCD member countries. *Tufts Center for the Study of Drug Development,* p. 11.

23. Ibid., p. 12.

24. Beam, Current U.S. Food and Drug Administration requirements, p. 11.

25. Gosse et al., Effects of U.S. regulatory policies, p. 12.

26. Ibid., p. 13.

27. S.R. Shulman et al. The Food and Drug Administration's early access and fast track approval initiatives: How have they worked? *Food and Drug Law,* 50(4), pp. 503-532.

28. Gosse et al., Effects of U.S. regulatory policies, p. 13.

29. Ibid.

30. Ibid.

31. Ibid.

32. S.R. Shulman and K.I. Kaitin. 1993. The Prescription Drug User Fee Act of 1992: A five year experiment for industry and the FDA. *Pharmacoeconomics,* 9(2), pp. 121-133.

33. Gosse et al., Effects of U.S. regulatory policies, p. 14.

34. CDER 1999 report to the nation, p. 17.

35. Ibid.

36. Ibid., p. 19.

37. P.B. Hutt. 1998. A guide to the FDA Modernization Act of 1997. *Food Technology,* 52(5), p. 54.

38. The FDA Modernization Act of 1997, *FDA Backgrounder,* November 21, 1997. Available: <http://www.fda.gov/opacom/backgrounders/modact.htm>.

39. J. Wechsler. 1999. FDAMA implementation policies to spur drug development, streamline FDA approval process. *Formulary,* 34, pp. 176-177.

40. Ibid.

41. Ibid.

42. Wechsler, FDAMA implementation policies to spur drug development, p. 177.

43. CDER home page. International activities. Available: <http://www.fda.gov/cder/audiences/iact/iachome.htm>, p. 2.

44. Ibid., p. 3.

45. Ibid., p. 3.

46. ICH M4 Organization of Common Technical Document for the Registration of Pharmaceuticals for Human Use, ICH Step 2, Draft Consensus Guideline, London, July 27, 2000, p. 3.

47. A. Giaquinto. 1997. A common technical document for applications. *Proceedings of the Fourth International Conference on Harmonization,* eds. P.F. D'Arcy and D.W.L. Harron. Brussels: Queen's University of Belfast, pp. 554-558.

Chapter 7

1. W.D. Reekie. 1977. *Pricing new pharmaceutical products.* London: Croom Helm.

2. F.N. Brand, R.T. Smith, and P.A. Brand. 1977. Effect of economic barriers to medical care on patients' non-compliance. *Public Health Reports,* 92(1), pp. 72-78.

3. N.B. Shulman, B. Martinez, D. Brogan, A.A. Carr, and C.C. Miles. 1986. Financial cost as an obstacle to hypertension therapy. *American Journal of Public Health,* 76(9), pp. 1105-1108.

4. D.E. Morisky. 1987. Nonadherence to medical recommendations for hypertensive patients: Problems and potential solutions. *Journal of Compliance in Health Care,* 1(1), pp. 5-20.

5. D.M. Black, R.J. Brand, M. Greenlick, G. Hughes, and J. Smith. 1987. Compliance to treatment for hypertension in elderly patients: The SHEP pilot study. *Journal of Gerontology,* 42(5), pp. 552-557.

6. Shulman et al., Financial cost as an obstacle to hypertension therapy, pp. 1105-1108.

7. E.M. Kolassa and M.C. Smith. 1993. *1992 national survey of hospital pharmacies: Hospital pharmacy directors' ability to use and understand pharmaceutical economic outcomes research.* University, MS: Research Institute of Pharmaceutical Sciences, University of Mississippi, March.

8. P.W. Abramowitz, E.G. Nold, and S.M. Hatfield. 1982. Use of clinical pharmacists to reduce cefamandole, cefoxitin, and ticarcillin costs. *American Journal of Hospital Pharmacy,* 39, pp. 1176-1180.

9. D.A. Hess, C.D. Mahony, P.N. Johnson, W.M. Corrao, and A.E. Fisher. 1990. Integration of clinical and administrative strategies to reduce expenditures for antimicrobial agents. *American Journal of Hospital Pharmacy,* 47(March), pp. 585-591.

10. C.I. Miyagawa and J.O. Rivera. 1986. Effect of clinical pharmacists' interventions on drug therapy costs in a surgical intensive care unit. *American Journal of Hospital Pharmacy,* 43(December), pp. 3008-3013.

11. E.A. Chrischilles, D.K. Helling, and C.R. Aschoff. 1989. Effect of clinical pharmacy services on the quality of family practice physician prescribing and medication costs, DICP. *The Annals of Pharmacotherapy,* 23(May), pp. 417-421.

12. H. Lazarus and M.C. Smith. 1988. After the order is written: Pharmacists' interventions in hospital drug therapy. *Medical Marketing and Media,* May, pp. 76-80.

13. S. Greenfield, E.C. Nelson, M. Zubkoff, W. Manning, W. Rogers, R.L. Kravitz, A. Keller, A.R. Tarlov, and J.E. Ware. 1992. Variations in resource utilization among medical specialties and systems of care: Results from the medical outcomes study. *JAMA,* 257(12), pp. 1624-1630.

14. A.H. Taubman and N.N. Mason. 1989. How to price a retail pharmacy's goods and services. In W. Tindall, ed., *Retail pharmacy practices.* Alexandria, VA: National Association of Retail Druggists, pp. 465-505.

15. E.M. Kolassa. 1995. Physicians' perceptions of drug prices and their effect on the prescribing decision. *Journal of Research in Pharmaceutical Economics,* 6(1), pp. 23-37.

16. R.F. Holcombe and J. Griffin. 1993. Effects of insurance status on pain medication prescriptions in a hematology/oncology practice. *Southern Medical Journal,* 86, pp. 151-156.

17. R.N. Zelnio and J.P. Gagnon. 1979. The effects of price information on prescription drug product selection. *Drug Intelligence and Clinical Pharmacy,* 13, pp. 156-159.

18. E.M. Kolassa. 1993. The new environment for pharmaceutical pricing. *Product Management Today,* 4(1), pp. 21-22.

Chapter 8

1. B.F. Banahan, J.P. Bentley, L. Sun, and K.I. Lee. 1999. *Physicians' attitudes toward and response to direct-to-consumer advertising.* Paper presented at the An-

nual Conference of the American Association of Pharmaceutical Scientists, New Orleans, November.

Chapter 9

1. R. Corey. 1983. *Industrial marketing: Cases and concepts,* Third edition. Englewood Cliffs, NJ: Prentice-Hall, p. 311.

Chapter 10

1. Economists talk about various forms of utility in terms of varying usefulness. An antibiotic has more utility when it has been formulated into a finished-dosage form than when it is a bulk powder, more usefulness if it is the drug needed than just any antibiotic, and a higher value when it is available for use right away. Utility theory helps explain how markets form and evolve—that is, to provide various types of utility (usefulness) to customers.

2. G.D. Havell and G.L. Frazier. 1997. *Marketing: Connecting with consumers.* Upper Saddle River, NJ: Prentice-Hall, pp. 14-15.

3. Such retailers typically maintain fixed business addresses, but they are not open to the public in that sales are not made at these base locations.

Chapter 11

1. The illegal or illicit drug market is not part of this discussion, except to the extent that some legitimate drugs are diverted into illicit markets for nonmedical purposes.

2. It took community pharmacy ninety years (1900-1989) to reach 2 billion prescriptions dispensed in a year. Reaching 3 billion prescriptions took ten years (1990-1999). The 4 billion mark will require only five years (2000-2004).

3. Different markets address the question of package size quite differently. In Europe, the market has evolved a much different model of packaging: pharmaceuticals are available from manufacturers in more package sizes, most of which are designed to be dispensed intact (as unit-of-use or course-of-therapy sizes).

4. GMPs are now referred to as cGMPs. The addition of a small "c" refers to "current," reflecting the fact that FDA requirements change over time and that the registrant is responsible for complying with the most current FDA requirements.

5. If a manufacturer, for instance, shipped 100 orders to 100 different customers without the required records, the DEA could fine the manufacturer up to $25,000 for *each* of the 100 orders.

Chapter 12

1. The illegal or illicit drug market is not part of this discussion, except to the extent that some legitimate drugs are diverted into illicit markets for nonmedical purposes.

2. Finished-dose pharmaceuticals are those which are ready for use by patients or administration by health care providers. Three antecedent pharmaceutical forms—intermediate dosage forms, purified active ingredients, and raw materials—

are important components of the U.S. drug industry but fall outside the scope of this discussion.

3. In this context, the term *rights* refers to trademark and patent protections conveyed by individual governments that give the manufacturer limited marketing exclusivity.

4. Pharmacists, as part of pharmaceutical services, repackage when they dispense in quantities less than a trade package. Repackagers in this context do not provide requisite pharmaceutical services or attempt to meet state board of pharmacy professional requirements but are interested solely in changing package size.

5. The package size indicator portion of the NDC number will be different; the labeler identification and product identifier remain the same as before.

6. Note that issuance of a patent (and/or trademark) precedes and is unrelated to FDA marketing approval. Often a significant part of the patent's life is used up before the manufacturer receives FDA approval. This puts additional pressure on the manufacturer to recover its costs in a shorter period of time, i.e., before its patent expires and others can apply for FDA approval to market.

7. NDAs are required for the initial FDA application. Generic developers can file a shorter application, known as an abbreviated NDA, or ANDA.

8. Despite aspirations and efforts to transform the practice of pharmacy into an information-based, pharmaceutical care concept that some view as separate and distinct from dispensing/distributive activities, pharmacists will continue to be responsible for safeguarding and at least overseeing, if not participating directly in, dispensing.

9. Few separate Internet pharmacies, started since 1999, are still operating. Whether the business model and/or implementation was flawed or the timing was wrong remains to be determined.

10. A buying group is a commercially allowable collaboration among competing but like buyers (businesses, organizations, and/or government agencies) that increases their combined buying power in order to get better prices and terms of sale from sellers.

Chapter 13

1. B.H. Herxheimer. 1978. In *The scientific basis of official regulations of drug research and development,* Ghent, Belgium: Heymans Foundation.

2. F. Hughes. 1999. *Medicine avenue: The story of medical advertising in America.* Huntington, NY: Medical Advertising Hall of Fame.

3. E. Moench. 1986. American Writers Association and the Pharmaceutical Advertising Council symposium. Printed in the *Journal of Pharmaceutical Marketing and Management,* 1(2), pp. 51-56.

4. K. Schueler. 1986. American Writers Association and the Pharmaceutical Advertising Council symposium. Printed in the *Journal of Pharmaceutical Marketing and Management,* 1(2), pp. 57-66.

5. Q.H. Douden. 1980. In *Medical Marketing and Media,* 15(3), p. 26.

6. National Analysts. 1986. Study conducted for the Pharmaceutical Manufacturers Association (now PhARMA). Philadelphia, PA: Author.

7. G. Papazian. 1985. Media selection as a fine art. *Pharmaceutical Executive,* 5(3), p. 50.

8. J. Palshaw. 1982. Are you mining the wealth? *Medical Marketing and Media,* 17(10), p. 47.

Chapter 14

1. B.G. McMillian, P.R. Bergamo, and L.C. Wyatt. 2000. In *Pharmaceutical Executive,* April, p. 104.

2. Ibid.

3. M.C. Smith. 1977. Where are the blacks in prescription drug advertising? *Medical Marketing and Media,* 12(May), pp. 47-48.

Chapter 15

1. F. Hughes and J. Kallir. 1994. *Medicine avenue: The story of medical advertising in America.* Huntington, NY: Medical Advertising Hall of Fame.

2. G. Carson. 1961. *One for a man, two for a horse.* New York: Doubleday.

3. S. Engle. 1999. Latest in the pipeline. *R & D Directions,* 5(3), p. 20.

4. A. Ries and J. Trout. *Positioning: The battle for your mind.* New York: Warner Books.

5. R. Girondi. 1993. Applying relative media values to the pharmaceutical promotion planning process. *Product Management Today,* 4(4), pp. 21-23.

6. *Med Ad News,* September 2001, p. 14.

Chapter 16

1. The Boston Consulting Group. 1993. The changing environment for US pharmaceuticals [internal corporate report]. New York: Author, April, p. 20.

2. C.B. Luce. 1988. Cost-effectiveness studies of pharmaceuticals: Methodological considerations. In ed. W. Van Eimeren, *Socioeconomic aspects of drug therapy.* Berlin: Springer-Verlag, p. 87.

3. D. Neuhauser. 1981. *Survey of research results and current status of CBA/CEA in technology assessment: Cimetidine as a model.* Philadelphia, PA: Leonard Davis Institute of Health Economics, University of Pennsylvania.

4. National Wholesale Druggists' Association annual report, 1993.

5. J. Avorn, K. Harvey, S.B. Soumerai, A. Herxheimer, R. Plumridge, and G. Bardelay. 1987. Information and education as determinants of anitibiotic use: Report of Task Force5. *Review of Infectious Diseases,* 9(3), pp. S286-S296.

6. K. Johnson. 1991. MM&M interview. AMA guidelines: "We'll stay the course." Here's why. *Medical Marketing and Media* 26, pp. 82-88.

7. D. Kessler. 1991. Drug promotions and scientific exchange. *New England Journal of Medicine,* 325(3), pp. 201-203.

8. T.D. Rucker. 1976. Drug information for prescribers and dispensers: Toward a model system. *Medical Care,* 14(2), pp. 156-165.

9. J. Radam, McAdams Medical Advertising and Promotion, personal communication, 1993.

10. P.H. Rubin. 1991. Economics of prescription drug advertising. *Journal of Research in Pharmaceutical Economics,* 3(4), p. 29.

11. Ibid., p. 30.

12. A. Masson and P.H. Rubin. 1985. Matching prescription drugs and consumers: The benefits of direct advertising. *New England Journal of Medicine,* 313(8), pp. 513-515.

Index

Page numbers followed by the letter "f" indicate figures; those followed by the letter "t" indicate tables.